Field
Inter
Medicine

DAVID S. SMITH, M.D.
Associate Clinical Professor of Medicine
Department of Internal Medicine
Yale University School of Medicine
New Haven, Connecticut

LYNN E. SULLIVAN, M.D.
Assistant Professor of Medicine
Department of Internal Medicine
Yale University School of Medicine
New Haven, Connecticut

SEONAID F. HAY, M.D.
Assistant Professor of Medicine
Department of Internal Medicine
Yale University School of Medicine
New Haven, Connecticut

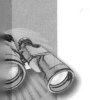

 LIPPINCOTT WILLIAMS & WILKINS
A **Wolters Kluwer** Company
Philadelphia · Baltimore · New York · London
Buenos Aires · Hong Kong · Sydney · Tokyo

Acquisitions Editor: Danette Somers
Developmental Editor: Tanya Lazar
Supervising Editor: Nicole Walz
Production Editor: Erica Broennle Nelson, Silverchair Science + Communications
Senior Manufacturing Manager: Benjamin Rivera
Cover Designer: Larry Didona
Compositor: Silverchair Science + Communications
Printer: R.R. Donnelley, Crawfordsville

Library of Congress Cataloging-in-Publication Data

Field guide to internal medicine / edited by David S. Smith, Lynn
E. Sullivan, Seonaid F. Hay.
  p. ; cm. – (Field guide series)
Includes bibliographical references and index.
ISBN 0-7817-2828-2
  1. Internal medicine–Handbooks, manuals, etc. I. Smith, David
S. (David Scott), 1954- II. Sullivan, Lynn E. III. Hay, Seonaid F. IV.
Series: Field guide (Philadelphia, Pa.)
  [DNLM: 1. Internal Medicine–Handbooks. WB 39 F453 2004]
RC55.F455 2004
616–dc22

                                    2004014463

Care has been taken to confirm the accuracy of the information presented and to describe generally accepted practices. However, the authors, editors, and publisher are not responsible for errors or omissions or for any consequences from application of the information in this book and make no warranty, expressed or implied, with respect to the currency, completeness, or accuracy of the contents of the publication. Application of this information in a particular situation remains the professional responsibility of the practitioner.

The authors, editors, and publisher have exerted every effort to ensure that drug selection and dosage set forth in this text are in accordance with current recommendations and practice at the time of publication. However, in view of ongoing research, changes in government regulations, and the constant flow of information relating to drug therapy and drug reactions, the reader is urged to check the package insert for each drug for any change in indications and dosage and for added warnings and precautions. This is particularly important when the recommended agent is a new or infrequently employed drug.

Some drugs and medical devices presented in this publication have Food and Drug Administration (FDA) clearance for limited use in restricted research settings. It is the responsibility of health care providers to ascertain the FDA status of each drug or device planned for use in their clinical practice.

10 9 8 7 6 5 4 3 2 1

CONTENTS

SECTION 2 ▪ CARDIOLOGY

SECTION 4 ▪ GASTROENTEROLOGY

SECTION 6 ■ NEUROLOGY AND PSYCHIATRY

SECTION 7 ▪ RHEUMATOLOGY AND ALLERGY

SECTION 9 ▪ RENAL AND ELECTROLYTE

CONTRIBUTING AUTHORS

Joseph V. Agostini, M.D.
Assistant Professor of Medicine
Department of Internal Medicine
Section of Geriatrics
Yale University School of Medicine
New Haven, Connecticut

Haider A. Akmal, M.D.
Fellow
Department of Medicine
Division of Digestive Diseases
Yale University School of
  Medicine
Yale–New Haven Hospital
New Haven, Connecticut

Christopher S. Alia, M.D.
Fellow
Department of Pulmonary and
  Critical Care Medicine
Yale–New Haven Hospital
New Haven, Connecticut

Ashwin Balagopal, M.D.
Chief Resident
Department of Internal Medicine
Yale–New Haven Hospital
New Haven, Connecticut

Beth Anne Biggee, M.D.
Fellow in Rheumatology
Tufts University School of Medicine
New England Medical Center
Boston, Massachusetts

Douglas W. Bowerman, M.D.
Attending Staff Physician
Department of Internal
  Medicine
F.F. Thompson Hospital
Canandaigua, New York

Ursula C. Brewster, M.D.
Clinical Instructor of Medicine
Department of Internal Medicine
Section of Nephrology
Yale University School of
  Medicine
New Haven, Connecticut

Vadjista Broumand, M.D.
Fellow
Renal Division
Brigham and Women's Hospital
Boston, Massachusetts

Catherine Chiles, M.D.
Associate Clinical Professor
Department of Psychiatry
Yale University School of Medicine
New Haven, Connecticut

Vladimir Coric, M.D.
Assistant Clinical Professor of
  Psychiatry
Department of Psychiatry
Yale University School of Medicine
New Haven, Connecticut

Holly Craig, M.D.
Whitney Internal Medicine
Hamden, Connecticut

Xinqi Dong, M.D.
Instructor of Medicine
Department of Internal Medicine
University of Chicago Pritzker
  School of Medicine
Chicago, Illinois

Craig G. Gunderson, M.D.
Instructor in Medicine
Department of Internal Medicine
Yale University School of Medicine
New Haven, Connecticut

Anya C. Harry, M.D., Ph.D.
Fellow
Department of Pulmonary and
  Critical Care Medicine
University of Pennsylvania School
  of Medicine
Philadelphia, Pennsylvania

Seonaid F. Hay, M.D.
Assistant Professor of Medicine
Department of Internal Medicine
Yale University School of Medicine
New Haven, Connecticut

David J. Horne, M.D.
Clinical Instructor
Department of Internal Medicine
Yale University School of Medicine
Chief Resident
Department of Internal Medicine
Yale–New Haven Hospital
New Haven, Connecticut

Avlin B. Imaeda, M.D., Ph.D.
Chief Resident in Medicine
Department of Internal Medicine
Yale University School of Medicine
Yale–New Haven Hospital
New Haven, Connecticut

Vinni Juneja, M.D.
Fellow
Department of Medical Oncology/
    Hematology
Yale University School of Medicine
New Haven, Connecticut

Devan L. Kansagara, M.D.
Primary Care Internal Medicine
    Resident
Department of Medicine
Yale University School of Medicine
New Haven, Connecticut

N. Christopher Kelley, M.D.
Fellow
Department of Internal Medicine
Section of Cardiovascular Medicine
Yale University School of Medicine
New Haven, Connecticut

James N. Kirkpatrick, M.D.
Fellow
MacLean Center for Medical Ethics
Chicago, Illinois

Jeffrey D. Kravetz, M.D.
Assistant Professor of Medicine
Department of Internal Medicine
Yale University School of Medicine
New Haven, Connecticut
VA Connecticut Healthcare
    System
West Haven, Connecticut

Michelle Lee, M.D.
Yale University School of Medicine
New Haven, Connecticut

Joseph K. Lim, M.D.
Clinical and Research Fellow
Division of Gastroenterology and
    Hepatology
Stanford University School of
    Medicine
Stanford, California

David Litvak, M.D.
Fellow
Department of Cardiology
Yale University School of Medicine
New Haven, Connecticut

Caroline Loeser, M.D.
Fellow
Department of Internal Medicine
Section of Digestive Diseases
Yale University School of Medicine
New Haven, Connecticut

Daus Mahnke, M.D.
Fellow
Department of Gastroenterology
University of Colorado Health
    Sciences Center
Denver, Colorado

Bridget Ann Martell, M.D., M.S.
Associate Research Scientist
Department of Medicine
Yale University School of Medicine
New Haven, Connecticut
VA Connecticut Healthcare System
West Haven, Connecticut

Melinda M. Mesmer, M.D.
Yale University School of Medicine
New Haven, Connecticut

Michael A. Nelson, M.D.
Department of Internal Medicine
Yale–New Haven Hospital
New Haven, Connecticut

Nha-Ai Nguyen-Duc, M.D.
Staff Physician
Division of General Internal Medicine
Stanford University School of
    Medicine
Stanford, California
Palo Alto VA Healthcare System
    General Medicine Clinic
Palo Alto, California

Amy M. Nuernberg, M.D.
Clinical Instructor
Department of Internal Medicine
Yale–New Haven Hospital
New Haven, Connecticut

Mark Nyce, M.D.
Fellow
Division of Digestive Diseases
University of Virginia Health System
Charlottesville, Virginia

Stephen E. Possick, M.D.
Fellow in Cardiovascular Medicine
Department of Internal Medicine
Section of Cardiology
Yale University School of Medicine
New Haven, Connecticut

Joseph Quaranta, M.D.
Attending Physician
Department of Internal Medicine
Yale University School of Medicine
New Haven, Connecticut

Jeffrey T. Reynolds, M.D.
Nephrologist
New Haven, Connecticut

Stephanie Rosborough, M.D.
Resident in Emergency Medicine
Department of Emergency Medicine
Yale University School of Medicine
New Haven, Connecticut

Julie R. Rosenbaum, M.D.
Assistant Professor of Medicine
Department of Medicine
Yale University School of Medicine
New Haven, Connecticut

Christopher B. Ruser, M.D.
Assistant Professor of Medicine
Department of Internal Medicine
Yale University School of Medicine
New Haven, Connecticut
VA Connecticut Healthcare System
West Haven, Connecticut

Lisa Sanders, M.D.
Clinical Instructor
Department of Internal Medicine
Yale University School of Medicine
New Haven, Connecticut

Louis C. Sanfilippo, M.D.
Assistant Clinical Professor
Department of Psychiatry
Yale University School of Medicine
New Haven, Connecticut

Rachel Schoss, M.D.
Department of Internal Medicine
Yale University School of Medicine
New Haven, Connecticut

Jared G. Selter, M.D.
Postdoctoral Fellow in Cardiovas-
    cular Medicine
Department of Internal Medicine
Section of Cardiovascular
    Medicine
Yale University School of Medicine
New Haven, Connecticut

Rhuna Shen, M.D.
Department of Medicine
Robert Wood Johnson University
    Hospital
New Brunswick, New Jersey

Melissa A. Simon, M.D., M.P.H.
Chief Resident
Department of Obstetrics and
    Gynecology
Yale–New Haven Medical Center
New Haven, Connecticut

David N. Smith, M.D.
Fellow
Department of Internal Medicine
Section of Cardiology
Yale–New Haven Hospital
New Haven, Connecticut

David S. Smith, M.D.
Associate Clinical Professor of
    Medicine
Department of Internal Medicine
Yale University School of Medicine
New Haven, Connecticut

Sandra A. Springer, M.D.
Clinical Instructor of Medicine
Department of Internal Medicine
Section of Infectious Diseases
Yale University School of Medicine
Yale–New Haven Hospital
New Haven, Connecticut

Kathleen Stergiopoulos, M.D., Ph.D.
Fellow
Department of Internal Medicine
Section of Cardiology
Yale University School of Medicine
New Haven, Connecticut

Lynn E. Sullivan, M.D.
Assistant Professor of Medicine
Department of Internal Medicine
Yale University School of
    Medicine
New Haven, Connecticut

Lisa Gale Suter, M.D.
Yale Robert Wood Johnson Clinical
    Scholar
Department of Internal Medicine
Section of Rheumatology and Gen-
    eral Internal Medicine
Yale University School of Medicine
New Haven, Connecticut

E. Scott Swenson, M.D., Ph.D.
Fellow
Department of Internal Medicine
Division of Digestive Diseases
Yale University School of
    Medicine
New Haven, Connecticut

Meredith Talbot, M.D.
Staff Physician
Yale–New Haven Hospital
New Haven, Connecticut

Karen S. Taraszka, M.D., Ph.D.
Fellow
Department of Dermatology
Yale University School of Medicine
New Haven, Connecticut

Eric N. Taylor, M.D.
Clinical and Research Fellow in
    Nephrology
Brigham and Women's Hospital
Boston, Massachusetts

John Toksoy, M.D.
Assistant Clinical Professor
Department of Internal Medicine
Yale University School of Medicine
New Haven, Connecticut

Gaby Weissman, M.D.
Fellow in Cardiology
Department of Internal Medicine
Section of Cardiovascular Medicine
Yale University School of Medicine
New Haven, Connecticut

Richard Mark White, M.D., Ph.D.
Fellow
Department of Medical Oncology
Dana-Farber Cancer Institute
Massachusetts General Hospital
Boston, Massachusetts

Henry Klar Yaggi, M.D.
Assistant Professor of Medicine
Department of Internal Medicine
Section of Pulmonary and Critical
    Care Medicine
Yale University School of Medicine
New Haven, Connecticut
VA Connecticut Healthcare System
West Haven, Connecticut

Jennifer L. Yeh, M.D.
Cardiology Fellow
Department of Cardiology
Yale University School of Medicine
Yale–New Haven Hospital
New Haven, Connecticut

PREFACE

Field Guide to Internal Medicine arises out of recognition of the need for a comprehensive yet concise book to guide medical students on their internal medicine rotation and to be a valuable rapid source of information to medical residents. Internal medicine is a broad and deep specialty. The classic textbooks, including newer electronic resources, are exquisitely detailed references that are thousands of pages in length, which make them superb sources for gaining an in-depth perspective on a single problem, yet poor sources for developing a balanced overview of the whole field of internal medicine during a time-limited clinical rotation. We envision students being able to read this book cover to cover during their time on medicine. We wanted it to be readable, not just a list or outline of facts, like so many other handbooks. In addition, we see it as a condensed source of high-value clinical information, where the student or resident can read about a disease in the 5 minutes before seeing a patient or making rounds.

In balancing the text between being compact and comprehensive, we have focused on the 121 most important internal medicine conditions, particularly medical emergencies and common diseases seen in hospitalized patients. These comprise the core internal medicine diseases and syndromes that a medical student should master. For familiarity, we have organized the text along traditional internal medicine specialty lines. Each chapter begins with an overview of why that disease is important (helping to see the forest as well as the trees) and the key challenges to effective diagnosis and treatment. The discussion then focuses in turn on the salient features of clinical presentation, pathophysiology, diagnosis, and management. A comprehensive color atlas of more than 200 diagnostic images was selected to complement the text, representing the broad spectrum of diagnostic modalities and classic findings in key diseases.

The text is written through the perspective and experience of Yale senior residents, who are extremely current in their clinical knowledge, yet proximate to the learning experience. Each chapter was further reviewed and edited by a general internist and a subspecialist. The principal editors are all active teachers of Yale medical students and residents and, additionally, bring their collective experience as recent medicine chief residents, former clerkship director, and current practicing general internists. The field of internal medicine evolves rapidly, so this book of necessity captures a snapshot in time, but we attempted to be current while focusing on timeless principles.

Field Guide to Internal Medicine is unique in simultaneously being a comprehensive, concise, portable, and visual medicine text. It is our hope that it will become an indispensable companion to the learner seeking mastery of the rich field of internal medicine.

D.S.S.
L.E.S.
S.F.H.
New Haven, Connecticut
July 2004

ACKNOWLEDGMENTS

The editors gratefully acknowledge the Yale medical subspecialty reviewers:

Infectious Diseases: David L. Coleman, M.D., Professor of Medicine
Cardiology: Lawrence H. Young, M.D., Professor of Medicine
Pulmonary and Critical Care Medicine: Mark D. Siegel, M.D., Associate Professor of Medicine
Gastroenterology: Deborah D. Proctor, M.D., Associate Professor of Medicine
Hematology and Oncology: Michal G. Rose, M.D., Assistant Professor of Medicine
Neurology: Sujai D. Nath, M.D., Assistant Clinical Professor, Clinical Neurologist
Psychiatry: Catherine Chiles, M.D., Associate Clinical Professor of Psychiatry
Rheumatology and Allergy: Liana Frankel, M.D., Assistant Professor of Medicine
Endocrinology: Silvio E. Inzucchi, M.D., Associate Professor of Medicine
Renal and Electrolyte: Richard N. Formica, M.D., Assistant Professor of Medicine, and Aldo J. Peixoto, M.D., Assistant Professor of Medicine

We also thank Glen A. Vahjen, M.D., Assistant Clinical Professor of Diagnostic Radiology, for providing original radiographic images from his teaching collection.

Most of the clinical diagnostic images were provided by Lisa Kugelman, M.D., and Douglas Grossman, M.D., from the Yale Dermatology Resident's collection, and by Stephen Spencer, M.D., from the Dartmouth Dermatology collection.

Section 1

Infectious Diseases

Chapter 1

CELLULITIS

Kathleen Stergiopoulos

OVERVIEW

Cellulitis is an acute inflammatory response of the skin characterized by localized pain, erythema, swelling, and heat. The infection is usually limited to the dermis and subcutaneous tissues. Treatment is based on the empiric use of antibiotics, in most cases whose spectrum covers the typical offenders, *Streptococcus pyogenes* and *Staphylococcus aureus*. Immediate consultation to surgery is warranted in cases in which deep-seated infections are suspected, such as necrotizing fasciitis.

PATHOPHYSIOLOGY

Bacteria gain access to the epidermis through cracks in the skin, abrasions, cuts, burns, insect bites, surgical incisions, and intravenous catheters. Cellulitis caused by *S. aureus* usually spreads from a central localized infection (an abscess, folliculitis, or an infected catheter). Cellulitis caused by *S. pyogenes* tends to be more rapidly spreading, however, and is frequently associated with lymphangitis and fever. Patients with recurrent cellulitis may have chronic venous stasis, impaired lymphatic drainage of the extremity (previous axillary node dissection for breast carcinoma or radical pelvic surgery), or previous saphenous venectomy for coronary bypass surgery. Moreover, acute streptococcal cellulitis, at times associated with bacteremia, may also occur in association with the parenteral injection of illicit drugs. Less common causes of cellulitis include *Streptococcus pneumoniae*, *Haemophilus influenzae* (periorbital cellulitis in children), *Vibrio* (handling raw seafood), *Pseudomonas* (in hospitalized, immunocompromised host), and *Clostridia* species. Lower extremity cellulitis associated with cutaneous ulcers in diabetic patients may be polymicrobial in origin.

CLINICAL PRESENTATION

As noted above, cellulitis is characterized by localized pain, erythema, swelling, and heat. Borders of the infection are usually not well demarcated. In addition, patients may have lymphadenitis (proximal erythematous streaking) and regional lymphadenopathy. Systemic features, such as fever, malaise, and chills, may develop.

DIAGNOSIS

When there is open drainage, an open wound, or an obvious portal of entry, Gram stain and culture can provide a definitive diagnosis. More often, in their absence, the bacterial etiology is often difficult to establish. Even with needle aspiration at the leading edge or punch biopsy of the cellulitis tissue itself, cultures are positive in only 20% of cases. Blood cultures have a yield of less than 5%.

MANAGEMENT

Oral penicillinase-resistant penicillins or first-generation cephalosporins are the agents of choice. If penicillin-allergic, a macrolide or vancomycin may be used. In more severe cases of cellulitis and in populations at higher risk for disseminated disease (elderly patients with multiple medical problems, diabetics, immunocompromised), use of parenteral antibiotics is preferred. Symptomatic relief can be achieved with leg elevation and use of nonsteroidal antiinflammatory agents.

Chapter 2

FEVER OF UNKNOWN ORIGIN

Sandra A. Springer

OVERVIEW

The term *fever of unknown origin* (FUO) has been used to describe a specific subset of fevers that are persistent and require extensive evaluation in order to diagnose. Initially, classic FUO was described by Petersdorf and Beeson in 1961 in a landmark paper titled *Fever of Unknown Origin: Report on 100 Cases.* It was defined as a temperature of 101°F (38.3°C) or higher lasting for 3 weeks or longer that remained undiagnosed after 1 week of hospitalization. Since that time, there have been several additional defined subtypes of FUO, including the nosocomial FUO, which is controversial and refers to a fever that manifests in a patient within the first 24 hours of hospitalization; the immunodeficient FUO; and the human immunodeficiency virus (HIV)–related FUO.

PATHOPHYSIOLOGY

Fever, often mistaken as a sign of infection, is actually a sign of inflammation. A fever is a response by the hypothalamus secondary to activation by pyrogens, or circulating cytokines, such as tumor necrosis factor or interleukin-1. Tissue injury is the most common cause of production of inflammatory cytokines that cause a febrile response. The primary causes of FUO include infections, neoplasm, connective tissue diseases, miscellaneous causes, and undiagnosed etiologies. More recent evaluation of causes of FUO has shown differences based on age. Although earlier studies listed infection as the most common cause of FUO (25–50% of cases) among all age groups, more recent studies have found connective tissue diseases, followed by infection and then malignancy, to be the most common cause of the FUO in patients older than age 65. In younger populations, infection is the third most common cause of FUO (21% of cases), after unknown causes (29%) and miscellaneous causes (26%). Notably, fewer patients older than age 65 have undiagnosed FUOs (8%), compared to patients younger than age 65 (30%).

Infectious Causes

Common infectious etiologies of FUO are abscesses, tuberculosis, complicated urinary tract infections, and endocarditis. The more common abscesses are intraabdominal, subdiaphragmatic, hepatic, and pelvic. Less common infectious causes include *Salmonella*, intraperinephric abscess, splenic abscesses, cytomegalovirus, and toxoplasmosis. Rarer infectious causes of FUO include HIV, dental abscesses, sinusitis, osteomyelitis, *Yersinia*, *Listeria*, brucellosis, Lyme disease, Q fever, leptospirosis, blastomycosis, and histoplasmosis. The likelihood of a specific infectious etiology depends on the medical history, demographics, and social and travel history of the patient.

Neoplastic Causes

Malignancies account for approximately 30% of all causes of FUO. They are the third most common cause of FUO in patients older than age 65 and the fifth leading cause of FUO in patients younger than 65 years old. The most common neoplastic causes are lymphomas, leukemias, renal cell carcinoma, and metastases to the liver and central nervous system. Less common neoplastic causes of FUO are hepatomas, pancreatic cancer, and colon cancer. Rare causes include atrial myxomas.

Rheumatologic Causes

Collagen vascular diseases account for 10% of cases of FUO and are the second most common causes of FUO in patients older than age 65 years and the fourth most common cause of FUO in patients younger than 65 years old. The most important causes are temporal arteritis and adult Still's disease. Other causes include periarteritis nodosa, rheumatoid arthritis, systemic lupus erythematosus, and vasculitis. Less common causes include noninfectious granulomatous diseases, such as sarcoidosis and granulomatous hepatitis.

Miscellaneous Causes

Drug fever is the primary miscellaneous cause. Less frequent causes include cirrhosis, alcohol hepatitis, Crohn's disease, hypertriglyceridemia, and recurrent pulmonary emboli. Factitious or self-induced illness secondary to self-injections of pyrogen-causing substances must be included as a possible etiology. Twelve percent to 22% of FUOs remain undiagnosed.

CLINICAL PRESENTATION

Patients with FUO present with a history of chronic or intermittent fevers. Associated symptoms include chills and tachycardia or other symptoms specific to certain diseases, such as weight loss, night sweats, and fatigue in persons with tuberculosis or lymphoma.

DIAGNOSIS

A thorough history of the patient's present illness, as well as his or her social, sexual, travel, and family histories, must be obtained. A history of intravenous drug or alcohol use and consumption of specific foods, including unpasteurized milk or raw meat, as well as exposures to animals and new medications, is important. The history should be repeated multiple times while the patient is hospitalized. A complete physical examination should be performed, including evaluation of fundi, skin, and lymph nodes and careful auscultation of the heart for murmurs and evaluation of the joints for signs of inflammation.

Laboratory studies obtained should be tailored to the individual patient but should include a complete blood count with a differential, chemistries, erythrocyte sedimentation rate, and urinalysis, including microscopy. Blood cultures should be collected from several different sites and should be held for at least 2 weeks for slow-growing organisms. Specific serologic studies should be done if the history and physical examination suggest a specific diagnosis, such as cytomegalovirus or toxoplasmosis. Rheumatologic analyses, such as antinuclear antibodies, rheumatoid factor, and complement levels, should be obtained if a connective tissue disorder is suspected based on the history and physical examination. HIV status should be determined after the patient has given consent. Other body fluids should be cultured if there are symptoms suspicious for a specific disease, including urine, sputum, stool, cerebrospinal fluid, and direct evaluation of blood smears for malaria or *Borrelia*. A purified protein derivative with controls should be placed to rule out tuberculosis.

All patients should have a chest radiograph. If indicated, computed axial tomography (CAT) scan of the chest, abdomen, and pelvis can also be very useful. A negative CAT scan does not rule out disease; however, a positive CAT scan showing an abnormality increases the yield by identifying a specific site to biopsy. A cardiac echocardiogram is indicated if endocarditis or atrial myxoma is suspected. Magnetic resonance imaging can be used to evaluate for osteomyelitis. Radionucleotide scans, including indium or technetium-labeled white blood cell scans to detect chronic infections and gallium scans to detect both infectious and neoplastic causes, can also be helpful. These tests have a high rate of false-positive and false-negative results, however. Invasive procedures, such as lumbar puncture or biopsies of the skin, lymph nodes, bone marrow, or liver, may be necessary to obtain a definitive diagnosis and should be performed based on the patient's history, physical examination, and laboratory data.

MANAGEMENT

Empiric antibiotics should not be used in patients with FUO except in the case of culture-negative endocarditis. It is reasonable to begin patients on treatment for tuberculosis if there is a high suspicion for tuberculosis, with the goal to stop such therapy if there is no clinical evidence of the disease within a certain time period. If the patient is deteriorating rapidly or is neutropenic, empiric antibiotics should be initiated. Corticosteroids are not generally accepted as empiric treatment for FUO unless the patient has a biopsy-proven vasculitis, such as temporal arteritis. Some data have suggested low-dose naproxen (Naprosyn) (250 mg b.i.d.) for control of fever if malignancy is suspected; however, there are no confirmatory data.

Chapter 3

HUMAN IMMUNODEFICIENCY VIRUS AND ACQUIRED IMMUNODEFICIENCY SYNDROME

Sandra A. Springer

OVERVIEW

Human immunodeficiency virus (HIV) is a retrovirus that predominantly infects cells with the CD4 surface marker, which over many years causes depletion of the immune system, leading to the acquired immunodeficiency syndrome (AIDS). AIDS encompasses numerous opportunistic infections (OIs) and neoplasms, including *Pneumocystis carinii* pneumonia (PCP) and Kaposi's sarcoma. There are two strains of HIV, the more common type 1 (HIV-1) and the less well-known type 2 (HIV-2). Type 1 is transmitted via exchange of bodily fluids, predominately blood and semen. The modes of transmission are sexual contact, blood transfusions, intravenous drug use, and vertical spread from mother to fetus. Without highly active antiretroviral treatment (HAART), most persons infected with HIV-1 progress to death secondary to AIDS within 8 to 10 years after infection. More than 16 million people died from AIDS in 1999, and almost one-half of the deaths occurred in sub-Saharan Africans alone.

PATHOPHYSIOLOGY

HIV is a member of the lentiviruses. The structure of HIV-1 has been identified as having two copies of single-stranded RNA genome inside a core that is surrounded by a lipid envelope. The envelope has glycoproteins studding the outside, including gp120, gp41, and p24. Gp120 and gp41 with other necessary coreceptors form a binding site for the human CD4 receptor on the host cells, thereby allowing invasion of the virus into the host cell. The p24 antigen can be assayed for diagnostic purposes. Once the virus is inside the cell, it is uncoated and forms multiple copies of enzymes, such as reverse transcriptase (RT), protease, and integrase, that are released into the cytoplasm. RT performs important functions, such as RNA-dependent DNA polymerization and DNA polymerization for a single-stranded DNA intermediate. The product is a DNA copy of the RNA virus that is then transported into the host cell nucleus and integrated into the host genome as a provirus by the integrase enzyme. The host cell then uses its own cellular RNA polymerases to form viral messenger RNA that is then translated into viral proteins. Important regulatory proteins of the HIV-1 genome include *rev*, *tat*, *gag*, *env*, and *pol*. The protease enzyme functions by cleaving the viral capsid proteins and transcriptional enzymes. The new viral components with new RNA copies of the HIV genome then bud out of the host cell and create a new infectious product, repeating the process.

HIV usually enters the body through a vulnerable mucosal surface, is entrapped by the follicular dendritic cells, and is carried to lymphoid tissues and exposed to the CD4 T-helper cells. It is initially contained by cellular and humoral immune responses. Cellular immunity includes cytotoxic T-cell (CD8) activation and killing of infected CD4 cells, whereas the humoral immunity response to HIV includes immune complex formation and complement activation, as well as neutralizing antibody formation. The host's cytokine cascade activation is the primary phenomenon that leads follicular dendritic cells to transmit the virus to CD4 T-cells. Once seroconversion occurs, usually within 6 to 12 months, chronic HIV infection is established. The CD4 T-cells are the predominant cells that are infected, and their levels begin to be depressed. Immunosuppression is secondary to a combination of multiple factors, including cell-mediated and humoral immune response depletion. These multiple factors include: (i) direct lysis of the CD4 lymphocyte after viral replication, which can lead to depletion; (ii) direct programmed cell death, known as *apoptosis*, which is triggered by the binding of a primed T-cell to gp120; (iii) autoimmune-mediated attack of the host's cytotoxic killer cells against the CD4 T-cells; (iv) HIV itself can infect the CD34 bone marrow cells, which are a group of cells that contain the myeloid progenitor cell, and, therefore, the host may be unable to generate new immunocompetent cells; and (v) HIV can infect developing thymocytes and thymic stromal cells, thereby further inhibiting the immune system's ability to regenerate. The HIV-1 virus also has been found to be a provirus in numerous other cells, providing a latent course of infection that is unaffected by HAART and provides a source for constant viral replication. Reservoirs that have been identified other than CD4 T-lymphocytes include macrophages, follicular dendritic cells, central nervous system (CNS) cells, and prostate cells. Currently, there is no effective means to completely remove the latent virus from these identified cellular reservoirs.

The rate of disease progression to AIDS and death is directly related to the plasma HIV RNA viral load. In one study, approximately 80% of patients infected with HIV-1 progressed to death secondary to AIDS within 6 years if the plasma HIV-1 RNA concentration was more than 30,000 copies per mL, as opposed to 0.9% of patients with plasma HIV-1 RNA concentrations of 500 copies per mL or less.

CLINICAL PRESENTATION

Acute retroviral syndrome, or *acute HIV-1 infection*, is a transient symptomatic illness associated with a sudden acute viral replication. Approximately 40% to 90% of people acutely infected with HIV-1 develop symptoms. Symptoms are associated with the acute dissemination of the virus to various deep lymphoid tissues and occur approximately 4 to 11 days after initial infection. Symptoms include fever, generalized lymphadenopathy, pharyngitis, an erythematous maculopapular rash, arthralgias, myalgias, headache, diarrhea, malaise, nausea, vomiting, oral or genital ulcerations, and primary neurologic manifestations, such as Guillain-Barré syndrome. The differential for acute HIV includes acute mononucleosis, cytomegalovirus (CMV), herpes simplex virus, rubella, toxoplasmosis, hepatitis, disseminated gonococcal infections, syphilis, Lyme disease, drug reactions, and connective tissue diseases.

Chronic HIV infection, usually seen 6 to 12 months after acute primary infection, may present with fatigue and evidence of OIs, such as PCP, oral candidiasis, tuberculosis (TB), and disseminated *Mycobacterium avium* complex. The appearance of OIs has been directly correlated to the total number and percentage of CD4 T-lymphocytes. The following OIs are more likely to develop at the following total CD4 T-cell counts; therefore, dependent of the CD4 count, patients should be evaluated for the symptoms of each of the following diseases:

Absolute cluster of CD4 count	Major OIs encountered
>500	Bacterial infections
	Oral candidiasis
	Oral hairy leukoplakia
	Mycobacterium TB infection
	Varicella zoster
250–500	Above plus:
	Esophageal candidiasis
	Kaposi's sarcoma
50–250	Above plus:
	PCP
	Toxoplasmosis
	Extra-CNS lymphomas
	HIV encephalopathy
	Progressive multifocal leukoencephalopathy
<50	Above plus:
	CMV retinitis
	Disseminated *Mycobacterium avium* complex
	Cryptococcal meningitis
	Protozoan enteritides
	Disseminated varicella-zoster virus disease
	Refractory oral esophageal candidiasis
	Invasive aspergillosis
	CNS lymphoma

DIAGNOSIS

A thorough history should be taken, including medical history, surgical history, sexual history, drug and alcohol history, psychiatric history, and travel history. Travel history is important because it helps to identify risk for certain endemic infections, such as histoplasmosis or coccidioidomycosis. A thorough physical examination should be performed, including examining fundi for retinitis, oropharynx for thrush, neck and axilla for lymphadenopathy, lungs for evidence of pneumonia, heart for murmurs, abdomen for hepatosplenomegaly, genital and rectal area for ulcers or evidence of other sexually transmitted diseases, extremities and skin for rashes, and an extensive neurologic and psychiatric evaluation.

Blood work must be obtained, including an enzyme-linked immunoassay for HIV antibodies, which do not appear in the serum until approximately 22 to 27 days after acute infection. A Western blot should be performed to confirm the results of the enzyme-linked immunoassay. A p24 antigen assay can be obtained, but 20% to 40% of patients with HIV-1 have a negative p24 assay. HIV RNA is more reliable and can detect the virus 1 to 3 weeks earlier than standard serologic tests, but it is also more expensive. A patient with suspected acute HIV but with low viral loads should be retested to rule out a false-positive result. Other laboratory analyses include complete blood count with differential. Within the first 2 weeks of HIV infection, lymphopenia is seen with reduction of both CD4 and CD8 subsets. Within 3 to 4 weeks after infection, a lymphocytosis develops, with a predominately larger increase in CD8 T-cells and, to a lesser degree, CD4 T-cells. A mild thrombocytopenia is also commonly seen.

MANAGEMENT

Once a patient is diagnosed with HIV infection, baseline screening laboratories to look for the presence of OIs should be obtained, including a purified protein derivative; hepatitis A, B, and C viral titers; VDRL and rapid plasma reagent; toxoplasmosis antibody; CMV antibody; electrolytes; blood urea nitrogen; creatinine;

and liver function tests. A complete blood count should be checked at baseline and then every 3 to 6 months. Baseline HIV RNA viral load and CD4 and CD8 subsets should be checked. A chest x-ray and eye examination should be performed, and all female patients should have a Papanicolaou smear initially and every 3 to 6 months, given the increased risk of cervical cancer in women with HIV disease. All patients need counseling regarding the prevention of the spread of HIV; avoidance of specific foods, such as raw meat, eggs, and nonfiltered water; and information concerning the various pharmacologic treatments available to them. Before the institution of HAART, the importance of medication adherence must be discussed, as the risk of developing drug resistance with medication noncompliance is a potential problem. Regardless of whether the patient is ready to start treatment with HAART, he or she should be started on appropriate prophylactic medications to prevent the development of OIs. The development of OIs is associated with the level of the CD4 T-cell count. The following are the recommendations for beginning prophylaxis for OIs and the medications to use:

PCP
> When CD4 <200 or a history of oropharyngeal candidiasis or a CD4 T-cell percentage of <14%:
>> Trimethoprim-sulfamethoxazole, 1 double-strength tablet per day or 3 times per week. Or 1 single-strength tablet qd *or*
>> Dapsone plus pyrimethamine plus leucovorin *or*
>> Aerosolized pentamidine *or*
>> Atovaquone, 1,500 mg PO qd

Toxoplasmosis
> When CD4 <100 in patients with a positive immunoglobulin G antibody to *toxoplasma gondii*:
>> Trimethoprim-sulfamethoxazole, 1 double-strength tablet per day *or*
>> Dapsone-pyrimethamine *or*
>> Atovaquone with or without pyrimethamine

TB
> All HIV-positive patients with a purified protein derivative reaction ≥5 mm of induration should have a chest radiograph and clinical evaluation to rule out active TB. If there is no evidence of active TB, prophylaxis should be given. All HIV-positive patients who are close contacts of persons with infectious TB should also be administered chemoprophylaxis. TB can affect the HIV-positive patient at any CD4 count level. Chemoprophylaxis options include:
>> Isoniazid daily or twice weekly for 9 months *or*
>> Isoniazid plus rifampin and pyrazinamide for 2 months *or*
>> Isoniazid plus rifabutin and pyrazinamide for 2 months
> All patients receiving isoniazid should be given pyridoxine (vitamin B_6) to prevent peripheral neuropathy.

Mycobacterium avium complex
> When CD4 <50:
>> Clarithromycin, 500 mg PO b.i.d. or
>> Azithromycin, 1,200 mg PO every week or
>> Rifabutin

CMV
> When CD4 <50 in patients who are CMV seropositive, the administration of oral ganciclovir must be considered.

Vaccinations include pneumococcus, influenza, and hepatitis A and B (if viral titers for these are negative).

Treatment using HAART includes the following classes of antiretroviral agents:

1. Nucleoside reverse transcriptase inhibitors (NRTIs) competitively inhibit RT, resulting in DNA chain termination and reduced viral replication.
   - Zidovudine or azidothymidine or Retrovir
   - Didanosine or Videx
   - Zalcitabine or HIVID
   - Stavudine (D4T) or Zerit
   - Lamivudine (3TC) or Epivir
   - Abacavir or Ziagen
   - Tenofovir or Viread
   - Emtricitabine (FTC) or Emtriva
2. Nonnucleoside reverse transcriptase inhibitors bind at distinct sites on the RT enzyme, noncompetitively inhibiting it.
   - Nevirapine or Viramune
   - Delavirdine or Rescriptor
   - Efavirenz or Sustiva
3. Protease inhibitors inhibit HIV protease, an enzyme required for the cleavage of viral polyprotein precursors, preventing the generation of functional HIV proteins.
   - Saquinavir or Invirase and Fortovase
   - Ritonavir or Norvir
   - Indinavir or Crixivan
   - Nelfinavir or Viracept
   - Amprenavir or Agenerase
   - Lopinavir/Ritonavir or Kaletra
   - Atazanavir or Reyataz
   - Fosamprenavir (F-APV) or Lexiva
4. Fusion membrane inhibitors.
   - Enfurvitide (T20) or Fuzeon

Treatment should be offered to symptomatic patients (patients with thrush, unexplained fever) and to asymptomatic patients with CD4 T-cells less than 350 or plasma HIV greater than 30,000 copies per mL (bDNA assay) or plasma HIV greater than 55,000 copies per mL (RT-polymerase chain reaction assay).

The recommended regimen for initial treatment of established HIV infection includes either three NRTIs or two NRTIs and a protease inhibitor or two NRTIs and a nonnucleoside reverse transcriptase inhibitor. When designing a regimen, the following aspects must be considered:
- Side-effect profile of each medication
- Number of pills to be taken
- Interactions with other non-HIV medications
- Previous antiretroviral exposure

The plasma HIV RNA viral load should be assayed 2 to 8 weeks after initiation of antiretroviral therapy and then every 3 to 4 months to evaluate the effectiveness of therapy. With optimal therapy, there should be a log 10 decrease in the viral load at 8 weeks of treatment and an undetectable viral load (<50 copies/mL) at 4 to 6 months of treatment. If the viral load has not decreased appropriately, then patient compliance and viral resistance should be assessed. One method of determining if a patient has developed resistance to specific antiretroviral therapy is to perform a genotypic or phenotypic assay of the patient's virus.

Genotyping and phenotyping of HIV is done to determine which antiretroviral agents should be used based on the resistance pattern of viral variants present for each individual patient. Genotypic assays determine the presence of specific mutations within antiretroviral target gene products. Genotyping identifies specific mutations that can confer cross-resistance to other antiretrovirals but does not offer information regarding the function of the changes. Phenotypic assays are *in vitro*, culture-based tests used to determine the relative ability of the virus to grow in the presence of varying concentrations of a drug. Phenotyping is useful because it can yield direct information about how well the specific antiretrovirals inhibit the replication of the patient's specific strain of HIV, similar to bacterial susceptibility tests. Typically, the viral load must be at least 3,000 to perform these assays with relative reliability. They are very expensive tests and should be used only on a case-by-case basis in patients suspected of having resistance to certain antiretrovirals to provide more information about tailoring specific antiretroviral therapy. They should not be ordered routinely on all HIV patients.

Postexposure prophylaxis should be considered after unprotected sexual exposures, such as receptive anal and vaginal intercourse, insertive vaginal and anal intercourse, and unprotected receptive fellatio with ejaculation. In addition, patients with a partner who is known to be HIV infected or is in a high HIV risk group should be offered prophylaxis. Treatment should be initiated within 72 hours of exposure. Health care providers or others who have been exposed to known HIV-positive blood or other bodily fluids from high-risk patients via needle stick or other puncture should also be offered prophylaxis. The recommended treatment protocol includes 4 weeks of therapy, including an NRTI with azidothymidine, D4T, 3TC, or didanosine. Nelfinavir or indinavir should be offered to anyone with exposure to a patient who has a high viral load of more than 50,000 copies per mL of HIV RNA, advanced HIV, or history of treatment with the aforementioned NRTIs.

Chapter 4

INFECTIOUS ARTHRITIS

N. Christopher Kelley

OVERVIEW

Septic arthritis, or joint space infection, is one of the most rapidly destructive joint diseases. Despite advances in antibiotic therapy and arthroscopy, the morbidity and mortality in this disorder have not changed in more than 30 years. Between 25% and 50% of patients with nongonococcal joint infections suffer long-term sequelae, and death occurs in 5% to 15% of cases. Because of the severity of the consequences of septic arthritis, any joint suspected of being infected requires prompt evaluation and therapy.

PATHOPHYSIOLOGY

Septic arthritis is usually secondary to the hematogenous seeding of the synovial membrane from a transient or persistent bacteremia. An acute inflammatory cell response develops within hours and involves the membrane and the synovial fluid. The synovial membrane responds to inflammation by proliferation; cytokine and protease release by the inflammatory cells produce cartilage and subchondral bone degradation and inhibit new cartilage synthesis. The end result of this inflammatory cascade is irreversible joint damage within a few days. Staphylococci are the most common causative organisms in adults (40–50% of all cases), followed by group A streptococci (10–30%), gram-negative bacilli (10–20%), and anaerobes (<5%). *Neisseria gonorrhoeae* is an important pathogen that should be considered in young, sexually active adults. Group B, C, and G streptococci infections are also common in diabetics. Joint infections are rarely polymicrobial, unless there is direct inoculation of the joint space from trauma. There is an increased incidence of septic arthritis in patients with preexisting joint disease, intravenous drug use, and decreased immunocompetence. Patients with an impaired immune response are more susceptible to unusual infections, such as fungi and mycobacteria, usually in the setting of disseminated infection. Prosthetic joint infections are characterized as *early*, usually due to perioperative wound contamination, and *late*, due to hematogenous spread, and vary widely in their presentation.

CLINICAL PRESENTATION

Patients with septic arthritis generally present acutely with a single swollen and painful joint. The knee is involved in more than 50% of cases, although wrists, ankles, and hips are also commonly affected. Approximately 10% to 20% of joint infections are polyarticular, most likely occurring in patients with rheumatoid arthritis or in patients with overwhelming sepsis. Most patients are febrile, although high spiking fevers and chills are uncommon. Disseminated gonococcal infection presents with an acute monoarthritis in less than 50% of cases. A more typical presentation is that of a migratory polyarthralgia affecting large joints, tenosynovitis, and a painless maculopapular or petechial rash.

DIAGNOSIS

The differential diagnosis for acute monoarthritis is broad and includes crystal-induced arthritis (gout, pseudogout), osteoarthritis, joint trauma with hemarthrosis, Lyme disease (acute monoarthritis can occur months after the initial rash), and any chronic inflammatory joint disease (especially the seronegative spondyloarthropathies, such as Reiter's syndrome, and rheumatoid arthritis). The definitive diagnosis of septic arthritis is obtained from synovial fluid aspiration and analysis by cell count, Gram stain, and culture. Fluid should be sent for crystal analysis to rule out urate or calcium pyrophosphate crystals. Synovial fluid in septic arthritis usually has a leukocytosis (50–150,000 white blood cells/mm^3) with a neutrophil predominance, although lower counts do not necessarily rule out infection (especially in the setting of an immunocompromised host). The Gram stain is only positive in 50% to 80% of all cases of bacterial arthritis. Synovial fluid culture is positive in more than 90% of cases of bacterial arthritis. Gonococci are difficult to culture from synovial fluid; cultures from the cervix or urethra provide better yields and should be obtained if there is suspicion for gonococcal joint infection. Other synovial fluid findings, such as decreased glucose, decreased viscosity, and elevated protein, are not sensitive. Cultures should be sent for unusual organisms based on the clinical scenario, such as a history of tuberculosis exposure or active tuberculosis, travel to or living in an area with fungal infection or Lyme disease, or, in the case of a monoarthritis, refractoriness to conventional therapy. It is important that blood cultures be obtained, given that they are positive in up to 50% of patients with bacterial arthritis.

MANAGEMENT

Antibiotic therapy should be initiated promptly and be guided by synovial fluid Gram stain and the clinical scenario. If gram-positive cocci are seen on the Gram stain, cefazolin or oxacillin (or vancomycin, if nosocomial infection is suspected) should be used. Gram-negative bacilli should be treated with a third-generation cephalosporin, aminoglycoside, or quinolone (especially if *Pseudomonas* is suspected). Ceftriaxone or ceftizoxime should be used if a gonococcal infection is suspected. Because the Gram stain is negative in a large proportion of cases, empiric antibiotic coverage is reasonable if there is a high index of suspicion for a joint space infection. Treatment should be tailored to culture results. Most sources advocate a treatment course of 14 days of parenteral antibiotics followed by 14 days of oral therapy, if possible. To minimize inflammatory sequelae, all infected joints should be tapped until no fluid is evident. This can be accomplished in most joints with serial needle aspiration. Arthroscopic drainage, which is becoming more popular because of better irrigation and joint visualization, or open drainage may be necessary if response to therapy is poor or drainage is inadequate. If the patient has an inadequate response to standard therapy, a search for more unusual organisms should be initiated. Infection of bioprosthetic joints generally requires surgical removal of the infected joint.

Chapter 5

INFECTIOUS DIARRHEA

Avlin B. Imaeda

OVERVIEW

Diarrhea is an extremely common cause of outpatient and inpatient hospital visits and commonly occurs as a nosocomial process. Several hundred children die each year from diarrhea, even in the United States. There are approximately 200,000 hospitalizations and 1.5 million outpatient visits attributed to diarrhea among children and adults in the United States. Diarrhea, mostly infectious, is the second leading cause of death worldwide. Although noninfectious diarrhea is common in the United States, frequent travel, immigration, human immunodeficiency virus (HIV) and acquired immunodeficiency syndrome, and other immunocompromised states have changed the differential diagnosis of diarrhea that must be considered in developed countries.

PATHOPHYSIOLOGY

Diarrhea is defined as greater than 200 to 250 g of stool per day with an increase in stool liquidity and frequency. Generally, diarrhea is categorized as *acute* if it has lasted for up to 7 to 10 days, *persistent* if it has lasted 14 or more days, and *chronic* if it has lasted 1 month or more. The mechanisms of diarrhea depend on the infecting organism and the site of the gastrointestinal tract that is involved. The small bowel functions as a secretory and nutrient-absorptive organ. Infection of this part of the bowel tends to cause a profuse watery diarrhea, associated with cramping, bloating, and significant weight loss if water is not replenished or if diarrhea is long-standing. The large bowel stores concentrated waste and is a muscular excretory organ. Diarrhea caused by large-bowel infection is more likely to be small volume and associated with pain and tenesmus. Blood, mucous, and white blood cells are much more likely to be found in the stool, and fever is more common with large-bowel diarrhea.

Vibrio cholerae, *Staphylococcus aureus*, *Bacillus cereus*, and *Clostridium perfringens* all produce toxins that act within hours of ingestion. *Salmonella*, *Shigella*, *Campylobacter*, and *Yersinia* multiply and invade the lining of the gastrointestinal tract before causing symptoms; thus, onset of symptoms can take days. *Salmonella* species are relatively sensitive to gastric pH and require a large bacterial load in a host with a normal gastric pH, whereas *Shigella* species are quite resistant, and as few as ten organisms are capable of causing infection.

CLINICAL PRESENTATION

Clinical presentation varies by the organism and the site of infection (Tables 5–1 through 5–3). Although most pathogens cause self-limited acute diarrhea, parasites such as *Giardia* and the intestinal spore-forming protozoa *Cryptosporidia*, *Microsporidia*, *Isospora*, and *Cyclospora* can cause diarrhea lasting a few months, even in immunocompetent hosts. Diarrhea is usually much more severe and more likely to become chronic in immunocompromised hosts.

TABLE 5–1 Small-Bowel Pathogens

Pathogen	Historic Clues	Onset	Course
Escherichia coli			
EHEC	Beef, pork, cider	3–5 d	Acute
ETEC	Developing world	>14 h	Acute
Clostridium perfringens	Home canning, beef, pork, poultry	8–14 h	Acute
Staphylococcus aureus	Beef, pork, poultry, eggs	1–7 h	Acute
Bacillus cereus	Beef, pork, rice, vegetables	1–7 h	Acute
Vibrio cholerae	Gulf coast, United States	Hours to 5 d	Acute
Rotavirus	Daycare, nurseries, infantile diarrhea	>14 h	Acute
Norwalk agent	Outbreaks, food-borne, shellfish	>14 h	Acute
Cryptosporidium	Daycare, pools, AIDS, drinking water	—	Asymptomatic, protracted
Microsporium	AIDS, travelers	—	Asymptomatic, protracted
Isospora belli	Haiti, HIV	—	Asymptomatic, protracted
Cyclospora	Raspberries, outbreak, HIV	—	Asymptomatic, protracted
Giardia lamblia	Daycare, pools, camping, beavers	—	Acute, protracted

AIDS, acquired immunodeficiency virus; EHEC, enterohemorrhagic *E. coli*; ETEC, enterotoxigenic *E. coli*.; HIV, human immunodeficiency virus.

TABLE 5-2 Small-Bowel and Large-Bowel Pathogens

Pathogen	Historical Clues	Onset	Course
Salmonella	Beef, pork, poultry, eggs, milk, reptiles	6–72 h	Acute
Shigella	Daycare centers, vegetables	1–7 d	Acute
Campylobacter	Poultry, milk, Guillain-Barré	1–7 d	Acute
Yersinia	Pork, beef, milk, iron overload, sore throat, pseudoappendicitis	1–11 d	Acute to protracted
Cytomegalovirus	Acquired immunodeficiency syndrome, CD4 <50	—	Chronic

DIAGNOSIS

A careful symptom, exposure, and travel history must be obtained. No diagnostic workup is necessary for a young healthy individual in whom the diarrhea resolves within 3 to 7 days. Patients at extremes of age, those who show signs of dehydration, are immunocompromised, have other comorbid illnesses, or who have had prolonged symptoms should be considered for further workup and possibly inpatient treatment. A gross examination of the stool for blood and mucus and a microscopic examination for stool white cells can be useful for differentiating large- and small-bowel diarrhea or differentiating invasive from noninvasive organisms. A history of antibiotic use is important to evaluate for *Clostridium difficile* colitis or antibiotic-associated diarrhea. *C. difficile* is evaluated by enzyme-immunoassay antigen tests or the more sensitive and specific cell culture toxin assay. Stool samples can be sent for routine bacterial culture for *Shigella, Salmonella,* and *Campylobacter.* Special requests should be made if there is suspicion of *Yersinia, V. cholerae,* or *Escherichia coli* O157:H7. Sending stool for parasite evaluation and even routine stool cultures is usually not indicated for patients in whom diarrhea began more than 3 days into hospitalization. In patients with HIV, stool should be sent for staining for the intestinal spore-forming protozoa. Endoscopic biopsy may be needed in HIV-infected patients,

TABLE 5-3 Large-Bowel Pathogens

Pathogen	Historic Clues	Course
Clostridium difficile	Antibiotic use Days up to >1 mo	Acute to protracted
Vibrio parahaemolyticus	Coastal United States, shellfish	Acute
Enteroinvasive *Escherichia coli*	Milk, cheese	Acute
Adenovirus	AIDS, organ transplant	Acute to chronic
Mycobacterium avium-intra-cellulare	AIDS, CD4 <50, organ transplant	Chronic
Entamoeba histolytica	Travel to Mexico, anal sex, institutions	Acute to chronic

AIDS, acquired immunodeficiency virus.

particularly for diagnosis of cytomegalovirus (colon) and some of the intestinal spore-forming protozoa (small bowel).

An important differential diagnosis for small-bowel diarrhea includes malabsorption syndromes; Crohn's disease; secretory diarrheas, such as antibiotic-associated diarrhea; and, importantly, osmotic diarrhea. Osmotic diarrhea can be surreptitiously self-induced but is often nosocomial, caused by such agents as sorbitol found in acetaminophen elixir and tube-feedings. A gap of more than 10 osmoles between the measured osmolarity and the calculated [2([Na] + [K])] stool osmolarity can help to diagnose an osmotic diarrhea.

Finally, infections caused by *Salmonella typhi* and *Brucella* sp. can be found in the United States and should be considered with recent travel to or from developing countries or exposure to certain animals, respectively. These organisms may require repeated blood cultures for identification; bone marrow biopsy is the most sensitive diagnostic test. *Strongyloides stercoralis* can be seen even in patients who have not traveled recently, as its life cycle allows it to persistently infect a host for years. Symptomatic infection may occur with steroid use or other immunosuppression. A stool parasite examination identifies this organism.

MANAGEMENT

Most acute infectious diarrhea does not require therapy. Maintaining adequate hydration is the most important therapy, and oral hydration is often adequate. World Health Organization oral rehydration therapy is very effective, and there are some similar commercially prepared products for this purpose. Fruit juices, soda, and Gatorade are not as effective and can worsen diarrhea, as they are often hyperosmolar and do not adequately replete electrolytes. Empiric antibiotic therapy for bacterial diarrhea is usually not indicated but should be used in severely ill and bacteremic patients. Ciprofloxacin is the drug of choice for empiric therapy, and this can be tailored if the organism is identified. Bismuth subsalicylate can be used adjunctively for its antibacterial and toxin-binding effects. Some evidence suggests that *Salmonella* infection can be worsened by antibiotic therapy, likely due to the decrease in normal intestinal flora. Evidence also exists that antibiotic therapy may increase the risk of hemolytic-uremic syndrome in enterohemorrhagic *E. coli* infection. Treatment of acquired immunodeficiency syndrome–related infectious diarrhea is complicated and requires organism-specific therapy. Immunosuppressed patients may require chronic suppressive therapy for infections with *Mycobacterium avium-intracellulare* and some of the intestinal spore-forming protozoa.

Chapter 6

INFECTIVE ENDOCARDITIS

David S. Smith

OVERVIEW

Endocarditis is an infection of the endocardial surface of the heart. Although potentially deadly, diagnosis is not always obvious. Patients may present with a nonlocalizing fever and a subtle murmur, or with manifestations of septic emboli, such as stroke or splinter hemorrhages under the nails. If considered in the differential, diagnosis is usually readily established by blood culture.

PATHOPHYSIOLOGY

Left-sided (aortic or mitral valve) endocarditis usually develops on a valve previously damaged by rheumatic fever, congenital malformation, or myxomatous degeneration. Right-sided (tricuspid or pulmonic valve) endocarditis usually occurs in an injection drug user or on a valve previously damaged by a right heart catheter.

The characteristic lesion, a vegetation, is composed of platelets, fibrin, bacteria, and inflammatory cells. Mitral valve prolapse is the most common underlying factor, especially in patients with mitral regurgitation and thickened leaflets.

Native valve endocarditis is most often caused by streptococci, with *Streptococcus viridans* causing 35% of cases, usually entering the circulation through the mouth. The finding of *Streptococcus bovis* is associated with colon cancer in 20% of cases. *Staphylococcus aureus* causes 30% of cases, arising from cutaneous infections. Enterococci from a gastrointestinal source cause 10% of cases. *Haemophilus, Actinobacilli, Cardiobacterium, Eikenella,* and *Kingella* (HACEK) organisms are nonenteric, gram-negative organisms causing less than 10% of cases. Prosthetic valve endocarditis within 2 months of surgery (early) is caused by *Staphylococcus epidermidis* or *S. aureus* in the majority. Cases occurring more than 1 year after surgery (late) are due to community-acquired organisms. Nosocomial infections are increasingly common at tertiary care hospitals, arising from an infected intravascular device. An injection drug user usually has *S. aureus* endocarditis, but *S. viridans, Pseudomonas aeruginosa,* and *Candida parapsilosis* or polymicrobial infections are also seen.

CLINICAL PRESENTATION

The onset of endocarditis is often subacute and subtle, with low-grade fever (maximally, 38–39°C) and fatigue. Murmur is present in 85% but may not be loud. Other symptoms of a subacute presentation include anorexia, weight loss, and night sweats. Osler's nodes, found in 25% of patients with a subacute presentation, are raised, red, tender lesions on the pads of the fingers or toes, representing immune complex deposition. Janeway lesions are flat, red, nontender lesions on the palms or soles, representing septic emboli. Petechiae may be seen on the palate or conjunctivae. Retinal hemorrhages with a pale center, Roth spots, strongly suggest endocarditis. Longitudinal splinter hemorrhages in the nails are commonly found but are nonspecific and also caused by minor trauma. Splenomegaly is found in 50% of patients with sub-acute endocarditis. Associated left upper quadrant pain and a friction rub suggest splenic infarction or abscess.

Congestive heart failure and neurologic complications have the greatest impact on outcome. Congestive heart failure is usually caused by valvular damage, less commonly by embolic myocardial infarction. Extension of the infection into the septum may cause heart block of varying degrees. The most common neurologic manifestations are cerebral emboli and aseptic meningitis. These may be complicated by stroke, mycotic aneurysm with subsequent subarachnoid hemorrhage, brain abscess, or purulent meningitis. Renal manifestations are common, ranging from microscopic hematuria caused by emboli to proliferative glomerulonephritis due to circulating antigen-antibody complexes.

DIAGNOSIS

Thinking of the diagnosis of endocarditis is usually the most difficult part. Continuous bacteremia is a hallmark of infection and can be readily identified with blood cultures. Fastidious organisms or concurrent antibiotic therapy may make organisms more difficult to recover. Two sets of blood cultures collected by separate venipunctures should be collected within 2 hours of presentation. Echocardiography can identify vegetations and abscess, as well as assess the severity of valve damage. Transesophageal echocardiography is more sensitive than transthoracic echocardiography in detecting vegetations and abscesses, especially in prosthetic valve endocarditis (positive in 85–90% of cases). The Duke criteria have aided accurate diagnosis, with a specificity of 0.99 (0.97–10) (Table 6–1).

TABLE 6-1   Duke Criteria for the Diagnosis of Infective Endocarditis[a]

Major criteria

    Typical microorganism isolated from two separate blood cultures (*Streptococcus viridans*, *Streptococcus bovis*, HACEK group, *Staphylococcus aureus*, or community-acquired enterococcal bacteremia without a primary focus)

    Microorganism consistent with infective endocarditis isolated from persistently positive blood cultures

    Single positive blood culture for *Coxiella burnetti* or phase I immunoglobulin G antibody titer to *C. burnetti* >1:800

    New valvular regurgitation (increase or change in preexisting murmur not sufficient)

    Positive echocardiogram (transesophageal echocardiogram recommended)

Minor criteria

    Predisposing conditions (high risk: previous endocarditis, aortic valve disease, rheumatic heart disease, prosthetic valve, coarctation of the aorta, congenital cyanotic heart disease; moderate risk: mitral valve prolapse with regurgitation or leaflet thickening, mitral stenosis, pulmonic stenosis, tricuspid valve disease, hypertrophic cardiomyopathy)

    Fever >38°C (100.4°F)

    Vascular phenomena (not petechiae or splinter hemorrhages)

    Immunologic phenomena (rheumatoid factor, glomerulonephritis, Osler's nodes, or Roth spots)

    Positive blood cultures that do not meet major criteria (except single isolates of coagulase-negative staphylococci) or serologic evidence of active infection

---

HACEK, *Haemophilus aphrophilus, Actinobacillus actinomycetemcomitans, Cardiobacterium hominis, Eikenella corrodens,* and *Kingella kingae.*

[a]Clinically definite if two major, one major and three minor, or five minor criteria are present. Possible if one major and one minor or three minor criteria are present.

MANAGEMENT

Antibiotics should be started only when the diagnosis is secure or when there is evidence of aggressive tissue destruction. Initial empiric therapy is based on the clinical circumstances, that is, using vancomycin and gentamicin in prosthetic valve endocarditis to cover *S. aureus* and *S. epidermidis*. Treatment regimens must be bactericidal to be effective and may require further synergism, as between a penicillin and an aminoglycoside, for resistant streptococci and enterococci. Streptococci are treated with penicillin and gentamicin, enterococci with ampicillin and gentamicin, *S. aureus* with oxacillin and gentamicin, *S. epidermidis* with vancomycin and gentamicin, and HACEK organisms with ceftriaxone. Uncomplicated native valve endocarditis due to a penicillin-sensitive organism and right-sided endocarditis can be cured in 2 to 4 weeks. Patients with streptococcus, suppurative complications, or prosthetic valve endocarditis should be treated for 4 to 6 weeks.

Initially, the patient should be monitored closely for complications, such as a changing murmur; emboli to joints, skin, or brain; heart block due to valve ring abscess; or congestive heart failure. Acute heart failure from valve destruction or rupture of the sinus of Valsalva is the most certain indication for surgical intervention.

Antibiotic prophylaxis is used for procedures producing bacteremia in patients with a prosthetic valve, congenital or acquired valve malformations, and mitral valve prolapse with mitral regurgitation as evidenced by a murmur. Prophylaxis for procedures above the diaphragm is aimed at *S. viridans*; for those below the diaphragm, it is aimed at enterococci.

Chapter 7

MENINGITIS

Lynn E. Sullivan

OVERVIEW

Meningitis is an inflammation of the meninges and subarachnoid space. There are myriad causes of meningitis, but it is a diagnosis that must be considered in any patient that presents with fever and mental status changes. In the case of acute bacterial meningitis, missing this diagnosis could lead to a catastrophic outcome.

PATHOPHYSIOLOGY

Bacterial meningitis evolves from nasopharyngeal colonization and mucosal invasion or from bacteremia from sources other than the nasopharynx. The bacteria survive in the bloodstream because they evade the complement pathway, cross the blood–brain barrier, and enter the cerebrospinal fluid (CSF). Potential sites of invasion include the cribriform plate area, the choroid plexus, and the dural venous sinuses. Low levels of complement, immuno-globulin, and opsonic activity contribute to decreased host defenses, thereby facilitating invasion by bacteria. The presence of bacteria causes white blood cells to enter the CSF. In viral meningitis, viruses enter the CSF through the gastrointestinal, respiratory, or urogenital tracts or through injection into the skin by mosquitoes or ticks, as in the case of the arboviruses. Replication of the virus occurs outside the central nervous system (CNS), followed by subse-quent hematogenous spread to the CNS. The severity of the infection is dependent on the host's immune system as well as the virulence of the spe-cific virus. Certain viruses preferentially attack specific cell types in the CNS; therefore, different pathogens can result in different clinical presentations. In most cases of fungal meningitis, pulmonary exposure followed by hema-togenous spread is the primary pathogenetic mechanism. Decreased host defenses or an immunocompromised host increases the likelihood of devel-oping a fungal CNS infection.

CLINICAL PRESENTATION

Generally, patients with meningitis present with complaints of generalized headache, steady or throbbing, intensified by sudden head movements. They often also report fever, photophobia, mental status changes, and, occasion-ally, seizures. On examination, they can exhibit signs of meningeal irritation, including nuchal rigidity and a positive Kernig or Brudzinski sign. *Neisseria meningitidis* causes meningococcal meningitis and classically presents with a rash characterized by pink tender maculopapules and petechial hemorrhages involving the trunk and extremities. *Streptococcus pneumoniae* is the most likely cause of bacterial meningitis in which seizures develop. Likewise, there is an increased likelihood of neurologic findings, such as seizures, in meningitis secondary to *Listeria monocytogenes*. *Borrelia burgdorferi*, the spirochete responsi-ble for causing Lyme disease, can produce meningitis with disseminated dis-ease. Headache is the primary symptom, but facial nerve palsies can be seen.

DIAGNOSIS

Obtaining a microbiologic diagnosis is important to tailor antimicrobial ther-apy, but delaying treatment could have serious consequences. If pyogenic men-ingitis is suspected, empiric antibiotics should be started immediately, even before proceeding to the lumbar puncture (LP). If the patient has a focal neu-rologic examination or evidence of papilledema by funduscopic examination, they should undergo computed tomography of the head before the LP is per-formed to rule out the presence of increased intracranial pressure. When per-forming an LP, an opening pressure should be checked, with the normal range being 100 to 200 mm Hg. An increased pressure suggests an intracranial suppu-rative foci or cerebral edema. Evaluation of the CSF includes looking at the color, with xanthochromic or yellow-colored fluid indicating a possible previ-ous subarachnoid hemorrhage, pink fluid indicating a traumatic LP, and turbid fluid indicating that white blood cells are present, indicative of infection. Pleo-cytosis signifies that there is an increased number of one cell type, and the pre-dominance of a certain cell type is dependent on the specific pathogen. CSF should be collected in sterile tubes and sent to the laboratory for analysis for protein, glucose, cell count, Gram stain, culture and sensitivity, and cytology to rule out malignancy. If an increased number of red blood cells is found in the first tube and it persists in the cell count in subsequent tubes, it indicates that there may be a subarachnoid hemorrhage present. If there is a decrease in the number of red blood cells in subsequent tubes, the LP was likely traumatic. In addition, several samples of fluid should be sent for smear and culture for acid-fast bacilli to rule out tuberculosis, India ink stain to rule out cryptococcus, VDRL to rule out syphilis, and fungal and viral studies, including herpes simplex virus (HSV).

In bacterial infections, there is typically an elevated opening pressure, and the CSF reveals a leukocytosis with a neutrophilic predominance. In addition, CSF analysis shows a decreased glucose with a CSF-serum glucose ratio of less than 0.31, an increased protein, and increased lactate level. Performing latex agglutination diagnoses *Haemophilus influenzae, S. pneumoniae, N. meningitidis, Escherichia coli,* and Group B streptococcus. Polymerase chain reaction (PCR) analysis identifies *L. monocytogenes* and *N. meningitidis.* The CSF in the setting of *Mycobacterium tuberculosis* typically reveals a moderate pleocytosis, predominantly neutrophils or lymphocytes, moderately decreased glucose, and increased protein. With the enteroviruses, CSF reveals a pleocytosis with predominantly neutrophils evolving to lymphocytes. There is mildly increased protein and decreased glucose. CNS infections with the herpesviruses—HSV 1 and 2, varicella-zoster virus, cytomegalovirus, Epstein-Barr virus, human herpesvirus 6, and human herpesvirus 7—manifest with the most significant neurologic complications. CSF analysis reveals a lymphocytic predominance with normal glucose. CSF samples should be sent for PCR analysis to rule out HSV.

CSF in patients with human immunodeficiency virus (HIV) shows a mild lymphocytic pleocytosis with mildly increased protein and low-normal glucose. In *B. burgdorferi,* CSF has a lymphocytic pleocytosis with increased protein and normal glucose. A Lyme titer or PCR for DNA can be sent to confirm a diagnosis of Lyme disease. CSF in cryptococcal meningitis typically shows a pleocytosis with neutrophils of less than 50%, increased protein, and low-normal glucose. Samples should be sent for India ink stain and a latex agglutination test. The serum should be sent for cryptococcal antigen. CSF in patients with coccidioidomycosis reveals a pleocytosis with eosinophils, increased protein, and decreased glucose. Complement-fixing antibodies should be checked.

Certain host factors, including current medical conditions, have a significant impact on the likelihood of a certain pathogen causing the CNS infection. *H. influenzae* affects infants and young children or adults with sinusitis, otitis, or pneumonia or who are immunocompromised. *N. meningitidis* affects children and young adults and individuals with complement deficiencies. Pneumococcal meningitis affects adults with pneumonia, otitis, mastoiditis, sinusitis, or endocarditis secondary to *S. pneumoniae.* In addition, patients who are immunocompromised or have a CSF leak in the setting of a basilar skull fracture are at a greater risk of developing pneumococcal meningitis. Neonates, the elderly, alcoholics, or immunocompromised patients are more likely to develop meningitis secondary to *L. monocytogenes, Streptococcus agalactiae,* or group B streptococcus. Of the staphylococcus sp., *Staphylococcus. aureus* is seen in postneurosurgical patients and posttrauma patients, as well as in the setting of CSF shunts. *Staphylococcus epidermidis* is most commonly seen in patients with shunts in place. The gram-negative bacilli *Klebsiella* sp., *E. coli, Serratia marcescens, Pseudomonas aeruginosa,* and *Salmonella* sp., are most commonly seen in neonates, the elderly, postneurosurgical and posttrauma patients, and immunocompromised hosts.

The enteroviruses, such as echovirus and coxsackievirus, are primarily seen in infants and children during warm weather months and are transmitted via the fecal-oral route.

Meningitis secondary to the mumps virus is seen in unimmunized populations during winter months. The risk of infection with *Treponema pallidum,* the pathogen that causes neurosyphilis, is increased in patients with a signifi-

TABLE 7-1 Antibiotic Therapy in the Management of Meningitis

Pathogen	Choice of Antibiotic
Haemophilus influenzae	Third-generation cephalosporin
Neisseria meningitidis	Penicillin G, third-generation cephalosporin, or ampicillin
Streptococcus pneumoniae	Third-generation cephalosporin; very resistant: third-generation cephalosporin + vancomycin (vancomycin has variable cerebrospinal fluid penetration)
Listeria monocytogenes	Ampicillin or penicillin G ± aminoglycoside
Streptococcus agalactiae	Ampicillin + aminoglycoside
Staphylococcus sp.	Oxacillin or nafcillin; vancomycin for resistant organisms; add rifampin if not responding
Pseudomonas aeruginosa, Acinetobacter, Enterobacteriaceae	Broad-spectrum cephalosporin + aminoglycoside
Myobacterium tuberculosis	Isoniazid, rifampin, pyrazinamide
Herpesviruses	Acyclovir
Treponema pallidum	Penicillin G
Borrelia burgdorferi	Ceftriaxone
Cryptococcus neoformans	Amphotericin B
Coccidioides immitis	Amphotericin B

cant sexual history. Lyme meningitis secondary to *B. burgdorferi* is seen more frequently in patients with a history of exposure to deer ticks or wooded areas. *Cryptococcus neoformans*, one of the fungal infections that can cause meningitis, is associated with bird droppings and is also seen in immunocompromised patients, especially those with HIV. Coccidioides immitis, a second cause of fungal meningitis, is primarily seen in immunocompromised patients or patients with HIV.

MANAGEMENT

Antibiotic therapy is a key component in the management of meningitis and the appropriate antibiotic, whether chosen based on Gram stain results or on an empiric basis, should be administered in a prompt fashion (Table 7-1).

Use of corticosteroids in adults with meningitis is controversial. Tuberculous meningitis, which typically manifests with significant inflammation with an increased risk of hydrocephalus, warrants corticosteroid therapy. In addition, corticosteroids are indicated in certain cases of children with meningitis and to treat cerebral edema in adults with pyogenic meningitis.

Chapter 8

NECROTIZING FASCIITIS

Kathleen Stergiopoulos

OVERVIEW

Necrotizing fasciitis is an uncommon infection of the subcutaneous tissue that results in the progressive destruction of superficial or deep fascia, causing destruction of arteries (via thrombosis) and nerves, leading to gangrene. These infections are classified as types I and II. A subtype of necrotizing fasciitis of the perineal area, usually in men, is known as *Fournier's gangrene*. These infections are commonly associated with early onset of shock and organ failure. The distinction between cellulitis and necrotizing fasciitis is crucial, because cellulitis is amenable to antimicrobial therapy, whereas necrotizing fasciitis requires urgent surgical débridement of necrotic tissue, in addition to the use of antimicrobial agents.

PATHOPHYSIOLOGY

Type I necrotizing fasciitis is a mixed infection caused by aerobic and anaerobic bacteria and occurs most commonly after surgical procedures and in patients with diabetes and peripheral vascular disease. Bacterial isolates are commonly polymicrobial, including *Staphylococcus aureus*, *Escherichia coli*, group A streptococci, *Peptostreptococcus* sp., *Prevotella* and *Porphyromonas* sp., *Bacteroides fragilis*, and *Clostridium* sp. Necrotizing fasciitis should be considered in patients with cellulitis who have signs of systemic infection, such as tachycardia, leukocytosis, marked hyperglycemia, or acidosis.

Type II necrotizing fasciitis is caused by group A streptococcus and was previously named *streptococcal gangrene*. Most cases are community-acquired, but 20% are nosocomial or acquired in a nursing home. Type II infections can occur in any age group and among patients without comorbid illnesses. Predisposing factors include a history of blunt trauma, varicella infection, intravenous drug abuse, and a penetrating injury, such as in the setting of a laceration, surgical procedure, or childbirth. The skin is the portal of entry in patients after trauma or surgery. Hematogenous translocation in patients in whom no obvious portal of entry exists, originating in the throat with asymptomatic or symptomatic pharyngitis, to the site of blunt trauma or muscle strain results in the development of necrotizing fasciitis and associated myonecrosis. The M protein of group A streptococcus is a filamentous protein anchored to the cell membrane, which has antiphagocytic properties. Types 1 and 3 M proteins are most commonly associated with necrotizing fasciitis, as these strains can produce one or more pyrogenic exotoxins. Necrotizing fasciitis caused by these strains is frequently associated with streptococcal toxic shock syndrome characterized by the early onset of shock and multiorgan failure.

CLINICAL PRESENTATION

Early recognition of necrotizing fasciitis is important, as there may be a rapid progression from an apparently mild process to one associated with extensive destruction of tissue, systemic toxicity, loss of limb, or death. Necrotizing fasciitis is more likely to develop in the setting of diabetes, alcoholism, and parenteral drug abuse. The affected area is initially erythematous, swollen, without sharp margins, hot, shiny, and exquisitely tender. The process progresses rapidly over several days, with sequential skin color changes from red to purple to patches of blue-gray. Within 3 to 5 days of onset, skin breakdown occurs with bullae containing thick or purple fluid, termed *violaceous bullae*, and frank cutaneous gangrene. Once the bullous stage is reached, there is already extensive deep soft tissue destruction, such as necrotizing fasciitis or myonecrosis. At this time, the area is no longer tender, but hypoesthesia develops secondary to thrombosis of small blood vessels and destruction of superficial nerves. Marked swelling and edema may produce a compartment syndrome. Pressures greater than 40 mm Hg require immediate fasciotomy. Leukocytosis is commonly present, as well as fevers to 102° to 105°F. Other symptoms, such as malaise, myalgias, diarrhea, and anorexia, may develop in the first 24 hours. Hypotension may be initially present or develop over time. Blood cultures are frequently positive. Hypocalcemia without tetany may occur when necrosis of subcutaneous fat is extensive. Other findings include azotemia, thrombocytopenia, and elevated creatine phosphokinase levels.

In type I infections, characteristic locations are feet, head and neck, perineum, abdominal wall, and postoperative wounds. Severe pain may not be present secondary to diabetic neuropathy. An obvious portal of entry is usually present, such as a site of trauma, a laparotomy performed in the presence of peritoneal soiling, perirectal abscess, decubitus ulcer, or an intestinal perforation secondary to neoplasm or foreign body. Gas may be present within subcutaneous tissue, particularly in patients with diabetes. In type II infections, common features are fever, severe local pain, and systemic toxicity. Gas in the soft tissues is usually absent, and in 50% of cases, there is no obvious portal of entry. Erythema may be present diffusely or locally, but in some patients, excruciating pain in the absence of any cutaneous findings is the only clue of infection.

DIAGNOSIS

A high degree of clinical suspicion is necessary, as it is often difficult to differentiate cellulitis from necrotizing fasciitis at early stages. Rising creatine phosphokinase levels may serve as an indication of progression of streptococcal cellulitis to necrotizing fasciitis and myositis. Plain radiograph of the site can be useful in demonstrating soft tissue gas, although if not present, the diagnosis of necrotizing fasciitis is still possible. Computed axial tomography or magnetic resonance imaging is useful in locating the site and extent of infection. The need for imaging should be balanced with appreciation of the rapidity with which infection progresses and should not delay urgent surgical débridement when the diagnosis is made on clinical grounds. Computed axial tomography or magnetic resonance imaging may be most useful early in the process when pain and swelling are evident but cutaneous changes are absent and the diagnosis is uncertain. Imaging may also be useful after surgery when further surgery needs to be considered. Gram-stained smears of superficial exudates may reveal the etiologic organism and guide antimicrobial therapy. Frozen section biopsy, Gram stain, and culture performed at the time of surgery provide a definitive diagnosis. If severe pain and swelling are present without the onset of cutaneous features and compartment syndrome is suspected, measurements of muscle compartment pressure are useful.

MANAGEMENT

Early and aggressive surgical exploration is essential in patients with suspected necrotizing fasciitis, myositis, or gangrene to visualize the deeper structures, remove necrotic tissue, reduce compartment pressure via fasciotomy, and obtain material for culture. In patients in whom the diagnosis is suspected on clinical grounds based on deep pain with patchy areas of surface hypoesthesia, crepitus, bullae, and skin necrosis, surgery should be performed with extensive incisions made through the skin and subcutaneous tissues until areas of normal tissue are found. Direct observation of the nature and extent of the pathologic process guides the decision regarding the necessity for simple drainage, radical débridement, or guillotine amputation. A second procedure is frequently necessary 24 hours later to ensure adequacy of the initial débridement.

In type I necrotizing fasciitis, early empiric antibiotic treatment usually includes ampicillin or ampicillin-sulbactam combined with clindamycin or metronidazole for anaerobic coverage. Broader gram-negative coverage is necessary if the patient has had a prior hospitalization or if antibiotics have been used recently, in which case ticarcillin-clavulanate or piperacillin-tazobactam should be substituted for ampicillin, or a fluoroquinolone or an aminoglycoside should be added. Studies suggest that clindamycin is superior to penicillin in the treatment of experimental type II necrotizing fasciitis/myonecrosis, supporting data by Eagle that were termed the *Eagle effect*. The failure of penicillin in this setting is likely secondary to a reduction in bacterial expression of critical penicillin-binding proteins during the stationary phase. Clindamycin may be more effective because it is not affected by inoculum size or the stage of growth. In addition, it suppresses toxin production and facilitates phagocytosis of *Streptococcus pyogenes* by inhibiting M-protein synthesis by decreasing adherence of bacteria to host cells and enhancing intracellular killing. Furthermore, it suppresses production of regulatory elements controlling cell wall synthesis and has a long postantibiotic effect that may be attributed to persistence of the drug at the ribosomal binding site. Although there are no data from clinical trials, it is recommended that type II infections be treated with penicillin G (4 million U IV q4h) in combination with clindamycin (600–900 mg IV q8h).

Chapter 9

NEUTROPENIC FEVER

Julie R. Rosenbaum

OVERVIEW

Neutropenia is a common occurrence in cancer patients, either as a result of the malignancy itself or as a result of its treatment. Without appropriate management, patients with neutropenia and fever, especially when the fever is due to gram-negative bacterial infection, have a high rate of mortality. It should be treated as an emergency, with prompt initiation of antimicrobial therapy. Better treatment has resulted in improved survival rates for these patients, as well as for patients who are immunosuppressed from organ or bone marrow transplant or human immunodeficiency virus. Infection as the cause of fever can be documented in approximately 40% of cases of neutropenic fever. Of these cases, an organism can be identified approximately 60% of the time.

PATHOPHYSIOLOGY

Early studies have shown that the frequency of infectious complications is related to the duration and degree of neutropenia. The frequency of infection increases as the absolute neutrophil count [(ANC); calculated as total white blood cell count times the percentage of neutrophils plus bands] falls below 1,000 per mm^3. The common definition of neutropenia is an ANC less than 500, and the likelihood of infection again increases when the ANC falls below 100. Other factors also affect the risk of patients with neutropenia, such as the use of intravascular devices, the presence of mucositis, leukemia (as opposed to solid malignancies), corticosteroid therapy, a history of antimicrobial prophylaxis, and some specific chemotherapeutic regimens. These regimens may include agents such as cytarabine, daunorubicin, doxorubicin, 5-fluorouracil, 6-mercaptopurine, and methotrexate. When a specific etiology of infection can be identified, gram-positive organisms, including coagulase-negative staphylococci, *Staphylococcus aureus*, and *Streptococcus viridans*, are the most common cause, accounting for 55% to 65% of infections associated with neutropenic fever. Gram-negative organisms, especially *Escherichia coli*, *Klebsiella* sp., and *Pseudomonas aeruginosa*, are the predominant species. These organisms were previously the major cause of neutropenic fever, but empiric treatment and prophylaxis, as well as the use of indwelling intravenous catheters, have now shifted the prevalence from these organisms to the gram-positive organisms. In the past decade, fungi, including *Candida* sp. and *Aspergillus* sp., have become frequent causes of primary infection and superinfection. Viral illnesses are increasingly being recognized, including herpes simplex virus, varicella-zoster virus, respiratory syncytial virus, cytomegalovirus, and influenza. Eighty percent of identified infections are believed to arise from the patient's own flora.

CLINICAL PRESENTATION

Patients with neutropenic fever often have no other signs of illness or infection besides an elevated temperature. Because of their compromised immune status, they cannot mount adequate inflammatory responses and may not show signs or symptoms in the face of extensive infection. Therefore, they may have pneumonia with a normal physical examination and normal chest x-ray at the start of the infection. In addition, patients with neutropenia who are infected may not mount a fever, especially if they are receiving corticosteroids or are elderly. Patients with temperatures less than 38.3°C may need to be treated with antibiotics if they have signs and symptoms of infection or appear to be acutely ill. Although patients with neutropenic fever may develop infection anywhere, the most common sites include cutaneous sites (cellulitis, ulcers, ecthyma gangrenosum), bacteremia, pneumonitis, sinusitis, oropharyngeal (stomatitis), or gastrointestinal tract (stomatitis, esophagitis, diarrhea, typhlitis, perirectal).

DIAGNOSIS

Initial examination of the patient should include a thorough examination, including focused assessment of such areas as the nose, retina, oropharynx, periodontal tissue, catheter sites, axilla, perianal area, and groin. Although perirectal evaluation is important, a digital rectal examination and rectal temperatures are not recommended. If a perirectal abscess or prostatitis is suspected, a rectal examination can be performed after the administration of appropriate antibiotic therapy. Any obvious signs of infection should be cultured. If significant diarrhea is present, stool samples should be assessed for *Clostridium difficile* toxin. Suspicious skin lesions should be biopsied. A chest x-ray should be performed but is often normal. Patients with pneumonitis may develop increasing signs of infection clinically and radiographically as the neutropenia resolves. Sputum and urine cultures should be obtained when clinically appropriate. Lumbar punctures should be performed if there are signs of CNS infection, including mental status changes. Blood cultures should be performed to evaluate for bacteremia. Cultures should be taken from both peripheral sites and central venous catheters. Some sources suggest that because of the low yield of daily blood cultures, specimens should be collected daily for the first 3 days and then every 2 to 3 days afterwards for the duration of the fever. For persistent pulmonary symptoms without diagnosis, bronchoscopy and bronchoalveolar lavage should be considered. Further imaging, including magnetic resonance imaging, computed axial tomography, and ultrasound, may be useful to look for specific infections.

MANAGEMENT

Although the definition of neutropenic fever varies according to source, guidelines from the Infectious Disease Society of America state that antimicrobial therapy should be initiated for a single temperature greater than 38.3°C orally or 38.0°C for more than 1 hour. Patients undergoing chemotherapy should be clearly instructed regarding the importance of receiving immediate care under these circumstances. Empiric broad-spectrum antibiotics should include coverage for gram-positive and gram-negative bacteria. Treatment should include combination therapy, such as a beta-lactam with antipseudomonal coverage and an aminoglycoside or double beta-lactams. Alternatively, monotherapy can also be safely used, as demonstrated in several studies, particularly in patients with either an ANC in the 50 to 500 range or those without indwelling intravenous devices. Antibiotics that may be safe to use as monotherapy include ceftazidime, imipenem, meropenem, and cefepime. Antimicrobial choices should be made according to the particular infection and susceptibility patterns of the institution. If cultures reveal a particular cause of the infection, one should ensure that therapy covers that organism appropriately, while maintaining broad-spectrum coverage through the duration of the neutropenia. Regarding the use of aminoglycosides, early data suggest that single-day dosing is safe in neutropenia, although some specialists are awaiting further data before accepting that practice. Specific anaerobic coverage should be considered in cases of necrotizing mucositis, sinus or periodontal abscess, perirectal abscess, pelvic or intraabdominal infection, or typhlitis.

Despite the importance of gram-positive organisms as agents in neutropenic fever, vancomycin is not recommended as part of initial empiric therapy because of the risk of causing resistant organisms. Addition of vancomycin should be considered if the patient presents with infected skin or catheter sites, hypotension, mucositis, history of methicillin-resistant gram-positive infection, or recent quinolone prophylaxis.

If patients have persistent fever after 5 to 7 days, antifungal agents should be added because the incidence of such infections increases with the duration of neutropenia and the use of broad-spectrum antibiotics. Amphotericin B has the longest history of use, but liposomal amphotericin and fluconazole are emerging alternatives with lower toxicities, although efficacy data are still evolving in the case of neutropenic patients. Fluconazole is ineffective against some fungi, including *Aspergillus* and some *Candida* sp. Its use may also promote shifts in fungal patterns at institutions. The use of liposomal amphotericin, although as effective as and with fewer side effects than traditional amphotericin, may be limited because of its expense.

Antimicrobial therapy should be continued as appropriate for an identified source, such as 14 days for bacteremia. When no source is identified, previous practice was to treat with antibiotics until the ANC was greater than 500, even if the patient had defervesced. More recent evaluations have shown that, especially in low-risk patients, patients can be changed to oral antibiotics, and, if tolerated, the patient can be safely discharged from the hospital. Using risk stratification, selected low-risk patients with febrile neutropenia are beginning to be treated with oral antimicrobials on an outpatient basis. This practice should be limited to patients who are reliable and have an anticipated return of a normal ANC within a few days, who reside near the hospital, who are hemodynamically stable, and not seriously ill. They should be observed for 6 to 8 hours after the first dose of therapy and should be followed closely during their course.

Growth factors, including granulocyte colony-stimulating factor and granulocyte-macrophage colony-stimulating factor, have also been used in the treatment of neutropenic fever. They reduce the severity and duration of neutropenia and reduce the frequency of fever and infection. Although studies demonstrated these benefits, as well as reduced need for antifungal therapy and better outcomes in patients with serious infections, the benefits were modest, mortality was not reduced, and routine use of these agents was not supported. Although granulocyte-macrophage colony-stimulating factor may be preferable in cases of fungal infection because monocytes and macrophages play an important role in host defense in these circumstances, it should generally be used with caution because it may increase the growth of leukemic cell lines and has been associated with leukemic transformation in patients with myelodysplastic syndromes. In general, growth factor use should be limited to patients with septic shock, organ dysfunction, or who are expected to experience prolonged neutropenia.

Chapter 10

OSTEOMYELITIS

N. Christopher Kelley

OVERVIEW

Osteomyelitis is an infection of the bone that results in inflammation with destruction of bone and eventual bony necrosis. It is a difficult infection to diagnose and treat; classification on the basis of the route of inoculation, duration of infection, and causative agent provides a guideline for the use of diagnostic tools, as well as for planning treatment.

PATHOPHYSIOLOGY

Infectious agents enter bone by hematogenous spread, from a contiguous focus of infection, or by trauma. Phagocytes attempt to contain the microorganisms and, in the process, release proteolytic enzymes and other proinflammatory mediators, which lyse surrounding bone and are toxic to tissues. Inflammatory debris enters the vascular channels, and the subsequent thrombosis and increased intraosseous pressure impede blood flow. As the infection becomes chronic, ischemic necrosis of bone ensues, resulting in devascularized bone fragments, which are called *sequestra*. Bacteria adhere tightly to damaged bone, which may explain their refractoriness to medical therapy. Healthy bone is highly resistant to infection; predisposing factors, such as prior trauma, foreign bodies, or vascular insufficiency, are frequently present in adults.

CLINICAL PRESENTATION

Presentation of osteomyelitis varies, depending on the acuity of the infection, the host's immune response, and the route of inoculation. Hematogenous osteomyelitis is more common in children, although it can be seen in the elderly, injection drug users, and patients with bacteremia from any cause, including indwelling vascular catheters. In adults, the primary site of infection is the vertebral column. Patients generally complain of vague, dull, constant back pain with tenderness over the involved vertebra paravertebral muscle spasm, which is usually insidious in onset over a period of 3 weeks to 3 months; by this time, the infection is usually chronic. The lumbar spine is involved in more than 50% of cases. A history of urinary tract infection or injection drug use is often present; other sources include soft tissue, infected indwelling catheters, endocarditis, and dental infections. Spread to adjacent vertebral bodies is common through the rich venous networks in the spine. Infection often penetrates the cortex to produce soft tissue abscesses posteriorly (epidural, subdural) or anteriorly (retroperitoneal, paravertebral, mediastinal, psoas). A single organism is usually implicated; *Staphylococcus aureus* accounts for the majority of pathogens isolated, but gram-negative rods are found in up to 30% of cases.

Osteomyelitis from a contiguous focus is the most prevalent type and is usually associated with an open fracture, surgical reconstruction of bone, prostheses, or chronic soft tissue infections. Infection usually manifests within 1 month of inoculation of the organisms with low-grade fever and pain. Sinus tracts can form but usually take more than 1 month from the time of inoculation. Although multiple organisms are usually involved, *S. aureus* and *Streptococcus* species are most common. A special subset of contiguous focus osteomyelitis occurs in patients with vascular insufficiency and in the small bones of the feet of diabetic patients. Diabetic neuropathy predisposes the foot to unrecognized repeated trauma and pressure sores, and if the affected area becomes infected, poor tissue perfusion may blunt the normal inflammatory response and create an environment conducive to anaerobic infections. The patient may present with an apparently localized infection, such as cellulitis, ulcer, or an ingrown toenail, unaware that the infection has spread into the adjacent bone. Systemic signs of infection are often absent. Again, multiple organisms are usually involved, including *Staphylococcus, Streptococcus, Enterococcus*, and anaerobic species.

Subsequent recurrences of osteomyelitis constitute chronic osteomyelitis. The hallmark of chronic osteomyelitis is the presence of dead bone, called a *sequestrum*. Patients generally present with chronic pain, persistent drainage, and sinus tracts to the skin surface that, if they become obstructed, can result in soft tissue infections or abscess formation.

DIAGNOSIS

Early diagnosis of osteomyelitis is critical, as prompt antibiotic therapy may prevent widespread bone necrosis. The erythrocyte sedimentation rate is usually elevated but is a nonspecific finding. Blood cultures are positive in many cases of acute osteomyelitis, but this finding depends on whether the source of infection is bacteremia, trauma, or contiguous spread. Plain films that may show soft tissue swelling, bone destruction, and periosteal thickening can take up to 2 to 3 weeks of infection before showing evidence of bone changes. The three-phase bone scan uses a radioactive tracer that accumulates in areas of increased osteoblast activity. The tagged white blood cell scan uses radiolabeled white blood cells that accumulate at sites of inflammation or infection and may be slightly more specific than a bone scan to detect acute osteomyelitis. Magnetic resonance imaging (MRI) gives detailed anatomic information and is especially useful in imaging the vertebral column and the diabetic foot but cannot always distinguish healing fractures and tumors from infection. When acute osteomyelitis is suspected, plain films should be obtained, then nuclear imaging, then MRI, if the diagnosis is still in doubt. When imaging the diabetic foot, MRI is the modality of choice. The gold standard for the diagnosis of osteomyelitis is open bone biopsy, which is usually required in vertebral body osteomyelitis or from other sites when medical therapy has failed. Needle biopsy is subject to sampling error and has a relatively low sensitivity. A high index of clinical suspicion, convincing radiologic studies, or positive blood cultures may eliminate the need for a surgical procedure.

MANAGEMENT

Intravenous antibiotic therapy for acute osteomyelitis should be initiated promptly and be based on the organisms isolated from blood or bone specimens. Empiric therapy should include agents active against gram-positive organisms (oxacillin, cefazolin, or vancomycin), and if gram-negative organisms are suspected, a third-generation cephalosporin, a quinolone, or an aminoglycoside should be used. The duration of intravenous antibiotic therapy is typically 4 to 6 weeks. Oral quinolones have been used after 2 weeks of intravenous therapy for the treatment of gram-negative infections. Vertebral body osteomyelitis rarely requires surgical débridement, except in cases of large soft tissue abscess or evidence of spinal instability or neurologic compromise. Surgical intervention for contiguous focus osteomyelitis is often necessary, in addition to prolonged antibiotic therapy. Patients with diabetes and vascular insufficiency are difficult to treat secondary to poor wound healing, and these patients are often managed with local débridement or amputation, in addition to parenteral antibiotics. Definitive treatment of chronic osteomyelitis requires extensive surgical débridement, which may result in substantial impairment depending on the location and extent of the infection. If surgery is not an option, patients can be managed with intermittent courses of antibiotics to suppress acute exacerbations. Long-term antibiotic therapy is often used, although its utility remains unproven.

Chapter 11

PNEUMONIA

David S. Smith

OVERVIEW

Bacterial pneumonia is the most common cause of death among infectious diseases in the United States, and pulmonary tuberculosis rivals human immunodeficiency virus worldwide as the greatest public health risk. Although pneumonia acquired by a healthy host is usually readily treated with oral antibiotics and resolves without sequelae, nosocomial pneumonia has a high mortality rate, up to 25% with intensive care unit admission. The physician is challenged to recognize these high-risk patients while not over-treating the great majority of patients who will do well with outpatient therapy.

PATHOPHYSIOLOGY

Host factors are key in etiology and diagnosis of pneumonia. Community-acquired pneumonia in a normal host is acquired by inhalation, with the most common organisms being *Streptococcus pneumoniae, Mycoplasma pneumoniae, Chlamydia pneumoniae,* and *influenzavirus.* Healthy younger adults are more likely to have mycoplasma infections, and older adults are more likely to have pneumococcal infections. Patients with altered B-cell function (e.g., myeloma) are more likely to have bacterial infections, whereas those with altered T-cell function (e.g., acquired immunodeficiency syndrome) are more susceptible to viral, fungal, or opportunistic infections, such as *Pneumocystis carinii.* Patients with underlying chronic obstructive pulmonary disease may have exacerbations leading to pneumonia caused by *Haemophilus influenzae, Branhamella catarrhalis,* or *Legionella* sp. Anaerobic organisms cause aspiration pneumonia and lung abscess. Antibiotic-resistant organisms, such as methicillin-resistant *Staphylococcus aureus,* and *Pseudomonas* sp., are becoming more common in hospital-acquired pneumonia.

CLINICAL PRESENTATION

The classic presentation of bacterial pneumonia is acute onset with a progressive course marked by cough (90%) productive of yellow or green sputum (66%), fever (100–104°F) with chills or rigors (15%), and pleuritic chest pain (50%). The patient often appears toxic. The affected lung often has coarse crackles and bronchial breath sounds, and there maybe localized percussive dullness. Viral pneumonia is associated with upper respiratory signs such as nasal congestion, sore throat, and a nonproductive cough. Elderly patients may present with confusion in the absence of fever.

Complications of pneumococcal pneumonia include bacteremia in 20% to 30%, parapneumonic effusion in a majority but empyema in only 2%, and meningitis rarely.

DIAGNOSIS

Diagnosis of pneumonia is made based on clinical suspicion combined with a chest x-ray showing a localized infiltrate. A lobar pattern suggests infection with *S. pneumoniae, Klebsiella pneumoniae, Legionella* sp., or a postobstructive pneumonia distal to a bronchogenic lung cancer. Cavitation caused by a necrotizing infection occurs with *S. aureus, Pseudomonas* sp., *Klebsiella* sp., and *Mycobacterium tuberculosis* infections, as well as lung cancers. Leukocytosis with a left shift is usually present. A high-resolution computed tomography scan is more sensitive than chest x-ray for interstitial disease, cavitation, empyema, and hilar adenopathy.

The specific organism can sometimes be identified by sputum Gram stain, sputum culture, or blood culture. On Gram-stained smear, look for predominant organisms associated with leukocytes. Gram-positive diplococci suggest *S. pneumoniae*, many small gram-negative coccobacilli suggest *H. influenzae*, and frequent leukocytes without organisms suggests atypical pneumonia caused by *Mycoplasma* sp., *Legionella* sp., or viruses. Specimens should be obtained by protected-brush bronchoscopy in critically ill patients, especially those who are immunocompromised. If the patient is critically ill and still not responding to therapy, an open-lung biopsy should be considered, as well as searching for clues to uncommon causes, such as severe acute respiratory syndrome. Blood cultures should be obtained on all hospitalized patients, and a diagnostic thoracentesis done when an effusion is present. A nasopharyngeal swab direct fluorescent antibody test can identify many of the common respiratory viruses. The etiologic pathogen may not be identified in up to 50% of cases, and any result must be viewed with skepticism if the patient fails to respond to directed therapy.

MANAGEMENT

Because of the nonspecificity of clinical, radiologic, and bacteriologic findings in the etiologic diagnosis of pneumonia, initial therapy is usually empiric, based on the expected organism, severity of illness, and comorbidity. Outpatient management of community-acquired pneumonia can be undertaken when the patient is not toxic or debilitated. The preferred outpatient treatment is erythromycin, which covers *S. pneumoniae, Branhamella catarrhalis*, and *M. pneumoniae*. If *H. influenzae* is suspected, clarithromycin, azithromycin, or levofloxacin should be used to extend the spectrum.

The decision to hospitalize depends on whether the patient is at increased risk for a complicated course or mortality. Factors influencing the decision include advanced age and comorbid conditions, such as chronic obstructive pulmonary disease, diabetes, congestive heart failure, postsplenectomy, and alcoholism. Clinical factors, such as hypoxemia (PaO$_2$ <60), multilobar pneumonia, or evidence of sepsis or shock, also mandate hospitalization. Large observational cohort studies have found that antibiotic coverage for typical and atypical organisms is associated with a lower risk of death than more narrow coverage. When the patient is hospitalized, therefore, treatment with a second-generation cephalosporin (e.g., cefuroxime) plus a macrolide, an antipneumococcal fluoroquinolone (e.g., levofloxacin or gatifloxacin), or a beta-lactam/beta-lactamase inhibitor (e.g., ampicillin-sulbactam) plus a macrolide is preferred.

Oxygen saturation should be measured and supplemental oxygen given if low. Pneumococcal and influenza vaccine should be used for primary prevention in all at-risk patients. Parapneumonic effusion should be sampled if empyema is suspected (especially if the patient appears toxic), and if found, chest tube drainage is indicated. Failure to respond to first-line treatment should prompt a search for nonbacterial organisms or noninfectious causes.

Chapter 12

SEPTIC SHOCK

Jared G. Selter

OVERVIEW

Septic shock involves derangements in the immune system and in individual organ systems. It is the thirteenth most common cause of death in the United States and the leading cause of death in noncoronary intensive care units. There are approximately 750,000 cases of sepsis each year in the United States, creating a financial burden of $5 billion to $10 billion. Reportedly, there has been a 140% increase in episodes of septic shock in the United States. The increase in septic shock is due to an aging and more immunocompromised population, with human immunodeficiency virus, diabetes, cancer, and renal failure as some of the contributing factors, as well as increased use of invasive treatment strategies.

PATHOPHYSIOLOGY

The inciting event in septic shock is the development of localized or disseminated infection followed by a biphasic immunologic response. Initially, an overwhelming inflammatory reaction occurs with the production of the proinflammatory mediators tumor necrosis factor and interleukin-1. These mediators affect the release of other potent inflammatory agents, including nitric oxide (NO). After this burst of inflammatory activity, an antiinflammatory state occurs, leaving the host susceptible to secondary infection, often with resistant, nosocomial pathogens, which can subsequently lead to death. Hemodynamic and cardiac compromise manifest with an increased cardiac index and decreased systemic vascular resistance (SVR) and blood pressure (BP) caused by increased levels of NO, leading to vasodilatation and decreased venous return. Pulmonary dysfunction is manifested by impaired oxygenation and ventilatory failure. Inflammatory mediators cause increased capillary permeability and pulmonary edema, leading to poor pulmonary compliance and increased work of breathing. Increased shunt fraction and ventilation/perfusion mismatch in the lungs from edema, as well as microthrombi in the pulmonary and peripheral circulations, alter oxygenation. The most serious pulmonary complication in sepsis is acute respiratory distress syndrome, which is a culmination of the above processes. Renal complications, such as oliguria and prerenal azotemia, are common in sepsis and likely due to hemodynamic alterations, elevated prostaglandins, and therapeutic strategies, but they are often reversible. Hemodialysis is needed in only approximately 5% of patients. Gastrointestinal dysfunction is manifested as decreased gastric pH, stress ulceration, motility dysfunction, and elevated liver enzymes. The hematologic disturbances of thrombocytopenia, impaired coagulation, and disseminated intravascular coagulation are seen as well.

CLINICAL PRESENTATION

Septic shock can progress rapidly, and therapy needs to be initiated before confirmatory test results are available. The clinician must rely on physical signs and a high level of suspicion to treat appropriately. Generally, the septic patient appears warm, flushed, and dry. These alterations are secondary to the vasodilatory nature of NO. Additionally, the patient has flat neck veins or negligible jugular venous distention. In combination with tachycardia, these signs are suggestive of high-output cardiac failure and are strongly suggestive of sepsis. In later stages, septic patients manifest profound hypotension. Patients with sepsis present with a primary respiratory alkalosis or with tachypnea to compensate for metabolic acidosis as well as hypoxemia. Normal or slow respiratory rates in patients who otherwise appear septic suggest impending ventilatory failure, and sepsis should not be discounted based on such findings. In all populations, particularly the elderly, sepsis presents with moderate or profound alterations in mental functioning, although focal central nervous system findings are rare. In hospitalized patients, decreasing urine output with adequate intake can signal impending sepsis. The physical presentation should also focus on the search for the cause of sepsis. Unilateral rales or decreased breath sounds suggest pneumonia or a pleural effusion; suprapubic or flank tenderness suggests genitourinary infections; and rashes, such as purpura fulminans or cellulitis, suggest other sources of infection.

DIAGNOSIS

The American College of Chest Physicians and the Society of Critical Care Medicine issued a consensus definition for sepsis and septic shock to assist in diagnosis (Table 12–1).

The workup for diagnosing sepsis should include a complete blood count; serum chemistries; blood urea nitrogen and creatinine; liver function tests; coagulation studies; blood, urine, sputum, and cerebrospinal fluid cultures with Gram staining; arterial blood gas analysis; and radiographic studies selected based on physical examination findings and clinical suspicion. Notably, blood cultures are only positive in 30% to 50% of sepsis cases. Chemistries should be analyzed for serum anion gap that, if present, suggests tissue hypoperfusion. In such cases, serum lactate levels should be obtained. Few studies, however, have shown a correlation between anion gap and severity of illness or mortality. The arterial blood gas should be analyzed closely for respiratory alkalosis, indicating early sepsis, or metabolic acidosis, indicating later sepsis, or both.

TABLE 12–1 American College of Chest Physicians and Society of Critical Care Medicine Definition of Sepsis

SIRS	Sepsis	Severe Sepsis	Sepsis with Hypotension	Septic Shock
Temp >38°C, <36°C HR >90 bpm RR >20, $PaCO_2$ <32 mm Hg WBC >12,000, <4,000, >10% immature forms (bands)	SIRS in response to infection	Sepsis with organ dysfunction	Sepsis with SBP <90 mm Hg, or a change of 40 mm Hg	Sepsis with hypotension despite adequate fluid resuscitation and perfusion abnormalities

HR, heart rate; RR, respiratory rate; SBP, systolic blood pressure; SIRS, systemic inflammatory response syndrome; WBC, white blood cell.

MANAGEMENT

Management of sepsis is three-pronged and includes supportive care, broad antibiotic coverage, and investigation for the source of infection. All therapies should be performed in an intensive care unit by trained, experienced personnel. Supportive care should begin with basic life support evaluation and treatment. If there is any sign of impending respiratory failure or if the patient's airway is at risk due to factors such as altered mentation, intubation and mechanical ventilation should be initiated. The ventilator should be managed so that underlying respiratory and metabolic abnormalities are corrected without undue trauma to the lungs. BP and perfusion support is also critical to reversing sepsis and improving the chances of survival. Patients with sepsis are universally intravascularly volume depleted from vasodilatation and increased losses. Initial support should be undertaken with crystalloid or colloid fluid solutions. If volume has been given in amounts exceeding 2 L and BP has not responded, vasopressor support is indicated. The agents most readily available are dopamine (DA), norepinephrine (NE), and phenylephrine (PE), with epinephrine rarely being used. DA is perhaps the most commonly used and best understood agent for treating shock. At low doses (3 µg/kg/minute), it has predominant dopaminergic activity leading to splanchnic dilation. At higher doses (3–8 µg/kg/minute or >8 µg/kg/minute), it has $beta_1$ and $alpha_1$ agonist activities, respectively. DA raises mean arterial pressure (MAP) via increases in SVR and cardiac index. Disadvantages of DA include tachycardia and resultant increased oxygen demand, as well as a theoretic increase in shunt fraction by increasing pulmonary blood flow. Renal dose DA remains controversial and unproved in clinical settings. NE is predominantly an alpha agonist and raises MAP via vasoconstriction and increased venous return. NE does not promote tachycardia as DA does and may decrease serum lactate levels. PE is purely alpha in its activity and raises MAP by increasing the SVR. This effect, in theory, reverses a pathophysiologic defect in sepsis and, as a result, is used increasingly in some centers. PE also increases urine output and oxygen delivery. Pressor support should be tailored to individual patient requirements and have a goal of a MAP greater than 60 or systolic BP greater than 90 mm Hg. Using lower dose combination, pressor therapy may also be of benefit to address the mixed dysfunction of sepsis and limit toxicity.

The administration of antibiotic therapy in sepsis and septic shock is critical and must be initiated early. Although all cultures should ideally be secured before delivering therapy, obtaining them should not delay treatment. Coverage should be broad initially and narrowed as culture results become available. Initial therapy should be directed at the most likely sources based on examination findings and epidemiologic data, keeping local resistance and infection patterns in mind. The most common sources for infection are lung (40–50%), abdominal/pelvic (20%), urinary tract (10%), and skin/soft tissue (5%) (Table 12–2).

Any closed fluid collections, such as effusions or abscesses, should be drained at the bedside or surgically because such collections are not well penetrated by parenteral antibiotics, and their acidic environment often negates the antibiotic's effectiveness. The role of pulmonary artery catheters (PACs) in the diagnosis and management of sepsis remains controversial. Although PACs can provide adjunctive information, a recent study did not show a survival benefit and even suggested worsened mortality in patients with PACs in place. Recently, investigators for the PROWESS study group reported on the use of recombinant human activated protein C (APC) in 1,690 patients with

TABLE 12–2 Typical Pathogens in Sepsis

Source	Community-Acquired Pathogens	Nosocomial Pathogens
Lung	*Streptococcus pneumoniae, Haemophilus influenzae, Legionella* sp., *Chlamydia pneumoniae, Pneumocystis carinii*	Aerobic gram-negative bacilli
Abdomen	*Escherichia coli, Bacteroides fragilis*	Gram-negative rods, anaerobes, *Candida*
Skin	Group A streptococcus, *Staphylococcus aureus, Clostridium* sp., polymicrobial (enteric gram-negative rods, *Pseudomonas aeruginosa*, anaerobes, staphylococcal sp.)	*S. aureus*, gram-negative rods
Genitourinary tract	*E. coli, Klebsiella* sp., *Enterobacter* sp., *Proteus*	Gram-negative rods, enterococci

severe sepsis. In this multicenter, randomized, double-blinded trial, investigators showed a 6.1% decreased absolute mortality rate and a 19.4% relative risk reduction (95% CI: 6.6, 30.8) in patients treated with APC, with only nonsignificant increases in serious bleeding events. Theoretically, APC corrects the pathophysiologic derangements in hemostasis described earlier and is recommended for patients who meet criteria for severe sepsis. Despite all the advances in the understanding and treatment of septic shock, outcome data are still disappointing, and current mortality rates for sepsis range between 35% and 55%.

Chapter 13

SEXUALLY TRANSMITTED DISEASES

Meredith Talbot

OVERVIEW

Sexually transmitted diseases (STDs) are a group of at least 25 diseases caused by bacteria, viruses, protozoa, and animals that are acquired through sexual transmission. Fifteen million people are infected annually, one-fourth of whom are teenagers. Although some STDs carry minimal risk, others cause infertility, ectopic pregnancy, chronic pelvic pain, preterm labor, and cervical cancer in females; penile cancer in males; and neurologic damage, pneumonia, and sepsis in newborns. All individuals with STDs are more susceptible to acquiring the human immunodeficiency virus and other STDs because of disruption of the epithelial surface.

PATHOPHYSIOLOGY

The mechanisms by which STDs induce injury vary by organism. Gonorrhea and chlamydia are caused by intracellular bacterial pathogens that gain access to their host via attachment receptors specific for genital epithelium. Heat shock protein is then produced, which directly damages epithelial cells and incites a local inflammatory reaction. Over time, STDs can lead to fibrosis in the genital tract in the form of pelvic inflammatory disease (PID) and can be oncogenic. Human papilloma virus (HPV) and herpes simplex virus (HSV) can cause cervical cancer. HPV-16 encodes two major oncogenic proteins, E6 and E7, which immortalize the target cell.

CLINICAL PRESENTATION

Perhaps the most important clinical presentation of STDs is that of the asymptomatic patient. When symptomatic, there are several classic findings. Women may complain of vaginal discharge, dysuria, ulcers, abdominal pain, or infertility. Abdominal pain in women, especially when accompanied by fever, is cause for concern for PID, which is most commonly caused by chlamydia or gonorrhea. PID can also cause cervical motion tenderness or adnexal tenderness. An important differential diagnosis for PID is ectopic pregnancy, tuboovarian abscess, and appendicitis.

Men tend to complain of dysuria, urethral discharge, painful or painless ulcers, testicular pain, or proctitis.

Chlamydia trachomatis is the most common bacterial STD. There are 3 million cases a year, and the prevalence is greater than 10% in teenage girls. Forty percent of untreated women develop PID. Most women and men are asymptomatic. When symptomatic, women typically complain of bilateral lower abdominal pain, vaginal discharge, abnormal menstrual bleeding pattern, dyspareunia, and infertility. Ascending infection can lead to right upper quadrant tenderness and liver function test elevations (Fitz-Hugh–Curtis syndrome). Men typically complain of dysuria and a watery mucoid discharge. *C. trachomatis* is also the most common organism producing a reactive arthritis (Reiter's syndrome).

There are 650,000 cases of *Neisseria gonorrhoeae* diagnosed yearly. As with chlamydia, most women are asymptomatic, but men tend to complain of urethritis. Both women and men can experience sterility. *N. gonorrhoeae* can also cause Fitz-Hugh–Curtis syndrome, Reiter's disease, pharyngitis, and proctitis.

Twenty million people are currently infected with HPV, and 5.5 million people are infected annually. Men and women typically present with painless warts on the genito-anal areas or with no symptoms at all. The main concern with HPV is that strains 16, 18, 31, and 45 account for 80% of all cervical cancers.

HSV II currently infects 45 million people, making it the most common STD in the United States. Patients present with painful vesicular lesions, but most people are without symptoms. HSV, like HPV, can increase the risk of cervical cancer.

Syphilis, caused by *Treponema pallidum*, is relatively rare in the developed world. In primary syphilis, patients present with a painless ulcer (chancre) that is contagious and lasts for approximately 1 month. In secondary syphilis, patients present with systemic symptoms, such as a fever, diffuse maculopapular rash that occurs on the palms and soles and looks like copper coins, and condylomata lata in the genital area. In tertiary syphilis, which can occur up to 20 years later, patients present with gumma, central nervous system effects, including tabes dorsalis, and vascular and bone lesions.

There are 5 million cases of *Trichomonas vaginalis* diagnosed annually. Infection places women at risk for preterm labor. Women typically complain of a green discharge with a fishy odor.

Bacterial vaginosis is caused by *Gardnerella vaginalis* and is associated with PID. Patients complain of malodorous vaginal discharge.

DIAGNOSIS

Diagnosis of chlamydia is made by testing cervical or urethral swabs with an enzyme-linked immunoassay (sensitivity, 80–95%) or with nucleic acid amplification (sensitivity, 95%). In women, the diagnosis of gonorrhea is most commonly made by Gram stain and culture (60–80% sensitive, 100% specific) of cervical, rectal, or throat swabs. In men, DNA probes (sensitivity, 99%; specificity, 99%) of urethral, rectal, or throat swabs are usually diagnostic. Diagnosis of HPV is made clinically by the typical dermatologic findings of pinhead papules to cauliflower-like lesions or by Papanicolaou smear. Diagnosis of HSV is made with a Tzanck smear or growth in cell culture. *T. pallidum* cannot be cultured, so the diagnosis is made by darkfield microscopy, revealing the presence of motile spirochetes, or by serology. Serologic tests include nontreponemal antibody tests, such as the VDRL or the rapid plasma reagin test, and treponemal antibody tests, such as the fluorescent treponemal antibody-absorption test. Diagnosis of trichomonas is suspected with an increased vaginal pH and confirmed by the presence of motile protozoa on wet mount. DNA probes are 90% sensitive and 99.8% specific. Presence of *G. vaginalis* is suspected with a high vaginal pH, and diagnosis is made by Gram stain, which shows clue cells (93% sensitive, 70% specific).

MANAGEMENT

When managing an STD, it is important to screen the patient for other STDs and to screen and treat the patient's partner(s). Follow-up and counseling are crucial aspects of management (Table 13–1).

TABLE 13–1 Treatment Information for Sexually Transmitted Diseases	
Chlamydia	Doxycycline, 100 mg PO b.i.d. × 7 d, or azithromycin, 1.0 g PO × one dose. Also treat for gonorrhea.
Gonorrhea	Ceftriaxone, 125 mg IM × one dose, or ciprofloxacin, 500 mg PO × one dose. Also treat for chlamydia.
Human papilloma virus infection	Visible lesions may be treated with topicals, such as liquid nitrogen or podophyllin. In women: cervical lesions followed with Papanicolaou smears. Colposcopy.
Herpes simplex virus infection	Acyclovir, 400 mg PO t.i.d. × 10 d, or valacyclovir, 1,000 mg PO t.i.d. × 10 d
Syphilis	Benzathine penicillin G, 2.4 mu IM × one dose (primary and secondary)
Trichomoniasis	Flagyl, 2.0 g × one dose or 500 mg PO b.i.d. × 7 d
Bacterial vaginosis	Flagyl, 0.5 g PO b.i.d. × 7 d

Chapter 14

TICK-BORNE DISEASES

Lisa Sanders

OVERVIEW

Ticks are the most common disease vectors in the United States and are second only to mosquitoes worldwide. Over the past 30 years, tick-borne diseases have taken on a greater importance, as people have increasingly invaded rural areas for living, working, and playing. At this time, ten tick-borne diseases have been described, three of them in the past three decades. In most cases, the diagnosis is made and therapy started based on clinical suspicion, and for many patients, early diagnosis and treatment can be lifesaving. History, geography, and presentation can be helpful in making these important and uncommon diagnoses.

PATHOPHYSIOLOGY

Lyme disease is the most common tick-borne disease in the United States. It is caused by a spirochete *Borrelia burgdorferi* and is carried by the *Ixodes scapularis* (or *dammini*) tick. It is endemic to the northern Atlantic states, a few states in the upper midwest, and northern California. Rocky Mountain spotted fever (RMSF) was first described in Idaho in the late nineteenth century and was shown to be an infectious illness spread by ticks in the early twentieth century. The agent, a *Rickettsia*, a tiny obligate intracellular bacteria, is harbored by the common dog tick and is endemic to the southern Atlantic and western states. The tick transmits the disease during a prolonged period of feeding that may last up to 2 weeks. The bite is painless and frequently unnoticed. The disease may also be transmitted during the removal of ticks from persons or animals, especially when the tick is crushed between fingers. Most cases are diagnosed during late spring or summer. In the south, the disease most commonly affects children, whereas in western states, it is most commonly found in adult men. *Rickettsieae* are introduced into the skin and spread via lymphatics and small blood vessels to the systemic and pulmonary circulation, where they infect the vascular endothelium. Infection causes increased vascular permeability, resulting in edema, hypovolemia, and hypotension. Endothelial damage triggers the coagulation cascade, although frank disseminated intravascular coagulation is uncommon. Two similar diseases recently have been described and attributed to a *Rickettsieae*-like, obligate, intracellular bacteria, known as *Ehrlichieae*, which are found within the cytoplasm of the host's white blood cells. Human monocytic ehrlichiosis (HME) is caused by *Ehrlichia chaffeensis*. Human granulocytic ehrlichiosis (HGE) has been more recently described, but its agents are not as fully described. HME is carried by the lone star tick and most commonly infects middle-aged men. Cases have been reported most commonly in central and southern Atlantic states. Similar to most tick-borne illnesses, HME most commonly is reported in spring and early summer. HGE was initially described in the midwest but has been reported in the northeast and California. *I. scapularis*, the same tick that carries Lyme disease, is the principle vector, and so co-infection has been reported. Babesiosis is the third described tick-borne illness and is caused by a malaria-like protozoan. *Babesia* sp.

has been recognized as a pathogen of erythrocytes in domestic and wild animals since biblical times but only recently was found to cause human illness as well. *I. scapularis*, the tick vector of Lyme disease and ehrlichiosis, transmits this disease. As in the animal host, red cells are the target of the organism. Once inside the red cell, the protozoa undergo asexual budding. These daughter organisms exit the red cell, damaging the membrane and leading to the hemolysis that characterizes the disease. Infection is most common in coastal areas and islands of the north Atlantic states but has also been reported in several mid-Atlantic, midwestern, and west coast states as well. Subclinical infection is common in endemic regions, and transfusion-associated transmission as well as transplacental infection have been reported.

CLINICAL PRESENTATION

Peak season for tick-borne illnesses is late spring to early summer, although in Lyme disease, the season continues into early fall. Patients with Lyme disease range in age from 2 to 88 years, with a bimodal distribution. The disease is most common in children and middle-aged adults. Men are as likely as women to be infected. As with other spirochetal infections, Lyme disease generally occurs in stages, with remissions alternating with exacerbations and different clinical manifestations at each stage. Stage 1 disease is characterized by an erythematous rash that originates at the tick bite and expands outward with a central clearing. This rash, known as *erythema migrans* (EM), is most commonly seen at the axilla, thigh, and groin. Up to 80% of patients recall the presence of this rash. Within several days of the development of EM, many patients develop additional ring-shaped lesions that characterize stage 2. EM in stages 1 and 2 is often accompanied by malaise, fatigue, headache, fever, myalgias, and, rarely, signs of meningeal irritation or encephalopathy. Neurologic involvement in Lyme disease, including meningitis, encephalitis, and cranial neuritis, particularly a facial palsy, is seen in up to 15% of untreated patients weeks to months after the onset of the infection. In addition, up to 5% of untreated patients develop cardiac involvement, with atrioventricular block as the most common manifestation. These symptoms resolve within a few days, and permanent pacemakers are not usually necessary. During stage 2, migratory musculoskeletal pains are common, usually affecting one or two joints at a time and resolving within hours to days. Approximately 20% of patients have evidence of a mild hepatitis early in the illness. Late infection in Lyme disease, or stage 3, is characterized by intermittent arthritis, primarily in large joints, especially the knee. Attacks generally last weeks to months, separated by periods of complete remission. Neurologic involvement, most commonly a subacute encephalitis affecting mood or memory, is often noted.

The classic triad for RMSF of fever, rash, and a history of a tick bite is not usually seen at the time of presentation. Most patients have fever and a severe headache, but the rash only appears in a small fraction of patients on the first day and in fewer than one-half of patients in the first 3 days. The rash is petechial and often starts at the wrists or ankles, spreading to the palms and soles as well as to the trunk. Focal neurologic signs, meningismus, and photophobia can be seen and are poor prognostic indicators. Renal failure, pneumonia, noncardiogenic pulmonary edema, and myocarditis are seen in fewer than 20% of patients. Death occurs in untreated patients within 8 to 15 days after the onset of disease. Characteristic laboratory data are not specific: the white cell count may be normal, anemia is seen in up to 30%, and thrombocytopenia has been frequently reported. Hyponatremia is seen in one-half of patients with RMSF. Prognosis is largely related to the timeliness of appropriate therapy.

The clinical presentation of ehrlichiosis includes fever, myalgia, headache, nausea, and other nonspecific symptoms. Rash is seen in approximately one-third of patients. Leukopenia, thrombocytopenia, and transaminitis are common. Intracellular inclusions in leukocytes, called *morulae*, are rarely seen. The clinical presentation and laboratory findings of HGE are similar to HME, except that in HGE, the rash is much less common. HGE can be more severe than HME, with a higher rate of morbidity and mortality when left untreated. Clinical infection with babesiosis is most commonly seen in patients 50 years of age or older. Up to one-third of patients are asplenic. Malaise, anorexia, shaking chills, fever, headache, abdominal pain, and dark urine are common features.

DIAGNOSIS

The diagnosis of Lyme disease is based primarily on the characteristic clinical picture and exposure to an endemic area. Elevated antibody response can be detected in 90% of patients 4 to 6 weeks after infection. If serologic testing is needed, the Centers for Disease Control and Prevention recommend two-tiered testing with first enzyme-linked immunoassay and then Western blot to confirm positive and equivocal tests. During the early, localized infection, EM may resemble a cellulitis. Later stages must be distinguished from chronic fatigue syndrome or fibromyalgia. The differential diagnosis of RMSF includes typhoid fever, measles, rubella, bacterial or viral upper respiratory infections, gastroenteritis, meningococcemia, vasculitis, idiopathic thrombocytopenia purpura, thrombotic thrombocytopenia purpura, or Epstein-Barr virus. The diagnosis is made based on clinical findings but can be confirmed by serologic evaluation. The diagnosis of ehrlichiosis (both HME and HGE) is based on clinical suspicion, but organism-specific nucleic acids in body fluids detected by polymerase chain reaction and serologic testing are available for confirmation of the diagnosis. Delay in diagnosis and appropriate therapy is associated with increased mortality. In babesiosis, a hemolytic anemia, sometimes severe, is commonly seen. Peripherally located ring forms, similar to those seen in *Plasmodium falciparum*, are often noted. The white blood cell count is normal or low, and thrombocytopenia is common. Untreated, the disease may last for months but is rarely fatal.

MANAGEMENT

Oral doxycycline is adequate therapy for most forms of Lyme disease, with the exception being Lyme disease with neurologic manifestations. In these cases, patients should be treated with intravenous antibiotics, specifically ceftriaxone. In rare cases, a second course of antibiotics may be necessary. In RMSF, oral doxycycline, tetracycline, and chloramphenicol are the antibiotics of choice, although mortality remains as high as 5%, even amongst those treated. Maintenance of intravascular fluid balance is key in the management of these patients. In ehrlichiosis, doxycycline is also the treatment of choice. When therapy for babesiosis is necessary, a combination of clindamycin and oral quinine for a 7-day to 10-day regimen is given. Co-infection with Lyme disease has been frequently reported.

Chapter 15

TOXIC SHOCK SYNDROMES

Lisa Sanders

OVERVIEW

Toxic shock syndrome (TSS) is a devastating illness that primarily strikes young, healthy individuals with intact immune systems. It is characterized by acute onset of fever, hypotension, and an erythrodermic rash. Incidence of TSS is sporadic, with a prevalence of up to 20 per 100,000, and morbidity and mortality can be high. This infectious syndrome can be caused by *Staphylococcus aureus* or *Streptococcus pyogenes*, and both present with signs of shock and multiorgan failure. TSS associated with *S. aureus* was first described in children in 1978. It was not until several years later that its most familiar presentation of young women during menstruation, and ultimately, its association with a single type of tampon, was recognized. Retrospective analysis has shown that from 1970 to 1982, more than 1,700 cases of TSS were reported to the Centers for Disease Control and Prevention, with 96% of cases involving women and 92% having onset during menses. After the removal of hyperabsorbent tampons from the market, the incidence dropped from six per 100,000 women between the ages of 19 and 40 to one per 100,000 women. TSS secondary to *S. pyogenes* has been reported in all age groups, although it is most frequently seen in adults. Unlike staphylococcal TSS, men are as likely as women to be infected. Although many patients with this syndrome are healthy, streptococcal TSS is more likely to be seen in patients with conditions that affect the immune system, such as diabetes mellitus, alcoholism, or varicella infection, or promote hematogenous spread, such as surgery or trauma, both penetrating and nonpenetrating. It is frequently a complication of an existing streptococcal infection, usually of the soft tissue, although up to 50% of patients have no identifiable source of infection.

PATHOPHYSIOLOGY

With the decline in menses-associated TSS, it has become apparent than nonmenstrual TSS is also important. Most of these infections are associated with vaginal colonization of toxin-secreting staphylococci occurring under conditions such as childbirth, abortions, or vaginal infections often associated with intrauterine (contraceptive) devices. Up to 40% of cases, however, are associated with wounds after a variety of surgical procedures, including mammoplasty, arthroscopy, and rhinoplasty. Influenza-associated TSS has also been described. The mechanism of the *S. aureus* infection in the menses-associated TSS is not understood. Symptoms are linked to an endotoxin, most commonly TSST-1, which has been identified in up to 75% of patients. Other associated toxins include enterotoxin B (23%) and C (2%). *S. aureus* exotoxins are "super-antigens"—molecules that activate large numbers of T cells—resulting in a massive release of cytokines, which cause fever, endothelial injury, fever, endothelial injury, capillary leak, and subsequent hypotension. The rash is thought to represent marked peripheral vasodilatation associated with toxic injury of endothelial cells. TSS secondary to *S. pyogenes* was first reported in the mid to late 1980s and is defined as any streptococcal infection associated with the sudden onset of shock and multiorgan failure. Entry of group A streptococcus (GAS) into deep tissues or the blood stream may occur as a result of a breached barrier, or the organism may penetrate intact mucous membranes. Once the deep tissue or the blood stream have been invaded, toxins (scarlatina toxin A, B, C) as well as certain strains of GAS (M-1, M-3) act in a way similar to staphylococcal TSS, acting as superantigens, activating cytokine synthesis, and triggering capillary leak and hypotension.

CLINICAL PRESENTATION

TSS secondary to *S. aureus* typically is seen in young women aged 15 to 25 years with a history of tampon use. Nonmenstrual cases are typically more difficult to identify because the surgical wound site often looks benign. Seventy-five percent of these cases also occur in women and are frequently associated with prior antibiotics use and nosocomial acquisition. Mortality is higher in nonmenstrual cases because the diagnosis is often overlooked. In both cases, onset is acute. In menses-related cases, onset occurs during the patient's menses, and in other cases, occurrence is typically within 2 days after a surgical procedure. Fever, shock, rash, and multiorgan involvement are the defining characteristics of this syndrome, but diarrhea is also common (98%), as is myalgia (96%), fever higher than 40°C (87%), headache (77%), and pharyngitis (75%). The characteristic rash, an erythematous, deep-red sunburn rash, develops within hours of the onset of symptoms. The rash progresses to subsequent desquamation, especially of palms and soles, within 7 to 14 days. TSS secondary to *S. pyogenes* may begin insidiously, with 20% of patients reporting an influenza-like prodrome 24 to 48 hours before the development of hypotension. Pain, the most common initial symptom of streptococcal TSS, frequently precedes any tenderness or physical evidence of infection. It is typically abrupt in onset, severe, and progressive in nature. Fever is the most common presenting sign and can be significantly elevated. Mental status changes are seen in up to 55% of cases. Evidence of soft tissue infection is often present when there is a cutaneous portal of entry. The appearance of bullae suggests a deep soft tissue infection, such as necrotizing fasciitis or myositis. Other streptococcal infections associated with TSS are endophthalmitis, peritonitis, puerperal sepsis, septic arthritis, and, rarely, pharyngitis. A diffuse erythrodermic rash may be visible, although this is less common in streptococcal TSS than staphylococcal TSS. Renal insufficiency is common (>80% of cases), as is a normal white cell count with a significant left shift. Hypotension is apparent, either at the time of admission or within 4 to 8 hours, and bacteremia is also common (60% of cases). In one series, the acute respiratory distress syndrome occurred in up to 55% of cases. Most cases have been sporadic, with a prevalence of five to ten cases per 100,000 population, and mortality, even in the antibiotics era, may be as high as 50% to 70%.

DIAGNOSIS

TSS secondary to *S. aureus* is a clinical diagnosis based on the presence of fever, hypotension, rash, and multiorgan failure. The differential diagnosis of fever, hypotension, and rash in a previously healthy individual includes Rocky Mountain spotted fever, measles, and leptospirosis. In patients with blunt trauma or muscle strain who subsequently develop streptococcal TSS, the most common mistaken diagnosis is deep vein thrombosis. High fever and progressive, excruciating pain can help distinguish these diagnoses. The diagnosis of TSS is a clinical one, based on the presence of hypotension and multiorgan failure, with at least two organ systems involved. It can be confirmed with the isolation of GAS from a normally sterile or a nonsterile site involved in the illness, such as the throat, sputum, vagina, or a skin lesion.

MANAGEMENT

In staphylococcal TSS, aggressive fluid resuscitation with saline, colloid, or both is essential. Vaginal examination should be performed immediately, and tampons, if present, should be removed and cultures obtained. In nonmenstrual staphylococcal TSS, cultures of any possible site of infection should be obtained, even if there is no evidence of infection. A beta-lactamase–resistant antistaphylococcal antibiotic, such as oxacillin or nafcillin, should be administered at a dose of 8 to 10 g per day for 10 to 15 days. Clindamycin has been shown to decrease TSST-1 production and is recommended, in addition to the antistaphylococcal penicillin, for at least the first few days of treatment. Mortality ranges from 3% to 5%. In streptococcal TSS, aggressive fluid resuscitation is also necessary, often in amounts of 10 to 20 L. Prompt antibiotic therapy with empiric broad-spectrum coverage for septic shock should be initiated early. Once infection with streptococcus has been confirmed, high-dose penicillin and clindamycin are the antibiotics of choice. Intravenous immunoglobulin has been used with some success, although definitive studies have not been done.

Chapter 16

TUBERCULOSIS

Stephen E. Possick

OVERVIEW

Mycobacterium tuberculosis (M.TB) is a rod-shaped, non–spore-forming aerobic bacterium. Tuberculosis (TB) is responsible for approximately 3 million deaths worldwide each year. The World Health Organization estimates that between 19% and 43% of the world's population is infected with M.TB, with approximately 15 million Americans infected with the bacterium. It is, therefore, a critical public health issue and a constant concern in the inpatient and outpatient settings.

PATHOPHYSIOLOGY

Transmission of the bacterium occurs via droplet nuclei produced when someone with active pulmonary or laryngeal TB coughs, sneezes, or speaks. These droplet nuclei, only 1 to 5 mm in diameter, can remain aerosolized for hours. Small bacteria are able to reach alveoli, whereas larger particles become trapped in the mucus of the upper airways and are expelled. The number of droplet nuclei, concentration of bacteria, length of exposure, and immune status of the individual influence the risk of transmission. After inhalation, droplet nuclei proceed to host alveoli, where they are ingested by alveolar macrophages. If the bacterium survives this process, it grows slowly within the macrophage. This slow growth continues for 2 to 12 weeks until enough organisms, 10^3 to 10^4, are present to provoke a cellular immune response that results in a positive tuberculin skin test. The bacterium then travel to regional lymph nodes and may disseminate hematogenously to different organs. Ten percent of those infected eventually develop active disease, whereas more than 50% of this group will develop active disease in the first 2 years. Persons infected with human immunodeficiency virus (HIV), particularly those with low CD4 counts, develop active disease more quickly and in much greater numbers. The natural history of the disease carries a 50% mortality at 5 years if left untreated.

CLINICAL PRESENTATION

Systemic manifestations of active TB are relatively nonspecific. Fever is present in 37% to 80% of patients. Fatigue, weight loss, night sweats, anorexia, and weakness may be seen in active TB. In immunocompetent hosts, pulmonary TB accounts for 85% of active disease. The most common symptom is a cough that often progresses from nonproductive to productive. Hemoptysis and dyspnea are rare as presenting symptoms. Rales and bronchial breath sounds may be present.

Extrapulmonary TB presents a difficult diagnostic challenge. Patients infected with HIV have a much higher rate of extrapulmonary disease. Many sites are subject to infection and may occur in any individual with active TB, regardless of his or her immune status. Tuberculous lymphadenitis results in the painless swelling of the involved node. It is often bilateral and most likely to involve the cervical and supraclavicular chains. Systemic symptoms are uncommon if the node is the only involved organ. Pleural TB results in pleuritis with or without an effusion. Pleuritis with empyema is a less common variant. Genitourinary TB may involve the genitalia, female reproductive organs, or kidneys. More than 90% of those with genitourinary involvement have an abnormal urinalysis, typically characterized by sterile pyuria. Local symptoms predominate in this group and may include dysuria, hematuria, flank pain, and a scrotal mass. Forty percent to 75% of these patients have abnormal chest films. Skeletal involvement is usually heralded by pain in the involved area. It is more common in children due to the highly vascularized nature of the epiphyseal region. TB may also involve the marrow, resulting in marrow suppression. The central nervous system is a particularly dangerous site of involvement. TB meningitis may result from direct meningeal seeding or from rupture of an old parameningeal focus. TB meningitis primarily attacks the base of the brain and presents with headache, neck stiffness, decreased consciousness, and cranial nerve abnormalities. A tuberculoma presents less dramatically, usually coming to light as a slow-growing focal lesion. TB can affect any portion of the gastrointestinal tract, although it more commonly affects the distal terminal ileum and proximal colon, with pain and obstruction as presenting symptoms. TB may involve other intraabdominal organs as well as the peritoneum. TB may also involve the pericardium, resulting in tuberculous pericarditis and peritonitis. The symptoms of pericardial TB include systemic symptoms as well as those of cardiac tamponade. Disseminated, or miliary, TB occurs when a host is unable to contain the infection. Multiorgan system involvement occurs, and the symptoms and signs are manifold and can be nonspecific. Most patients have an abnormal chest film. The presence of a choroidal tubercle, a granuloma found in the choroid of the retina, suggests disseminated disease.

DIAGNOSIS

On physical examination, posttussive rales may be heard, characterized by fine rales at the apices on deep inspiration, followed by full expiration and hard cough. A number of laboratory studies may be abnormal in the setting of active disease. Blood work commonly reveals anemia, leukocytosis, increased erythrocyte sedimentation rate, increased ferritin, and decreased albumin. Chest films typically reveal the classic cavitary lesion, focal airspace consolidation in a patchy or confluent manner, and, rarely, lymphadenopathy. The most familiar diagnostic study is the tuberculin skin test, or purified protein derivative (PPD). M.TB produces a delayed-type hypersensitivity reaction to antigens contained in the PPD. The reaction is the result of sensitized T-cell recruitment to the antigen. The reaction may begin as early as 5 to 6 hours after injection and usually peaks over 48 to 72 hours, at which time the extent of induration should be recorded. The criteria for a positive PPD based on the degree of induration is as follows:

- 5 mm or larger:
  - HIV positive
  - Recent contacts of known TB cases
  - Fibrotic changes on chest x-ray consistent with old TB
  - Organ transplant, immunosuppressed-receiving equivalent of 15 mg of prednisone per day
- 10 mm or larger:
  - Recent arrival (<5 years) from high-prevalence country
  - Intravenous drug user
  - Individual in high-risk setting: health care worker, prison inmate, resident of homeless shelter, laboratory personnel
  - Individual with high-risk medical condition: diabetes mellitus, silicosis, chronic renal insufficiency, leukemia/lymphoma, carcinoma of head or neck, weight loss >10% of ideal body weight, history of gastrectomy, child younger than 4 years of age, child with no other risk factors exposed to a high-risk adult
  - Recipient of BCG vaccine, particularly if from a country with a high prevalence or in a high-risk group
- 15 mm:
  - Individuals with no risk factors

The diagnostic criteria for active TB include at least one sputum (induced specimens are preferable) positive for acid-fast bacilli (AFB), preferably obtained on three different days, providing a 50% to 80% yield. Gastric aspiration done after an 8-hour to 10-hour fast has a 40% yield. Bronchial washings and bronchial biopsy may be negative in active disease, as the topical anesthetics used in bronchoscopy can be toxic to M.TB. The first voided urine specimen usually is acidic and reveals pyuria without bacteria. Urine for AFB has a low yield.

Cerebrospinal fluid shows an increased protein, lymphocytosis, and low glucose. AFB smears are usually negative, although culture may be positive. Nucleic acid amplification techniques have 95% sensitivity and 98% specificity when smears are positive for AFB. The sensitivity drops to approximately 50% with negative smears and a positive culture.

Sputum culture is the gold standard and can detect as few as 10 bacterium per mL. The sensitivity approaches 85%, with 98% specificity. Cultures take 1 to 6 weeks to grow in liquid media and offer the added advantage of testing for drug sensitivity and typing M.TB.

MANAGEMENT

Individuals suspected of having active pulmonary TB should be isolated in a negative pressure room. All close contacts should be screened with PPD testing initially and at 6 weeks if a positive diagnosis is confirmed in the index case. *Latent TB* is defined as a positive PPD with negative chest film. Treatment for latent TB is isoniazid (INH) for 9 months or, if INH resistant, pyrazinamide (PZA) and rifampin for 2 months or rifampin alone for 4 months. Patients with HIV should receive INH for 9 months. Any patient receiving INH should also receive pyridoxine (vitamin B_6) to prevent the neuropathy associated with INH. In addition, liver function tests should be routinely monitored, as patients can develop an INH-induced hepatitis.

The patient with active TB has a positive PPD with positive sputum for AFB, a positive culture, or positive chest radiograph. The level of drug resistance is an important factor in terms of the choice of medications and duration of treatment. In regions with less than 4% INH resistance, patients with active TB should receive INH and rifampin for 6 months and PZA for the first 2 months. In regions with higher than 4% INH resistance, patients should receive INH and rifampin for 6 months and PZA for the first 2 months, with the addition of ethambutol or streptomycin for 2 months. Asia, New York City, and portions of South America have high rates of INH resistance. In the case of multidrug-resistant TB, the goal is to administer at least three medications active against the bacteria. Additional medications used include amikacin, ciprofloxacin, and levofloxacin.

Chapter 17

URINARY TRACT INFECTION AND PYELONEPHRITIS

Joseph Quaranta

OVERVIEW

Infections of the urinary tract range from uncomplicated cystitis, treatable on an outpatient basis, to complicated cystitis and pyelonephritis that results in septicemia, which necessitates hospitalization. The vast majority is treatable on an outpatient basis, with oral antibiotics. Pyelonephritis and cystitis associated with signs of systemic illness often require hospitalization and intravenous antibiotics.

PATHOPHYSIOLOGY

The most common etiology of urinary tract infections (UTIs) is gram-negative rods; among these, *Escherichia coli* is by far the most common. *Staphylococcus saprophyticus* accounts for approximately 10% to 15% of UTIs in young women. Other staphylococci and enterococci species are less common in the outpatient setting. These organisms are more common in patients with urinary catheters, in whom the likelihood of UTIs is increased. Other risk factors include pregnancy, urinary tract obstruction, a history of UTIs, sexual activity, diabetes mellitus, and vesicoureteral reflux.

CLINICAL PRESENTATION

The prevalence of non–catheter-induced UTIs is greater in women than in men. The characteristic clinical features of acute cystitis, or infection localized to the bladder, include polyuria, dysuria, suprapubic tenderness, and sometimes fever. Pyelonephritis can include all of these symptoms, with the addition of flank or back pain, chills, and fever.

DIAGNOSIS

In cystitis, urinalysis reveals a leukocytosis and the presence of leukocyte esterase and nitrite. Urine cultures typically reveal more than 10^5 organisms in a symptomatic patient. Patients with pyelonephritis are more likely to have a systemic leukocytosis and fever, and approximately 50% of patients have white cell casts present in their urine.

Imaging studies usually are not necessary in diagnosing pyelonephritis, but when symptoms in the patient with acute pyelonephritis do not resolve within 48 to 72 hours of antibiotic treatment, further evaluation should be carried out with a renal ultrasound, intravenous pyelogram, or computed tomography. These modalities can help to identify obstruction and the presence of a focal process, such as a renal or perinephric abscess.

MANAGEMENT

In uncomplicated cystitis, most patients can be treated as outpatients with oral antibiotics. A 3-day course of trimethoprim-sulfamethoxazole or a flouroquinolone is an appropriate regimen. In uncomplicated pyelonephritis, these oral antibiotics can be given on an outpatient basis for a 7-day to 14-day course. In complicated UTIs involving obstruction, septicemia, or pregnancy, or an inability to take oral medications, intravenous antibiotics are necessary. If enterococci are not suspected, then intravenous ceftriaxone or ceftazidime is appropriate. If enterococci are suspected, ampicillin plus an aminoglycoside is a prudent option until a culture-documented etiology is found. Therapy should continue for a total of 2 weeks.

Chapter 18

VIRAL HEPATITIS

Stephen E. Possick

OVERVIEW

Viral infection is the most common form of hepatitis, although various toxins may also result in hepatic inflammation. Fulminant liver failure is rare in the setting of viral hepatitis, and treatment is largely supportive in the acute phase. Early diagnosis and classification of viral hepatitis are critical in preventing community outbreaks of hepatitis A (HAV) and transmission of hepatitis B and C (HBV and HCV, respectively), which can become chronic and lead to cirrhosis and hepatocellular carcinoma.

PATHOPHYSIOLOGY

HAV is an RNA virus transmitted through the fecal–oral route. Oral inoculation leads to transportation across an intact epithelium and uptake at the level of the hepatocyte. The mean incubation period is 30 days, but the virus is excreted in the feces for 1 to 2 weeks before the onset of clinical symptoms and for 1 week after resolution of symptoms. Typically, the virus is spread within households. Large families, overcrowding, poor waste disposal, and travel increase the risk of acquiring the virus. Approximately 33% of U.S. residents carry serologic evidence of prior infection. HAV immunoglobulin M (IgM) is present during acute infection and persists for 3 to 6 months. HAV immunoglobulin G (IgG) reflects resistance and recovery. It may be seen in acute infection and persists for decades.

HBV has a prevalence of 350 million cases worldwide and is responsible for as many as 1 million deaths each year. HBV is a partially double-stranded DNA virus and is transmitted via semen, saliva, cervical secretions, and leukocytes. Sexual contact, perinatal contact, blood transfusions, and intravenous drug abuse with shared needles are common sources of transmission. The mean incubation period ranges from 60 to 90 days.

HCV is a single-stranded RNA virus. It is predominantly acquired through contact with contaminated blood or blood products, although there is a small risk of transmission through sexual contact. The average incubation period is 50 days. Hepatitis D (HDV) is a defective single-stranded RNA virus that requires concurrent infection with HBV to replicate. The modes of transmission are similar to those for HBV. HDV infection that is acquired as a co-infection with HBV carries a higher risk of severe acute disease but a low risk of chronic infection, whereas superinfection with HDV carries a high risk of severe and chronic liver disease. Hepatitis E, a single-stranded RNA virus transmitted via the fecal–oral route, is clinically indistinguishable from HAV, although it has a high fatality rate of 10% to 20% in pregnant women.

CLINICAL PRESENTATION

HAV presents acutely with nonspecific constitutional and gastrointestinal symptoms. Fever, malaise, anorexia, nausea, vomiting, arthralgia, and myalgia may be present. These symptoms often abate with the onset of jaundice that is characteristically accompanied by anorexia, malaise, and weakness. Dark urine and mild pruritis often precede jaundice. Slight hepatomegaly and a tender liver may be seen. Splenomegaly is rare. Complications include acute liver failure in 0.1% of patients, mononeuritis multiplex, and necrotizing vasculitis. A cholestatic variant of HAV results in marked jaundice and pruritis that may persist for months rather than a few weeks. HAV can relapse within weeks to months of the initial disease's resolution. Relapse may be associated with arthritis, vasculitis, and cryoglobulinemia, but the prognosis remains excellent.

The presentation of HBV may be insidious or acute. Symptoms may be absent in acute HBV, but they may include a prodromal syndrome consisting of nausea, vomiting, fatigue, malaise, myalgia, and headache. These symptoms typically precede the onset of jaundice by 1 to 2 weeks and may resolve with the onset of jaundice. Hepatomegaly may be seen, and splenomegaly is present in 10% to 20% of patients. Clinical and laboratory recovery generally occurs 3 to 4 months after onset of jaundice. Complications of acute HBV include acute liver failure in 0.1% to 1%, superinfection with HDV, and chronic HBV infection. Polyarteritis nodosa, membranous or membranoproliferative glomerulonephritis, and leukocytoclastic vasculitis have been reported in association with HBV. Chronic HBV is the most common complication and affects 3% to 5% of infected adults and 90% of infected neonates. Chronic HBV can lead to cirrhosis and hepatocellular carcinoma. The relative risk of each ranges from 12 to 79 for cirrhosis and 30 to 148 for hepatocellular carcinoma.

HCV rarely presents acutely. Seventy-five percent of patients are anicteric. When HCV is manifest in the acute setting, it produces a clinical syndrome similar to that described for HBV. The rate of fulminant hepatitis is 0.1%. Fifty percent to 70% of those with acute HCV go on to develop chronic disease. Estimates are that 15% to 20% of those chronically infected go on to develop cirrhosis or hepatocellular carcinoma. The development of these complications may be related to genotype.

DIAGNOSIS

Viral hepatitis should be suspected when jaundice or other clinical findings are present, or there is a history of exposure to certain risk factors. Patients with suspected ingestions should be screened for hepatotoxins, especially acetaminophen, to rule out other causes of hepatitis. Initial laboratory tests should include alanine aminotransferase and aspartate aminotransferase levels, which can range between 500 and 5,000; prothrombin time and protein and albumin to evaluate hepatic synthetic function; indirect and direct bilirubin; complete blood count; and electrolytes. Viral serologies should be obtained, including HAV IgM and IgG, HBsAg (surface antigen), anti-HBsAb (surface antibody), HBeAg, anti-HBc IgM (core antibody), anti-HCV, and HCV RNA (Table 18–1).

MANAGEMENT

Treatment for acute hepatitis is largely supportive and should focus on monitoring for acute and chronic complications. Signs of encephalopathy, coagulopathy, and liver failure should prompt immediate hospitalization and evaluation, but most patients can be monitored in the outpatient setting. Alcohol and other hepatotoxins should be strictly avoided. There is some evidence to support treatment of acute HCV with interferon alpha and ribavirin in an effort to reduce rates of chronicity. Patients with HBV or HCV should be monitored for development of chronic disease, as pharmacologic treatment is now available for the chronic phases of both diseases.

Treatment for chronic HCV and HBV is currently reserved for those with evidence of ongoing viral replication (elevated viral load), elevated alanine ami-

TABLE 18-1   Viral Serologies of Hepatitis

Anti-HAV IgM	Anti-HAV IgG	HBsAg	Anti-HBs	Anti-HBc IgM
Acute HAV; persists 3–6 wk. Anti-HCV. May or may not be positive in acute HCV; detection may be delayed.	With IgM, indicates acute infection; without IgM, indicates past infection, recovery, and immunity. HCV RNA. May be detected before the emergence of anti-HCV antibodies.	Acute HBV infection or chronic carrier.	May be seen with vaccination or cleared HBV infection. Indicates immunity.	Appears shortly after HbsAg. In setting of acute hepatitis, indicates acute HBV.

HAV, hepatitis A virus; HBc, hepatitis B core antibody; HBs, hepatitis B surface antibody; HBsAg, hepatitis B surface antigen; HBV, hepatitis B virus; HCV, hepatitis C virus; IgG, immunoglobulin G; IgM, immunoglobulin M.

notransferase, and evidence of chronic hepatitis on liver biopsy. Interferon alpha is available for use for both chronic HBV and HCV and is typically administered in daily or thrice weekly dosing for 3 to 6 months. Interferon alpha monotherapy appears to be more efficacious in treating chronic HBV, with sustained virologic response rates of 30% to 40%. Lamivudine (3TC) offers an alternative in the treatment of chronic HBV and has a superior side effect profile and once daily oral dosing. Lamivudine has been approved for monotherapy for chronic HBV. Histologic regression has been seen in more than 50% of those treated with lamivudine monotherapy after 1 year. The addition of antiviral medications, such as famciclovir, to increase the efficacy of lamivudine is currently being investigated.

Interferon alpha has been shown to produce sustained virologic response in 10% of patients with chronic HCV after 6 months of therapy. A new pegylated version of interferon alpha results in slower absorption and allows weekly dosing. Pegylated interferon has been shown to produce a virologic response of more than 50% in chronic HCV when used in concert with ribavirin. Response rates vary with different HCV genotypes. None of the treatments described has been shown to appreciably affect the rates of cirrhosis or hepatocellular carcinoma in chronic HCV and HBV. Significant relapse rates can occur with discontinuation of each of the described therapies.

Immunization is a key part of the management of the viral hepatitides. Administration of immune globulin containing anti-HAV provides protection against the virus via passive transfer of the antibody and is used for both preexposure and postexposure prophylaxis. Inactivated HAV vaccine should be given to certain high-risk groups in two divided doses (at 0 and 6–12 months). HBV immuneglobulin provides temporary protection (3–6 months) and is used in cases of postexposure prophylaxis. HBV vaccine should be administered to everyone 18 years and younger and to adults older than age 18 who are at risk for HBV infection. It is administered in three divided doses (at 0, 1, and 6 months). There is no indication for the use of immuneglobulin for prophylaxis of HCV, and no vaccine for HCV is available.

ACUTE ARTERIAL OCCLUSION

Kathleen Stergiopoulos

OVERVIEW

Acute occlusion of the arterial supply to an extremity is a medical or surgical emergency, or both. In patients in whom an extensive collateral circulation has not developed, and in circumstances in which it is the sole vessel supplying the end organ, progression to irreversible ischemia may begin 6 hours after the event. Thus, prompt diagnosis and treatment are imperative, both to reestablish flow through the site of occlusion and to prevent propagation of the thrombus. The differential diagnosis of acute arterial occlusion includes embolism, trauma, and thrombosis. The etiology of the occlusion should be sought whenever feasible, as treatment options differ.

PATHOPHYSIOLOGY

Acute arterial occlusion results in anoxia of the tissues supplied by the involved arterial segment. Gangrene may develop in approximately 50% of patients with this condition, depending on the site and length of occlusion, and presence or absence of collateral vessels. The initial clinical manifestations of pain, paresthesia, and paralysis reflect a greater susceptibility of nerves to ischemia when compared to surrounding structures. Muscle pain soon occurs, heralding impending muscle necrosis.

It is desirable to differentiate between embolism and thrombosis as the underlying cause, because the treatment options may differ. Arterial emboli can be divided into two categories: emboli that lodge in large-diameter vessels (most often of cardiac origin) and atheroemboli to smaller vessels that originate from a plaque or thrombus. An embolus from the heart usually occurs in the setting of atrial fibrillation, myocardial infarction (2–3 weeks postinfarction in association with mural thrombus), or valvular heart disease (rheumatic disease associated with mitral stenosis and dilated left atrium with mural thrombi or valvular vegetations). Seventy percent of cardiac emboli lodge in the arteries of the lower extremities, 13% in those of the upper extremities, 10% in the cerebral circulation, and 5% to 10% in the visceral circulation. Emboli generally lodge at arterial branch points, where the vessel diameter is abruptly reduced. Common sites are the bifurcation of the abdominal aorta, the common iliac artery, the common femoral artery, and the popliteal artery. Of note, the ischemic insult is more severe when the bifurcation of a vessel is involved, because there is no opportunity for collateral circulation to supply blood to the ischemic area. Atheroemboli are fragments of an ulcerated atherosclerotic plaque that become dislodged and travel downstream. The artery of origin is usually the aorta or iliac or femoral vessels. The most com-

51

mon example of atheroemboli is the "blue-toe" syndrome, with severe ischemia of the toes and forefoot in the presence of palpable pulses.

Spontaneous acute arterial thrombosis occurs most commonly in the presence of an underlying stenosis by atherosclerotic disease, precipitated by plaque disruption and exposure of the thrombotic core or by hypoperfusion due to inadequate cardiac output. Acute arterial thrombosis may occur after diagnostic and therapeutic intraarterial procedures, such as cardiac catheterization and peripheral vascular arteriography, secondary to the creation of an intimal flap and resultant thrombosis. In addition, an aneurysm may produce distal embolization of thrombotic material that may occlude an already stenotic vessel. Hypercoagulable states, such as antiphospholipid syndrome; resistance to activated protein C; and deficiencies in protein C, S, or antithrombin III, may also cause acute arterial thrombosis.

CLINICAL PRESENTATION

The classic presentation of a limb-threatening acute arterial occlusion includes the six Ps: pain, pallor, paresthesias, paralysis, pulselessness, and poikilothermia (change in temperature or coolness). More than 75% of patients with acute arterial occlusion have pain as the presenting symptom. Pain may be absent from the clinical syndrome because of diabetic neuropathy, adequate collateral flow resulting in less severe ischemia, or rapid progression to advanced ischemia. Paralysis and paresthesias are the two most important clinical features, because they indicate anoxia to motor and sensory nerve endings of the extremity. A patient who exhibits these clinical features for at least 6 to 8 hours is more likely to develop gangrene. Tissue ischemia usually develops one joint level below the segment of the occluded artery. The absence of pulses in the occluded extremity (and presence of pulses in the other) supports the diagnosis but usually does not absolutely confirm it, because pulses may be absent chronically in a patient with peripheral vascular disease. In general, the occlusion can be localized to the segment of the arterial tree immediately proximal to the site of pulselessness. Evaluation of muscle turgor can be useful, as it yields important information regarding the severity of ischemia and the degree to which the changes are reversible after reperfusion. Initially, the muscle is soft after the onset of ischemia; then, edema develops and the muscles have a "doughy" feel; finally, the muscle is stiff and hard when necrosis sets in (ischemic changes are irreversible).

For patients with atherosclerotic peripheral vascular disease, claudication is associated with an ankle-brachial index between 0.40 and 0.95, rest pain of 0.2 to 0.5, and tissue loss of 0 to 0.4.

DIAGNOSIS

In some cases, the diagnosis of acute arterial occlusion can be made with relative certainty on the basis of the patient's history and physical examination, and no further workup is required before definitive treatment is initiated. A history of peripheral vascular disease (i.e., claudication), as well as involvement of the contralateral limb, is helpful in determining thrombotic disease (these are usually absent in embolic disease). Examination of pulses in the entire extremity aids in localization of the occlusion site. Noninvasive Doppler ultrasound techniques and pressure and waveform characteristics are useful in the preoperative setting. Arteriography is performed when additional information is required—for instance, to determine the appropriate sites of inflow and outflow for a bypass graft. If the ischemia is severe, however, the urgency of revascularization may preclude preoperative angiography. A diligent search for the source of embolic disease should be made with the use of electrocardiography, echocardiography, and Holter monitoring if necessary. For atheroemboli, a thorough arteriographic evaluation is required to confirm the diagnosis and to identify precisely the offending lesion in preparation for operative intervention.

MANAGEMENT

Regardless of the etiology of the acute arterial occlusion, systemic heparinization and early involvement of a vascular surgeon are required. In a patient with an embolic occlusion of an otherwise normal vessel, embolectomy may be required. Embolectomy should not be avoided on the basis of risk to the patient, as the development of extremity gangrene and amputation incurs far greater physiologic and operative stresses. Attempts should not be made to restore blood flow to nonviable limbs, as reperfusion may result in the return of toxic substances, such as potassium, lactic acid, and myoglobin, to the circulation. The embolus is extracted through the arteriotomy by passing an embolectomy catheter proximally and distally to remove all propagated thrombus. For a patient with thrombosis of an atherosclerotic artery, operative therapy is generally a combination of thrombus removal and bypass grafting around the involved segment. Intraoperative thrombolytic therapy may be used if there are thrombi in the distal vessels. The patient must be closely monitored for the development of a compartment syndrome, and, if one develops, a fasciotomy should be performed.

Thrombolytic therapy (i.e., urokinase) may be used instead of or in addition to standard operative techniques, depending on the nature of the occlusion, and is indicated in any patient with an acute native graft occlusion. It can be used to lyse thrombi that are inaccessible by operative methods. Disadvantages include exposing patients with occult lesions to a risk of hemorrhage (most commonly, gastrointestinal tract, and most devastatingly, intracerebral), and dissolution of the clot may cause embolization to distal vessels.

Limb loss rates as high as 30% and hospital mortality as high as 20% have been reported after acute occlusion, emphasizing the need to pay close attention to the underlying medical condition.

Chapter 20

ACUTE MYOCARDIAL INFARCTION

David S. Smith

OVERVIEW

Acute myocardial infarction (MI) results from tissue ischemia produced by the thrombotic occlusion of a coronary artery. Accurate recognition and treatment are essential, because the mortality rate is 10% to 20%, at least one-half of which may be prevented with medical intervention. The diagnosis may be obscured by the broad differential of acute chest pain, denial by the patient, and the limited sensitivity of tests, such as electrocardiograms (ECGs) and cardiac enzymes that are available when admission decisions are made.

PATHOPHYSIOLOGY

Coronary artery plaques form over time by interaction of vascular endothelium with monocytes and platelets, promoting subintimal lipid accumulation. Factors including hyperlipidemia, hypertension, and cigarette smoking contribute to plaque development and progression. MI occurs when a plaque fissures, ruptures, or ulcerates. A platelet monolayer forms, releasing collagen, adenosine diphosphate, serotonin, and epinephrine, leading to platelet activation, induction of the potent vasoconstrictor thromboxane, and fibrinogen cross-linking. Occlusion of an epicardial coronary artery results in downstream tissue ischemia.

CLINICAL PRESENTATION

Acute MI is recognized by pain that is deep and visceral, described as heaviness "like an elephant standing on my chest"; squeezing; or crushing. It is similar in character to prior angina but is more severe and lasts longer, usually more than 30 minutes. The location is usually substernal, and it may radiate to the shoulder, ulnar aspect of the left arm, or neck. Nausea and diaphoresis may be present, especially in inferior MI. Up to 25% of MIs go unrecognized owing to lack of chest pain or atypical symptoms, particularly with diabetes.

A patient with acute MI often is anxious or restlessly moving in bed and pale, with cool extremities. Anterior MI is frequently associated with signs of sympathetic activation, such as tachycardia, whereas inferior MI is accompanied by parasympathetic hyperactivity, such as bradycardia or hypotension. Physical signs of ventricular dysfunction include a third (S_3) or fourth (S_4) heart sound, congestive heart failure, or a late apical systolic murmur due to mitral regurgitation due to papillary muscle dysfunction.

Patients can be divided into prognostic categories based on clinical presentation:

- Killip I: no sign of pulmonary or venous congestion (0–5% mortality)
- Killip II: moderate left heart failure with bibasilar rales, S_3, tachypnea, jugular venous distention or edema (10– 20% mortality)
- Killip III: severe heart failure with pulmonary edema (35–45% mortality)
- Killip IV: cardiogenic shock with hypotension (≤90 systolic), peripheral vasoconstriction/cyanosis, confusion, and oliguria (85–95% mortality)

DIAGNOSIS

Total occlusion of a coronary artery produces acute ST segment elevation, which evolves over time to a Q-wave MI. Subtotal obstruction with collateral flow produces transient T-wave flattening or inversion, which is diagnosed as unstable angina, or non–ST segment elevation MI if serum markers are present with pain. ST elevation of 1 mm or more in contiguous leads is strong evidence of thrombotic occlusion in a patient with acute chest pain, and immediate reperfusion strategies should be considered. A normal ECG reduces the likelihood of acute MI but does not eliminate it.

Necrotic heart muscle releases creatine phosphokinase (CK-MB) and troponins, which aid in diagnosis when measured serially over 12 to 24 hours. CK-MB rises within 4 to 8 hours of acute MI and peaks at 20 hours. Cardiac troponins appear early, remain elevated for 7 to 14 days, and are quite sensitive to minor degrees of myocardial injury. Troponin is useful in determining whether low-level CK-MB elevations are false-positive and in detecting small MIs below the threshold of CK-MB. Observation in an emergency room holding unit with serial testing (ECG, CK-MB, and troponin) for 4 to 6 hours, followed by an exercise test with imaging, is an accurate method of identifying low-risk patients.

Wall motion abnormalities detectable on echocardiogram are present in most patients with acute MI. Left ventricular ejection fraction can be accurately estimated and used for prognosis. Echocardiogram is also useful for diagnosing ventricular aneurysm, pericardial effusion, left ventricular thrombus, and right ventricular infarction. Doppler can detect complications, such as mitral regurgitation and ventricular septal rupture.

MANAGEMENT

For acute ST segment elevation MI, the American College of Cardiology/American Heart Association guidelines recommend the following acute interventions: (i) relief of ischemic pain, (ii) assessment of hemodynamic state and correction of abnormalities, (iii) reperfusion with primary coronary angioplasty or thrombolysis, and (iv) antithrombotic therapy to prevent rethrombosis of an ulcerated plaque. Acute management is followed by therapy to improve long-term prognosis: (i) angiotensin-converting enzyme inhibitors to prevent left ventricular remodeling and dilation, producing decreased contractility; (ii) beta-blockers to prevent recurrent ischemia and ventricular arrhythmias; (iii) anticoagulation in the presence of left ventricular thrombus or atrial fibrillation to prevent embolism; and (iv) statin therapy to stabilize plaques and prevent progression.

Aspirin should be given immediately and daily. Heparin by continuous infusion can reduce the progression of unstable angina to MI. Sublingual nitroglycerin may abolish the chest pain by reducing preload and therefore myocardial demand, and by dilating the stenotic vessel as well as collaterals. Transient response should prompt use of continuous intravenous nitroglycerin. Morphine is an extremely effective analgesic in acute MI, in repetitive 2-mg to 4-mg IV doses. Hypotension is common with both agents, and, if it occurs, can be treated by elevating the legs and giving a bolus of intravenous fluid. Early reperfusion of ischemic myocardium can rescue tissue before it becomes irreversibly damaged. Recanalization of an occluded epicardial artery within the first hour of symptoms can reduce mortality by 50%. Primary angioplasty with or without stenting is the reperfusion treatment of choice. Heparin and aspirin are used immediately post procedure. A glycoprotein IIb/IIIa inhibitor is added by some interventional cardiologists and reserved for imperfect results (e.g., dissection, residual thrombus) by others.

Statins reduce the lipid content and strengthen the matrix of arterial plaques, making them less vulnerable to rupture. Post MI, the goal of treatment is to reduce the low-density lipoprotein cholesterol to below 100 mg per dL. Beta-blockers produce a 20% reduction in cardiac mortality, 25% reduction in reinfarction, and 30% reduction in sudden death. Angiotensin-converting enzyme inhibitors reduce mortality and the development of heart failure in patients with an ejection fraction less than 40%.

The outcome of acute MI is related to the occurrence of the complications of arrhythmia and pump failure. Ventricular fibrillation is the most common cause of death, usually occurring within the first 24 hours of the onset of symptoms—more than one-half within the first hour. All patients with acute MI should be placed on continuous cardiac monitoring for at least 24 hours to watch for the development of ventricular tachycardia or fibrillation, which often occurs without warning arrhythmia. Prophylactic lidocaine has not been shown to improve outcomes of acute MI. Sustained ventricular tachycardia in a hemodynamically stable patient is treated first with IV lidocaine or amiodarone. If it does not respond, or if hemodynamic compromise develops, 50-J to 100-J synchronized countershocks are used. Ventricular fibrillation is treated with immediate 200-J unsynchronized countershock, followed by cardiopulmonary resuscitation protocol if unsuccessful.

Pump failure is the primary cause of in-hospital death from acute MI. Clinical signs include bibasilar rales, development of S_3 and S_4, and pulmonary congestion on chest x-ray. Hemodynamic effects are seen with loss of 20% to 25% of the left ventricular muscle mass, and cardiogenic shock with 40% loss or more. Mild congestive heart failure without hypotension is usually managed by diuresis with furosemide, given intravenously if symptoms dictate urgency. Nitrates can lower preload, improving compliance and reducing ischemia. Hemodynamic monitoring, using a balloon flotation catheter in the pulmonary artery, can help direct therapy. Patients with markedly elevated filling pressures (>22 mm Hg) benefit from diuresis, whereas those with low filling pressures (<15 mm Hg) and low cardiac index [<2.6 L/(minute/m^2)] benefit from volume expansion. Cardiogenic shock is characterized by hypotension (systolic pressure <80 mm Hg), markedly reduced cardiac index [<1.8 L/(minute/m^2)], and high filling pressures (wedge pressure >18 mm Hg). Because the mortality of cardiogenic shock is high, these patients are candidates for early revascularization by angioplasty or bypass surgery.

Right ventricular infarction occurs in patients with inferoposterior MI and is recognized by jugular venous distention and ST elevation in lead V$_4$R. Hypotension is common, and volume expansion is needed to maintain right ventricular preload. *Ventricular septal rupture* occurs with sudden, severe left ventricular failure in association with a pansystolic murmur. The diagnosis can be made by demonstration of a step-up in oxygen saturation at the level of the right ventricle by pulmonary artery catheter, or by color flow Doppler echocardiography. *Acute mitral regurgitation* due to rupture of a papillary muscle presents with sudden appearance of a loud systolic murmur and pulmonary congestion. The diagnosis is confirmed by Doppler echocardiogaphy and treated by surgical repair or replacement of the mitral valve. *Pericarditis* is a cause of recurrent chest pain post MI, recognized by a localized friction rub and treated with a nonsteroidal antiinflammatory drug. *Thromboembolism* complicates 2% to 5% of cases, and risk should be anticipated when there is an anterior MI, severe left ventricular dysfunction, or peripheral manifestations. Left ventricular thrombus can usually be detected by echocardiogram and treated with anticoagulants.

Chapter 21

AORTIC DISSECTION

David N. Smith

OVERVIEW

Aortic dissection is a catastrophic illness, presenting with acute chest pain and caused by a tear in the aortic intima. The incidence is approximately 2,000 per year; 50% to 75% of those cases are men, usually in the 60-year-old to 80-year-old age group, but it is also seen in younger patients with Marfan's syndrome. The clinician must be ever vigilant for this uncommon diagnosis, as it requires prompt diagnosis and intervention to save the patient's life.

PATHOPHYSIOLOGY

Two mechanisms contribute to produce dissection. First, the arterial wall is weakened over time by hypertension, age, trauma, or cardiovascular surgery, or by inherent weakness of the wall in collagen-vascular diseases, such as Ehlers-Danlos syndrome, Marfan's syndrome, or spontaneous rupture of the vasovasorum. Second, an initiating insult to the aorta must occur. Relatively anchored areas of the aorta are predisposed to wall stress and intimal dissection. Regardless of the cause, aortic dissection results from cystic medionecrosis or tear of the artery's tunica media. Pathology reveals penetrating ulceration or intramural hematoma. Propagation of the dissection results from sympathetic surges that increase shear stress forces on the arterial wall, therefore dictating the basis of treatment strategies. In the original DeBakey classification, type I involves both the ascending and descending aorta (10%), type II involves only the ascending aorta (60%), and type III involves only the distal aorta after the origin of the left subclavian artery. The more widely used Stanford classification separates dissections into those involving the ascending aorta and arch (type A) versus those distal to the left subclavian artery only involving the descending aorta (type B), emphasizing the critical nature of the former.

CLINICAL PRESENTATION

The signs and symptoms usually correlate with the mechanical consequences of the dissection. Pain symptoms (e.g., anterior chest pain radiating to the back, abdominal pain) result from the acute tear injury. The majority of patients (96%) can be identified by some combination of three clinical features: (i) immediate onset of pain with a tearing or ripping character; (ii) mediastinal or aortic widening, or both, on chest x-ray; and (iii) variation in pulse or blood pressure (BP), or both, between the right and left arm. Proximal extension of dissections can lead to acute aortic regurgitation (one-half to two-thirds of patients) or adventitial rupture, which causes bleeding into either the pericardium, causing tamponade, or into the chest, causing hemothorax. Acute myocardial infarction, especially involving dissection of the right coronary artery, or syncope can also result. Mechanical compression by an expanding hematoma may cause superior vena cava syndrome, Horner's syndrome, or airway compromise. Dissection can occlude branches of the aorta, causing ischemia to the extremities (20%), brain (5%), kidneys, gut, or spinal cord. Physical examination may reveal hypertension or hypotension, wide pulse pressure, BP discrepancy between the arms or pulse deficits, fever, tamponade physiology, left lung effusion, or a new diastolic murmur.

DIAGNOSIS

The chest x-ray shows a widened superior mediastinum in many patients with ascending aorta dissection and may also show left-sided pleural effusion, enlarged or irregular aortic knob, cardiomegaly, or a rightward displacement of the aorta. The electrocardiogram may show left ventricular hypertrophy, ischemic changes, or signs of tamponade (low-voltage or electrical alternans). Transesophageal echocardiogram is the test of choice in a hemodynamically unstable patient, despite missing the aortic arch. Although transthoracic echocardiogram has approximately 75% and 40% sensitivity in type A and B dissections, respectively, the transesophageal echocardiogram's sensitivity and specificity may be as high as 98% to 99% for proximal and distal dissections. Usual findings include dilatation of the aortic root, effusion, increased aortic wall thickness (extravasated blood), and an oscillating intimal flap. In hemodynamically stable patients, contrast computed tomography (CT) or magnetic resonance imaging (MRI) or magnetic resonance angiography (MRA) of the chest and aorta is appropriate to differentiate two lumens formed in dissection, as well as possible hematoma formation with or without compression of the true lumen. The MRI can also distinguish the direction of blood flow. CT has a sensitivity of 94% and specificity of 87%, and has the advantage of being readily available in most hospitals and emergency departments.

MRI has a sensitivity and specificity of approximately 98%. Aortography is less sensitive and specific than other diagnostic modalities but is most useful when suspecting branch occlusion. Coronary artery catheterization is helpful when myocardial ischemia is associated or immediately before surgery graft for a type A dissection.

MANAGEMENT

The patient should be on complete bedrest in an intensive care setting, with a Foley catheter and continuous BP monitoring. In general, the stable patient with descending aortic dissection can be medically managed by decreasing the shearing BP with intravenous nitroprusside (monitoring cyanide levels in renal insufficiency) plus beta-blockade (propanolol, esmolol, or labetolol) if there are no absolute contraindications. The ganglion blocker trimethaphan is an alternative when beta-blockers cannot be used. Mental status or neurologic changes, urinary output, and evidence of end-organ damage are monitored.

If the dissection involves the ascending aorta, the management is surgical, because these patients are at a high risk for a life-threatening complication, such as aortic regurgitation, cardiac tamponade, or myocardial infarction. Complicated type B dissections, defined by inability to control BP, increasing hematoma, persisting bleeding, ischemia distal to the dissection, or refractory pain, are also candidates for surgery.

As most type B dissections persist as chronic disease, subsequent ambulatory care is crucial. The primary care physician's aim is to maintain low systolic BPs using a beta-blocker combined with afterload reduction using an angiotensin-converting enzyme inhibitor or hydralazine. Patients should be seen often, with meticulous attention to vital signs, complaints of chest or back pain, or neurologic changes. Auscultation of the heart at every visit with a low threshold for obtaining an echocardiogram is mandatory to monitor aortic insufficiency. Periodic chest x-rays and CT or MRI should be obtained to screen for development of aneurysms. Patients with Marfan's syndrome require early prophylactic surgical correction of dilated ascending aorta segments.

Hospital survival is 70% to 80% overall (50% 10-year survival in those who needed emergent surgery), although redissection occurs in approximately 13% in 5 years (23% in 10 years).

Chapter 22

ARRHYTHMIA

David Litvak

OVERVIEW

The reasons to evaluate and treat arrhythmias include relief of symptoms, prevention of hemodynamic collapse or death due to a life-threatening arrhythmia, and reduction of the long-term risk that a non–life-threatening arrhythmia may herald in a high-risk patient. Deciding whether the patient is hemodynamically stable is the most important task in determining the pace and course of evaluation and management. Risk assessment also includes a determination of whether the patient has underlying ischemia due to coronary artery disease or reduced ventricular function.

PATHOPHYSIOLOGY

Tachyarrhythmias

The three sites at which tachyarrhythmias occur are the atria (supraventricular), the atrioventricular (AV) node (junctional), and the ventricles. The two mechanisms that cause tachycardias are increased automaticity and reentry loops. Increased automaticity refers to a focus within the heart with an increased rate of impulse formation. It may be a pacemaker in the sinus node or AV node or an ectopic pacemaker in the atria or ventricle. Reentry loops consist of a tissue electrical circuit with two limbs. One arm has a slow refractory period and the other a fast refractory period. Most commonly, a premature beat initiates a reentry tachycardia by sending an impulse through the limb with a fast refractory period. The impulse is initially blocked in the limb with a slow refractory period, but by the time the impulse makes its circuit, the slow limb is no longer refractory, and a loop is established.

Bradyarrhythmias

Sinus dysfunction is most commonly caused by age-related degeneration of the sinus node. Other causes include drugs (beta-blockers, calcium channel blockers, digoxin, quinidine, amiodarone, lithium, cimetidine), hypothyroidism, ischemia to the sinus node (60% right coronary artery, 40% left circumflex), infiltrative diseases (amyloid, hemochromatosis, sarcoid), infections (typhoid, Lyme disease, brucellosis), end-stage liver disease, profound hypoxia, and acidosis. Sinus dysfunction may be manifested as sinus bradycardia, sinoatrial block, sinus arrest, or the bradycardia-tachycardia syndrome. In the latter, tachyarrhythmias (atrial fibrillation, atrial flutter, or atrial tachycardia) are often followed by prolonged sinus pauses. AV conduction disturbances can also lead to bradycardia. AV blocks are caused by the same factors affecting the sinoatrial node. First-degree AV block is characterized by a PR interval longer than 0.20 seconds. Second-degree heart block occurs when some atrial impulses fail to be conducted to the ventricles. In second-degree block, Mobitz type I, progressive PR prolongation occurs until an atrial impulse is not conducted. It is often transient and due to ischemia or drugs (beta-blockers or digoxin). Second degree, Mobitz type II occurs with constant PR intervals and then a sudden, nonconducted atrial impulse. The His-Purkinje system is often diseased with associated QRS prolongation. These can convert to third-degree complete heart block without warning. Third-degree block occurs when all atrial impulses are blocked. Second-degree Mobitz type II block and third-degree block require pacemaker placement.

CLINICAL PRESENTATION

Tachyarrhythmias

The spectrum of clinical manifestations is broad, from no symptoms to palpitations to sudden syncope. Clinical stability must be assessed rapidly. Serious symptoms include chest pain, shortness of breath, and depressed mental status. Physical signs indicating instability are hypotension, distended neck veins, crackles, and decreased level of consciousness.

Bradyarrhythmias

Patients may present with symptoms due to decreased cardiac output: weakness, dizziness, shortness of breath, presyncope, or syncope. Symptoms may

TABLE 22-1 Distinguishing Supraventricular Tachycardia (SVT) with Aberrancy from Ventricular Tachycardia

SVT with Aberrancy	Ventricular Tachycardia (VT)
P before each QRS	Atrioventricular dissociation.
No concordance	Concordance (all QRS complexes in precordial leads point in the same direction; in negative direction is right VT, and in positive direction is left VT).
Presence of RS complexes favors SVT	No RS complexes in precordial leads (QRS consists of single Q or R wave) favors VT. If RS present, then beginning of R to nadir of S is >0.10 sec.
No fusion or capture beats	Fusion beats (abnormally shaped QRS, part of QRS results from ventricular activation and part from atrial activation), capture beats (P wave precedes narrow complex QRS amidst the wide complex tachycardia).
QRS <0.14 sec	QRS >0.14 sec.

be present at rest or may become apparent during exercise or fever, when sinus dysfunction prohibits expected augmentation of cardiac output.

DIAGNOSIS

Tachyarrhythmias

In identifying the type of arrhythmia, the most essential features are QRS width and regularity, and P-wave morphology. In narrow complex rhythms, the origin is above the ventricles. In regular narrow complex rhythms, the differential diagnosis includes sinus tachycardia, AV nodal reentrant tachycardia, AV bypass tract tachycardia, and atrial flutter. Distinguishing these depends on P-wave morphology (Table 22-1). Irregular narrow complex rhythms include atrial fibrillation, atrial flutter with variable block, and multifocal atrial tachycardia. Wide complex tachycardias may be ventricular or supraventricular with aberrancy. Long-term management may require an echocardiogram to assess ejection fraction and chamber sizes, cardiac catheterization or stress test to assess for ischemia, and electrophysiologic study to assess for circuits amenable to ablation or inducibility of ventricular tachycardia.

Bradyarrhythmias

The admonition "treat the patient, not the monitor" emphasizes that the most important point in evaluation is distinguishing between symptomatic and asymptomatic patients. Those without symptoms may be followed expectantly. In symptomatic patients, it is essential to link symptoms with electrocardiographic (ECG) changes. The link may be evident with a resting ECG but more likely requires a Holter monitor or an event recorder to be established. Also, exercise testing is useful to establish chronotropic incompetence, an inability to increase heart rate appropriately. Electrophysiologic studies are only indicated in symptomatic patients in whom ECG evidence of sinus dysfunction cannot be found.

MANAGEMENT

Tachyarrhythmias

In treating tachyarrhythmias, the patient's stability is paramount. Unstable patients (chest pain, severe dyspnea, change in mental status, hypotension, or congestive heart failure) should be cardioverted. Exceptions include multifocal

TABLE 22-2 Differential Diagnosis and Treatment of Tachyarrhythmias

Arrhythmia	Cause	ECG Findings	Treatment of Stable Patients
Sinus tachycardia	Automaticity due to physiologic response, not cardiac pathology	Regular, upright P waves before each QRS.	Treat underlying pathology.
Multifocal atrial tachycardia	Automaticity often due to pulmonary disease	*Irregular*, atypical P waves before each QRS.	Treat lung disease; may require slowing with CCB or amiodarone. *No DC cardioversion.*
Atrial fibrillation	Macro reentry loop	*Irregular*, absent P waves.	Nl EF, no WPW: CCB, beta-blocker, digoxin. Low EF, no WPW: digoxin, CCB, amiodarone. WPW: amiodarone, procainamide, flecainide, propafenone, or sotalol.
Atrial flutter	Macro reentry loop	Regular or *irregular* depending if AV block is consistent or variable. Sawtooth P waves. Rate usually around 150 (2:1 block).	Same as above.
AV nodal reentry tachycardia	Reentry loop	Regular, retrograde P waves usually buried within QRS.	Nl EF: adenosine or vagal maneuvers may be diagnostic or therapeutic. Can also use beta-blocker, CCB, or amiodarone. Low EF: amiodarone, CCB, diltiazem, *no DC cardioversion.*
AV bypass tract	Macro reentry loop	Regular, retrograde P waves often just after QRS.	Use amiodarone and procainamide. Flecainide, propafenone, or sotatolol may be helpful.
Wide complex tachycardia of unknown type	?	?	Should assume ventricular tachycardia but may try vagal maneuvers and/or adenosine if aberrancy is considered. Use amiodarone or DC cardioversion for rate control.
VT	Macro reentry loop	AV dissociation; QRS may be regular or slightly irregular; QRS morphology may be monomorphic or polymorphic.	Polymorphic VT: consider drug overdose and check baseline QT interval. If prolonged, correct electrolytes, give magnesium, consider overdrive pacing or isoproterenol. If normal QT, use amiodarone, lidocaine, sotalol, or beta-blocker (with Nl EF). Monomorphic VT: use procainamide, sotalol, amiodarone, or lidocaine, then cardiovert.

AV, atrioventricular; CCB, calcium channel blocker; DC, direct current; ECG, electrocardiogram; EF, ejection fraction; Nl, normal; VT, ventricular tachycardia; WPW, Wolff-Parkinson-White.

atrial tachycardia and AV nodal reentrant tachycardia in patients with a low ejection fraction. Specific therapies depend on making the appropriate diagnosis from the ECG and knowledge of a patient's ejection fraction (Table 22–2). Atrial tachycardias due to sinoatrial nodal reentry may be slowed or aborted by the use of vagal maneuvers or parasympathomimetic drugs. These modalities have little effect on the atrial rate in other atrial tachycardias. It is important to remember that all antiarrhythmic drugs (particularly class IC) have the potential to increase ectopy or induce or aggravate ventricular tachycardia, torsades de pointes, ventricular fibrillation conduction disturbances, or bradycardia.

Bradyarrhythmias

Once all secondary causes of sinus dysfunction have been ruled out, the mainstay of treatment for symptomatic patients is pacemaker insertion. AV sequential pacing is often used, as it may prevent atrial fibrillation. In patients with *acute* symptomatic bradycardia (e.g., in acute myocardial infarction), atropine may be used. It should not be used, however, in third-degree block or Mobitz II second-degree block, or for wide complex ventricular escape beats. If it is not effective, transcutaneous pacing, dopamine, epinephrine, or isoproterenol may be tried.

Chapter 23

CARDIOGENIC SHOCK

Jared G. Selter

OVERVIEW

Coronary artery disease (CAD) remains the leading cause of death in the United States. Eleven million individuals are affected with coronary atherosclerosis, and there are 1.5 million myocardial infarctions (MIs) in this country each year. Cardiogenic shock (CGS) is a life-threatening complication of MI and, although the mortality from MI has dramatically decreased over the last decade, the incidence of CGS (5–10% of MIs) has remained stable. Mortality from CGS remains between 45% and 80% in varying surveys. Although therapies continue to advance (e.g., percutaneous transluminal coronary angioplasty/stenting), the aging U.S. population and increasing prevalence of diabetes mellitus suggest that CGS will remain a common entity in coming years.

PATHOPHYSIOLOGY

The most common cause of CGS is MI, and this discussion focuses on this presentation. Other causes include cardiomyopathy, myocarditis, sepsis, acute valvular failure, myocardial contusion, and outflow and inflow obstruction. Complications from MI can be divided into two broad categories: mechanical and pump failure. Mechanical failure is the easier of the complications to understand on a conceptual basis. During an acute MI, infarcted areas, such as the mitral valve (MV), the ventricular free wall, and the intraventricular septum, are at risk for mechanical compromise. The posterior papillary muscle of the MV has a single vascular supply. During inferior wall MI, the papillary muscle can infarct and is at risk for rupture. Even if rupture does not occur, transient muscle dysfunction from ischemia can occur. Both situations lead to acute MV incompetence, decreased cardiac output (CO), and increased pulmonary capillary wedge pressure (PCWP) as the left atrium is quickly overwhelmed by increased pressure. Similar events occur during both free and intraventricular wall ruptures. During acute MI, infarcted tissue no longer contracts in synchrony with the viable myocardium, and paradoxical movements occur. The region between infarcted and viable tissue, stressed from compromised vascular supply, is under mechanical strain and can rupture. If the free wall ruptures, cardiac tamponade results and CO declines, leading to CGS. In intraventricular wall rupture, a large left-to-right shunt is created, leading to hypotension and congestive heart failure.

In pump failure, CGS can be considered the end result of a downward spiral of systolic and diastolic dysfunction that is initiated with the index infarction. When an infarct occurs, the remaining viable myocardium is forced to work at greater capacity with a limited vascular supply and fewer functional myocytes to compensate. Increased oxygen demand from sympathetic stimulation can cause infarct extension, as already compromised tissue near the index infarct is forced to work harder. "Ischemia at a distance" occurs when tissue that is geographically remote from the index insult is compromised owing to increased demand. Eighty percent of patients who develop CGS have multivessel disease. Several maladaptive processes also induce CGS. Renal fluid retention to maintain systolic blood pressure leads to increased preload and intraventricular pressures. Sympathetic stimulation to maintain pressure elevates afterload. Both of these adaptations lead to greater oxygen demand. Elevated intraventricular pressures from fluid retention, as well as compensatory tachycardia, limit the pressure-dependent coronary vascular supply, further decreasing myocardial contractility. Depressed contractility leads to diastolic dysfunction and elevated right atrial pressure. All contribute to a spiraling depression of CO.

CLINICAL PRESENTATION

The clinical presentation of CGS varies depending on the underlying cause. The classic presentation after MI is that of ashen, mottled skin that is cool to palpation. Such presentations are due to peripheral vasoconstriction in an attempt to maintain CO. The jugular veins are markedly distended, reflecting elevated PCWP. Additionally, patients have rales on pulmonary ascultation. Such a presentation is in contrast to that of those with septic shock, who have warm, dry extremities, lack elevated jugular venous pressure, and do not have rales on examination. Those in hypovolemic shock (e.g., hemorrhage, profound diarrhea) have cool extremities as do those with CGS, but they have flat neck veins and lack rales. Patients who develop CGS soon after MI may still complain of chest discomfort from the index infarct, but lack of this symptom should not dissuade the clinician from a CGS diagnosis, as not all patients, particularly those with clouded sensorium or silent ischemia (e.g., diabetics), complain of pain. In fact, altered mental status in the elderly may be the only presenting feature of impending CGS.

DIAGNOSIS

CGS is defined as a depressed CO in the setting of adequate intravascular volume and evidence of tissue hypoxia. Hemodynamic parameters include prolonged hypotension (<80 mm Hg for >30 minutes), a reduced cardiac index (1.8 L/minute/m^2), and high PCWP (>18 mm Hg) (Table 23–1).

A high clinical suspicion for CGS is the most critical tool in diagnosis. Given an appropriate clinical situation, the clinician should be able to use a succinct his-

TABLE 23-1 Hemodynamic Parameters for Cardiogenic Shock

Shock Type	CI	PCWP	SVR
Cardiogenic	Low	High	High
Septic	High	Normal/low	Low
Hypovolemic	Low	Low	High

CI, cardiac index; PCWP, pulmonary capillary wedge pressure; SVR, systemic vascular resistance.

tory and physical examination and various diagnostic tools to diagnose CGS. In a patient with hypotension and a new murmur after MI, mechanical failure should be considered immediately. Additionally, distant heart sounds would suggest pericardial effusion. Electrocardiography (ECG) can show telltale signs of new infarction or cardiac tamponade (e.g., electrical alternans or decreased voltage). ECG is not a sensitive tool for CGS or its precipitant events, however. Chest radiography should be obtained in all patients in whom CGS is considered to evaluate for pulmonary vascular congestion. Echocardiography is an invaluable tool in early diagnosis of CGS. Echocardiography can show new areas of wall motion abnormality and pericardial effusion. When used in combination with Doppler ultrasonography, new valvular incompetence or wall perforation can be seen. Unlike septic shock, in which pulmonary artery catheterization is controversial, CGS often requires such invasive monitoring, for diagnosis and after treatment. Additionally, a pulmonary artery catheter can provide access to right atrial and ventricular circulations and can show step-ups in venous oxygenation, suggestive of septal defects.

MANAGEMENT

Initial management of CGS is the same as for that of other medical emergencies but should be localized in intensive care unit settings with specialized nurses and physicians. Initially, the patient's airway, breathing, and circulation must be assessed and supported. If there is any question that the patient cannot protect his or her own airway, then intubation and mechanical ventilation should be initiated. In addition to airway protection, mechanical ventilation decreases cardiac work and can prevent further infarction. Hypotension should be assessed with noninvasive and invasive techniques. In patients without overt pulmonary congestion, an isoosmotic fluid challenge should be initiated. In patients with rales and hypotension on presentation, intravenous fluids should be avoided and circulatory support provided by vasopressor agents. There is no ideal pressor agent for CGS, however. Dobutamine is effective in exacerbations of chronic heart failure but can precipitate hypotension in shock via beta$_1$ activity and can worsen ischemia by stimulating cardiac work. Norepinephrine and pseudoephedrine have substantial alpha-agonist activity and dramatically increase afterload and, therefore, cardiac work. Dopamine is initially useful, although it raises mean arterial pressure and tissue perfusion, has beta-adrenergic effects, and can exacerbate ischemia by increasing workload. Combination therapy may reduce some of the toxic side effects of higher-dose individual therapy. The most effective form of circulatory support with afterload reduction is intraaortic balloon counterpulsation and is efficacious in numerous causes of CGS, including pump failure, MV failure, and wall rupture. Once the circulation is supported, judicious diuretic therapy can be used to limit pulmonary congestion and improve oxygenation. Other support should include continuous ECG monitoring to avoid arrhythmic complications, supplemental oxygenation to prevent hypoxemia, and pain relief with or without anxiolytics.

Perhaps the only definitive treatment for CGS is a preventive strategy. Most episodes of CGS occur several hours after an MI has occurred. By aggressively treating each MI as if it may proceed to CGS, using prompt revascularization by angioplasty and stenting or thrombolysis, episodes of shock and ultimately death may be avoided.

Chapter 24

CARDIAC ARREST

David Litvak

OVERVIEW

Cardiac arrest inspires fear in medical residents, because lives can be saved or lost based on the decisions made by the individual running a code. The American Heart Association has developed algorithms to assist in making quick decisions in critical situations. This chapter focuses on the assessment and treatment of the patient without a pulse. Early defibrillation is the most important determinant of outcome, with chances of survival falling by 7% to 10% per minute.

DIAGNOSIS

In approaching the pulseless patient, the cardiac rhythm must be classified into one of four categories: ventricular tachycardia (VT), ventricular fibrillation (VF), pulseless electrical activity (PEA), or asystole. The most common causes leading to these rhythms include cardiac ischemia, metabolic disturbances (commonly hyperkalemia or acidosis), drug overdoses (commonly digoxin or tricyclic antidepressants), an abnormal cardiac substrate, or some combination of these. In VF, there are disorganized depolarizations of the ventricular myocardium, leading to total pump failure. In the setting of pulselessness, all wide complex tachycardias should be treated as VT. A unique form of VT is torsades de pointes, or twisting about the axis. This rhythm is frequently seen in patients with a prolonged QT interval. Narrow complex tachycardia with a ventricular response of greater than 150 beats per minute can produce profound hypotension secondary to shortened diastolic filling time and decreased myocardial contractility. PEA encompasses all other rhythms, including idioventricular rhythms, ventricular escape rhythms, and bradycardia. In PEA, the heart rhythm is often not the cause of pulselessness; other etiologies must be sought, using the mnemonic MATCHED: *m*yocardial infarction (MI), *a*cidosis, *t*ension pneumothorax, *c*ardiac tamponade, *h*ypovolemia, *h*yperkalemia, pulmonary *e*mboli, and *d*rugs. Asystole is marked by a complete absence of electrical activity. This rhythm has the poorest prognosis.

MANAGEMENT

On arrival, the person running the code should loudly announce that he or she is in charge. The first priority should be to determine whether the patient has a pulse and to establish the rhythm. The most important predictor of a successful resuscitation is the time between cardiac arrest and initiation of treatment, specifically defibrillation. If the patient is not already on a monitor, the defibrillator paddles should be used immediately to establish the rhythm. If intravenous access has not been established, atropine, lidocaine, and epinephrine (ALE) can be given through the endotracheal tube.

Ventricular Fibrillation

In the case of VF or pulseless wide complex tachycardia (assumed VT), three successive shocks should be given in the unsynchronized mode at 200, 300, and 360 J. When delivering shocks, remember to remove nitroglycerin patches and avoid placing paddles directly over implantable defibrillators. Between each shock, the rhythm should be reassessed, but neither cardiac compressions nor pulse checks should be done. After the three shocks, check the rhythm and pulse. Checking the pulse is crucial, because VF cannot sustain a pulse; if a pulse is felt and VF is seen on the monitor, it is likely artifact of lead misplacement. If VF/VT persists and pulselessness is confirmed, make sure that the patient is being oxygenated adequately via a bag-valve mask (Ambu-bag) or endotracheal tube, chest compressions are being done, intravenous access has been established, a monitor is connected, and epinephrine is given. Chest compressions will produce a peak blood pressure of 60 to 80 mm Hg, and a cardiac output of one-quarter to one-third normal. After giving epinephrine, 1 mg, repeat defibrillation at 360 J. At this point, medications should be alternated with shocks. After each intervention, check for a pulse. Antiarrhythmics can be given for shock-refractory VT/VF, although there is only fair evidence supporting their benefit, including lidocaine, amiodarone, magnesium (especially in torsades de pointes), and procainamide. If the patient's rhythm stabilizes, a bolus of lidocaine must be given and a lidocaine drip started before transporting the patient. In sum: shock, shock, shock, epinephrine, shock, lidocaine, shock, amiodarone, shock.

Pulseless Electrical Activity

PEA is present when a patient with electrical activity other than VF, wide complex tachycardia, or narrow complex tachycardia does not have a detectable pulse. PEA includes regular sinus, junctional, idioventricular, ventricular escape, and bradycardic rhythms. Wide complexes and a slow rhythm are seen in dying myocardium or are associated with hyperkalemia, hypothermia, hypoxia, acidosis, or drug overdose. Narrow complex rapid tachycardia is found in hypovolemia, infection, pulmonary embolism, or cardiac tamponade. Initially, ensure adequate oxygenation, call for intubation, start cardiopulmonary resuscitation, obtain intravenous access, and carefully assess for a pulse. If available, use a portable Doppler ultrasound to check for a femoral pulse. Start treatment by giving epinephrine, 1 mg, and normal saline boluses. If bradycardia is present, administer atropine, 1 mg, and initiate transcutaneous pacing (TCP). In TCP, pads are placed on the anterior chest to the left of the sternum and on the back to the left of the thoracic spine. Initially, the device should be turned to maximal stimulating current to assure capture. The best measure of capture is improved hemodynamics and consistent ST segments and T waves after each pacer spike. After treatment, if the patient regains a pulse but remains hypotensive, give dopamine. Secondary causes for hemodynamic instability must be sought. Call for an electrocardiogram to assess for an acute MI. Get an arterial blood gas to check for acidosis. Listen for bilateral breath sounds, feel for crepitus, and assess jugular venous distention to diagnose a tension pneumothorax. Think about cardiac tamponade in patients who have had a recent cardiac procedure (especially pacer placement) or MI, and in patients with cancer, end-stage renal disease (uremia), or certain infections (tuberculosis, viral myocarditis). Consider hypovolemia, the most common cause of PEA, and hyperkalemia in patients with renal disease. Rule out hypoxia by checking an oxygen saturation. Examine the lower extremities for swelling, suggesting thromboembolic disease. Last, think of drug overdoses, such as tricyclic antidepressants, digoxin, calcium channel blockers, or beta-blockers.

Narrow Complex Tachycardia

In pulseless patients with a narrow complex tachycardia, immediate synchronized cardioversion must be performed starting at 100 J, followed by 200 J, 300 J, and 360 J. Between each shock, quickly assess the pulse. If the patient is refractory to cardioversion and remains pulseless, adenosine may be given and cardioversion attempted again. Remember to ensure adequate oxygenation, establish intravenous access, and obtain an electrocardiogram. Secondary causes of pulselessness should be sought (remember MATCHED).

Bradycardia

Usually, bradycardia is associated with low output rather than cardiac arrest, but a code may be called for manifestations of it. Atropine is effective for symptomatic sinus bradycardia but should not be used if Mobitz II block is suspected. TCP or a transvenous pacemaker should be used in second-degree or third-degree block, or when bradycardia persists after atropine or catecholamines.

Asystole

Asystole must be confirmed in multiple leads to rule out fine VF. As this is being done, the patient should be intubated, cardiopulmonary resuscitation continued, and intravenous access obtained. Asystole is treated the same as PEA with bradycardia, using epinephrine followed by atropine. TCP also can be used in conjunction with epinephrine and atropine. When all else fails, aminophylline can be given. As in PEA, the same secondary causes need to be investigated (remember MATCHED).

Medicines in Cardiac Arrest

Epinephrine

Administer a 1-mg bolus of 1:10,000 solution. Second and third boluses can be escalated to 3 mg and 5 mg. Give every 3 to 5 minutes. Flush with 20 mL of normal saline. Provides an alpha and beta agonist activity. Avoid use with alkaline infusions (i.e., bicarbonate).

Atropine

Administer a 1-mg bolus, with a maximum of 3 mg. Give every 3 to 5 minutes; the maximum dose is 3 mg. Atropine is effective at decreasing vagal tone, thus increasing conduction through the atrioventricular node.

Lidocaine

Administer a 1 mg per kg bolus, followed by a 0.5 mg per kg bolus every 10 minutes. The maximum dose is 3 mg per kg. Always follow with a drip at 2 mg per minute. Lidocaine is a type IA antiarrhythmic. It is not to be used in a third-degree atrioventricular block, because ventricular escape rhythm may be suppressed. Watch for toxicity: agitation, paresthesias, twitching, seizures.

Amiodarone

Administer 150 mg over 10 minutes, then 1 mg per minute ×6 hours, then 0.5 mg per minute ×18 hours. Amiodarone is a type III antiarrhythmic. It may produce hypotension soon after administration and has many long-term toxicities affecting lungs, liver, thyroid, and eyes.

Bretylium

Administer a 5 mg per kg bolus; repeat with 10 mg per kg if VF/VT persists. Repeat at 5 minutes and 30 minutes if needed. The maximum dose is 35 mg per kg. Infuse at 2 mg per minute. Bretylium releases norepinephrine and may produce hypotension.

Sodium Bicarbonate

Give 1 amp (50 mEq) every 10 minutes. Sodium bicarbonate is most useful in hyperkalemia. Its use in acidemia is controversial.

Procainamide

Load with 20 to 30 mg per minute; follow with an infusion of 1 to 4 mg per minute. Stop loading dose if arrhythmia suppressed, hypotension develops, QRS widens by 50%, or 17 mg per kg is given. Procainamide is used in patients with Wolff-Parkinson-White who develop rapid atrial fibrillation to prevent or treat VF/VT.

Magnesium Sulfate

Provide 2 g IV over 1 to 2 minutes. Magnesium sulfate is most useful in torsades de pointes. It may produce hypotension.

Dopamine

In treating hypotension, start a dopamine drip at 5 μg per kg per minute, with a maximum dose of 20 μg per kg per minute. Dopamine is useful as an adjunctive drug to treat hypotension in patients with sinus, junctional, or escape rhythms that are not tachycardic. These rhythms often develop after VF/VT resuscitations. If tachycardia develops with worsening hemodynamics, stop dopamine.

Aminophylline

Administer 250 mg over 1 to 2 minutes. Aminophylline is used when all else fails in bradysystolic arrests.

Chapter 25

CHEST PAIN

James N. Kirkpatrick

OVERVIEW

Chest pain accounts for 2% to 6% of emergency room visits in the United States, translating into 5 million visits per year. In emergency room patients with chest pain, acute myocardial infarction (MI) will be diagnosed in 2% to 4%, with a short-term mortality of 10% to 20%. Thus, the primary concern in the evaluation of nontraumatic chest pain consists of determining the presence or absence of ischemic heart disease; however, coronary insufficiency is only one of the many etiologies of chest pain, and differentiating between them often proves difficult.

Besides coronary heart disease, aortic dissection, pulmonary embolism (PE), and esophageal rupture are chest pain syndromes with high associated mortality. Missed aortic dissection leads to mortality of 28% in the first 24 hours, 50% within 2 days, and 90% over 3 months; PE carries a mortality rate of 10%; and esophageal rupture is always fatal if undiagnosed within 24 hours.

PATHOPHYSIOLOGY

Chest pain etiologies involve nearly every structure in the chest or affecting the chest, including components of the cardiovascular, pulmonary, gastrointestinal, musculoskeletal, and neurologic systems. Pain sensation in the chest, as in the rest of the body, is mediated through somatic and visceral innervations. Stimulation of the somatic sensory fibers is usually perceived as sharp, piercing, and localized pain. Anatomic structures of the chest with somatic innervation include skin, muscles, bones, joints, parietal pericardium, and parietal pleura. Stimulation of visceral structures, such as the myocardium and esophagus, produces pain that is diffuse and described as a dull ache, pressure, or squeeze. This distinction cannot completely delineate affected structures. For instance, transmural MI can cause an inflammatory response involving the overlying parietal pericardium. Further complicating anatomic distinction is the overlapping nature of thoracic nerve root innervations. In particular, the heart and esophagus share nerve roots T1 to T4.

CLINICAL PRESENTATION

Given the potentially fatal consequences of failing to promptly and accurately diagnose coronary ischemia, aortic dissection, PE, and esophageal rupture, recognizing clinical signs becomes an important first step in evaluating patients presenting with chest pain.

Acute Myocardial Infarction

The "classic" symptom complex of acute MI includes the descriptions *dull, ache, crush, crescendo,* and *vice-like.* This type of pain was found to be associated with various types of coronary ischemia in 54% of cases. Sharp or stabbing pain can occur in 16% to 22% of ischemic chest pain; however, when sharp chest pain was associated with positional and reproducible components, there were no cases of acute coronary syndrome among 596 patients. The location is most often retrosternal with radiation to one or both arms, shoulders, sides of the neck and jaw, or to the back. A recent study suggested that radiation to both arms indicated a higher specificity for coronary ischemia. Associated symptoms include shortness of breath, diaphoresis, nausea, weakness, and palpitations, which can improve the predictive value of chest pain for acute MI. Various studies have found that 12% to 33% of patients with acute MI, particularly the elderly, present with symptoms other than chest pain, including dyspnea, syncope, nausea, fatigue, confusion, and abdominal pain. On physical examination, patients often appear restless, uncomfortable, pale, and diaphoretic, and may exhibit Levine's sign—a clenched fist held over the precordium. Pulmonary rales or a new systolic murmur signal high risk for complications, specifically congestive heart failure and ischemic mitral regurgitation. A third heart sound (S_3) predicts a threefold increased risk of acute MI and death.

Aortic Dissection

Patients with aortic dissection have pain characterized by a severe tearing sensation, but it may instead be crushing. The time course usually involves sudden onset of steady pain. The location is anterior chest or abdomen, with radiation to shoulders or back, depending on the location of the dissection. Associated symptoms include syncope, diaphoresis, nausea, weakness, and lower extremity ischemic pain. Common risk factors include hypertension, Marfan's syndrome, and coarctated aorta. Physical examination of patients with aortic dissection usually reveals hypertension. Blood pressure and pulse intensity differences between extremities may define proximal versus distal dissection (e.g., difference between the two arms equals proximal, legs distal). A dissection into the aortic valve apparatus often produces a diastolic murmur of aortic regurgitation.

Pulmonary Embolism

The chest pain of PE is usually pleuritic and lateralized, as the pain signals parietal pleural irritation from pulmonary infarction. Substernal pain may occur in massive embolus. Associated symptoms include apprehension, dyspnea (these two are present in more than 90% of cases), cough, hemoptysis (in pulmonary infarction), diaphoresis, syncope (in massive embolus), and palpitations. Risk factors include immobilization, surgery within the preceding 3 months, prior PE or deep venous thrombosis, neoplasm, pregnancy or postpartum, concurrent oral contraceptive and tobacco use, congestive heart failure, chronic obstructive pulmonary disease, obesity, coagulopathy, and history of stroke. Physical examination may only demonstrate tachycardia. In massive PE, hemodynamic compromise may occur, along with signs of right heart strain (parasternal heave, wide split S_2 with loud P_2 component, elevated jugular venous pressure, hepatojugular reflux). A pleural friction rub signals pulmonary infarction.

Esophageal Rupture

Esophageal rupture results in severe pleuritic chest pain increased by swallowing and neck extension. It is persistent and located along the esophagus, usually in the left chest. It is associated with fever, diaphoresis, dyspnea, and other symptoms of shock secondary to mediastinitis. Risk factors involved are alcoholism, caustic or foreign body ingestion, esophageal cancer, and instrumentation. Physical signs include hypotension and subcutaneous emphysema.

Other Causes

Many nonemergent causes of chest pain have distinctive clinical signatures as well. *Musculoskeletal* chest pain is often worsened by inspiration and localized to point tenderness over a rib or muscle. Most young, active patients with chest pain have a musculoskeletal etiology. *Pericarditis* pain is pleuritic and often increased with swallowing or lying supine. The most distinctive physical finding is a pericardial friction rub. *Aortic stenosis* causes exertional pain (but usually not rest pain) very similar to coronary insufficiency. It may precede the development of syncopal events and orthopnea in the elderly or those with history of bicuspid valve or rheumatic fever. The systolic murmur of aortic stenosis, with associated single S_2, *parvus et tardus* carotid upstroke, and sustained left ventricular lift give physical clues. *Pneumonia* often causes a productive cough with fever in patients with immunodeficiency, uremia, impaired swallowing, chest wall disorders, and diabetes mellitus. *Pleurisy* follows a viral illness. Patients with chronic obstructive pulmonary disease, tobacco users, and lung cancer patients are predisposed to both pneumonia and *pneumothorax*. The dull pain of *gastroesophageal reflux disease* (GERD) and *ulcers* may closely mimic ischemic heart pain but often occur within 30 minutes to 1 hour of meals or in association with foods or medications causing irritation of the gastrointestinal tract mucosa. Accompanying symptoms include bloating and regurgitation.

Neurologic causes include *cervical angina*, a persistent dull, aching, or stabbing chest pain that is increased with neck movement. It is caused by cervical nerve root, usually C7, compression and is associated with radicular arm pain. A history of neck trauma is common. *Herpes zoster* causes burning pain and skin hypersensitivity in a dermatomal distribution. The pain may occur before eruption of vesicles.

Psychogenic chest pain may be associated with *hyperventilation syndrome* or *panic disorder*, both of which cause retrosternal pressure or lateral chest discomfort. Young patients with depression and anxiety may develop cardiac phobia despite negative diagnostic tests.

DIAGNOSIS

Clinical presentation is often not sufficient to differentiate life-threatening causes of chest pain from the many less serious conditions, or from each other. Diagnostic tests and procedures are essential.

The electrocardiogram (ECG) quickly assesses for cardiac ischemia, indicated by ST segment depressions and elevations, T-wave inversion, and hyperacute T waves or Q waves. It lacks ideal sensitivity, as it is only a single picture in the dynamic process of cardiac ischemia, although a normal ECG on presentation has a likelihood ratio of 0.1 to 0.3 for acute MI. Benign early repolarization, associated with J-point elevation, deserves special mention, as it may be mistaken for ischemic ST elevation. It may be morphologically differentiated in that the initial ST segment is concave up, the latter segment is usually notched or slurred, and there is a concordant and large T wave. In addition, the ST segment elevations of benign early repolarization are diffuse and greatest in leads V_2 to V_5.

Abnormal cardiac specific markers should accompany the ECG in most cases of MI. The MB isoform of creatinine kinase rises 4 to 6 hours after acute MI, peaks at 10 to 12 hours, and begins to decline after 3 days. Troponin T and I are more sensitive and specific for cardiac injury and have been found to predict repeat MI or death in both low- and high-risk populations. The troponins rise in 3 to 8 hours but may remain elevated for days. Other helpful blood tests include hemoglobin/hematocrit [potentially decreased in aortic dissection, esophageal rupture, peptic ulcer disease (PUD), and pancreatitis], white blood cell counts (elevated in stressful states but more so in pneumonia, mediastinitis, and pancreatitis), and electrolytes (detect acidosis from infection or shock, levels of potassium or magnesium important to the electrical state of ischemic myocardium, and hyponatremia suggesting syndrome of inappropriate secretion of antidiuretic hormone from a pulmonary process).

Chest x-ray evaluates for pneumothorax and pneumonia. It is also useful in the initial assessment of PE, as unilateral pleural effusion, raised hemidiaphragm, and decreased lung volume all support this diagnosis. The chest x-ray is abnormal in 80% to 90% of cases of aortic dissection, including widened mediastinum found in 75%, tortuous aorta, rightward displacement of the trachea, and 5 mm or greater density outside of a calcified aortic lumen. Chest x-ray also demonstrates the left-sided effusions, mediastinal air, and soft tissue emphysema of esophageal rupture.

Cardiac imaging and assessment studies are most often used to detect coronary artery disease in patients with low-risk or negative ECG and cardiac markers. Their sensitivity has been augmented by nuclear perfusion imaging, specifically resting and exercise sestamibi in the acute setting. Although a negative test does not completely exclude coronary artery disease, it indicates a low risk for subsequent cardiac event or death.

Specialized tests can help in diagnosis under appropriate circumstances. Echocardiogram can detect regional wall motion abnormalities in ischemic states. These findings or decreased ejection fraction accurately predict major cardiac events. Transesophageal echocardiography serves in the assessment of aortic dissection, particularly in unstable patients who cannot be moved for radiographic tests, whereas contrast computed tomography (CT) is the usual modality for rapid assessment of aortic dissection in stable patients. CT is also useful in assessing pancreatitis and biliary disease and assessing the extent of mediastinitis in esophageal rupture. Spiral CT is gaining acceptance for the detection of PE but still lacks sensitivity for small filling defects in the lung periphery. Ventilation/perfusion scanning is perhaps more sensitive but lacks specificity in patients with underlying lung pathology, and its interpretation rests heavily on pretest probability (clinical suspicion). An esophagram shows extravasation of gastrografin into the lung or mediastinum in esophageal rupture. Esophagogastroduodenoscopy, however, can also detect esophageal tears and other lesions of the upper gastrointestinal tract that cause chest pain, including PUD, GERD, and hiatal hernia.

MANAGEMENT

Although chest pain management mostly depends on the correct diagnosis, there are certain key treatments to administer while awaiting diagnosis. Intravenous access, supplemental oxygen, and cardiac monitoring are first steps. Any suspicion of cardiac ischemia should lead to treatment with aspirin and pain management. Nitrates should be used with some caution. They cause dangerous hypotension in right heart dysfunction. Furthermore, they alleviate chest pain due to both cardiac ischemia and esophageal spasm. Beta-blockers play a crucial role in coronary syndromes, except for decompensated heart failure and spasm secondary to cocaine ingestion (nitrates and benzodiazepines are indicated instead). Anticoagulation should be reserved for unstable angina and high suspicion of MI in patients without evidence for aortic dissection, pericarditis, esophageal rupture, or PUD. Consideration of glycoprotein IIb/IIIa inhibitors and thrombolysis or urgent percutaneous coronary intervention are essential when the ECG and clinical picture are diagnostic of acute MI. Management of aortic dissection involves large-bore intravenous access, blood type and cross match, alleviation of pain, immediate surgical consultation, and, most important, control of blood pressure with nitroprusside, a beta-blocker, or labetalol. PE indicates need for anticoagulation, which may begin empirically while awaiting diagnostic tests. Esophageal rupture usually requires surgical repair, as well as irrigation and drainage of the mediastinal cavity. Broad-spectrum intravenous antibiotics covering gram-positives, gram-negatives, and anaerobes should be administered to control mediastinitis in the meantime, and they should continue after surgical intervention.

Acute management of the less serious causes of chest pain involve symptom control and remediation of the underlying process. Pericarditis is best managed with nonsteroidal antiinflammatory drugs (NSAIDs), but prednisone may be necessary in severe cases. Pneumothorax may require chest tube placement, depending on the size. Patients with GERD usually receive some immediate relief from oral antacids and H_2 blockers. PUD is also managed with acid-reducing agents and treatment for *Helicobacter pylori*, when appropriate. Musculoskeletal chest pain responds to NSAIDs and rest. Cervical angina may be treated by intermittent cervical traction, physical therapy, NSAIDs, and muscle relaxants. The diagnosis of psychogenic chest pain is usually one of exclusion, but after it is made, reassurance, counseling and antidepressant or antianxiety medications are warranted.

Chapter 26

CONGESTIVE HEART FAILURE

Rachel Schoss

OVERVIEW

Congestive heart failure (CHF) occurs when abnormal cardiac function results in decreased cardiac output and consequently inadequate tissue perfusion. CHF has a high mortality risk, 50% at 2 years and 60% to 70% at 3 years. It is the leading cause of hospital admissions. With advances in the treatment of acute myocardial infarction creating a large elderly population with ischemic heart disease, heart failure is becoming ever more prevalent.

PATHOPHYSIOLOGY

The pathophysiology of heart failure has evolved to include explanations involving hemodynamic changes, pump failure, and, most recently, neurohormonal changes. Heart failure begins when left ventricular function is impaired after an acute or chronic insult, most commonly ischemic heart disease. This results in a depressed cardiac output, with the hemodynamic response to shift the Frank-Starling curve and thus increase preload to help sustain cardiac performance. In addition, myocardial hypertrophy occurs, increasing the mass of contractile tissue that helps to augment cardiac performance. It has been recently recognized that the depressed cardiac function activates a cascade of neuroendocrine systems, including the norepinephrine, adrenergic, and renin-angiotensin-aldosterone systems. These systems help augment contractility and maintain arterial pressure and perfusion of vital organs. In addition, these systems cause pulmonary vasoconstriction, leading to increased preload and systemic vasoconstriction, leading to increased afterload. Neurohormonal activation can also cause tachycardia with a resultant increase in myocardial oxygen demand and reduced coronary perfusion. Approximately one-third of patients have heart failure with preserved left ventricular systolic function (diastolic dysfunction). It occurs when ventricular relaxation is impaired, disabling ventricular filling. The most common causes of systolic dysfunction are coronary (ischemic) disease, hypertension, valvular disease, and idiopathic dilated cardiomyopathy. The most common cause of diastolic dysfunction CHF is hypertension.

CLINICAL PRESENTATION

When intravascular and interstitial fluid accumulate secondary to renin-angiotensin-aldosterone and other neurohormonal activation, pulmonary and peripheral edema develop. The pulmonary changes result in dyspnea, occurring initially with exertion and then progressing to occur at rest. Dyspnea with recumbency (orthopnea) and paroxysmal nocturnal dyspnea, sometimes associated with wheezing (cardiac asthma), are also very common and progress with the severity of the heart failure. Auscultation of the lungs typically reveals crackles over both lower lung fields, although pulmonary venous capacitance increases in chronic heart failure, and rales may be absent. After the extracellular fluid is in excess of approximately 5 L, symmetric, dependent, and pitting peripheral edema develops, and, as intravascular fluid increases, jugular venous distention may be appreciated with or without a hepatojugular reflex (the increase of jugular venous distention after compression of the right upper quadrant). The cardiac examination is significant for a laterally displaced precordial impulse, if the heart is enlarged and a third heart sound (S_3) can occur. Pulsus alternans, characterized by regularly spaced strong and weak pulses, is rare but virtually pathognomonic for severe left ventricular failure.

DIAGNOSIS

The electrocardiogram may have changes indicating coronary artery disease with old or new ischemic Q waves or ST segment changes. Findings of left ventricular hypertrophy and left atrial enlargement may be notable. Bradyarrhythmias or tachyarrhythmias, especially atrial fibrillation, may also be found. Chest x-ray commonly shows interstitial pulmonary edema, as evidenced by pulmonary haziness, plump perihilar vessels, and Kerley A or B lines (which occur transiently with elevated pulmonary venous pressures). Bilateral or right-sided pleural effusions may occur, which usually resolve with treatment. Cardiomegaly may or may not be present. Echocardiogram often reveals a depressed left ventricular ejection fraction but can show preserved left ventricular ejection fraction in diastolic dysfunction heart failure. It is also capable of identifying valvular disorders and tamponade, and hypertrophic, restrictive, or dilated cardiomyopathy.

MANAGEMENT

If the cause of the heart failure is identified and has the potential for reversibility, such as with ischemia, infection, alcohol, or valvular disorder, it should be corrected. Pharmacologic or electrocardiogram stress testing should be done to detect ischemic heart disease, assess exercise capacity, risk stratify, and assess response to therapy. The mainstay of medical therapy for heart failure includes digoxin, diuretics, and angiotensin-converting enzyme (ACE) inhibitors. Digoxin, long used in the treatment of heart failure, decreases neurohormonal activation and decreases atrioventricular nodal conduction, thus controlling the ventricular rate in atrial fibrillation. Digoxin decreases morbidity in heart failure but produces little change in mortality. It does have significant benefits in patients with severe heart failure. Diuretics, particularly loop diuretics, decrease preload and provide symptomatic relief. Patients with severe heart failure or renal insufficiency may require very large doses to maintain a euvolemic state. Spironolactone, which blocks aldosterone receptors, has been shown to decrease both morbidity and mortality in patients with severe heart failure.

ACE inhibitors have been the only medication to decrease both morbidity and mortality in heart failure. They decrease both preload and afterload, have a mild negative inotropic effect, and improve ventricular remodeling. Their use is limited by worsening renal function (not contraindicated with chronic renal insufficiency) and low blood pressure, both of which should initially be followed closely. Angiotensin receptor blockers have less bradykinin activity than do ACE inhibitors and still have similar decreased mortality in the treatment of heart failure. They still have the same changes in renal function as have ACE inhibitors, however, and to date, they should only be tried for therapy when ACE inhibitors are not tolerated.

Hydralazine and nitrates have been shown to improve survival in class II and III heart failure and are indicated in patients who cannot tolerate or have contraindications to ACE inhibitors. Beta-blockers improve survival and prevent CHF exacerbations in heart failure by their neurohormonal effects and decrease in heart rate but should be started when patients are stable on other therapies.

Chapter 27

HYPERLIPIDEMIA

Gaby Weissman

OVERVIEW

Coronary artery disease (CAD) and peripheral vascular disease are exceedingly common ailments in the Western world, with CAD being the leading cause of death among adults in developed countries, second only to infectious causes in the developing world. Hyperlipidemia has been associated with an increased risk of arteriosclerosis, and treatments leading to a reduction of cholesterol levels improve the outcome of patients experiencing CAD.

PATHOPHYSIOLOGY

Cholesterol acts as an important component of all cell membranes, as well as a precursor of bile acids, steroid hormones, and vitamin D. It is synthesized in the hepatic and extrahepatic tissues, and is ingested and transported from the intestinal mucosa. Lipoproteins serve to transport the various lipids. These lipoproteins include chylomicrons, very-low-density lipoproteins, low-density lipoproteins (LDLs), and high-density lipoproteins (HDLs). The latter serves to transport cholesterol from the vasculature to the liver and is protective. Cholesterol is excreted as bile salts in the gastrointestinal tract. Inherited defects in production, transport, particle recognition, and excretion can lead to hyperlipidemia.

CLINICAL PRESENTATION

Hyperlipidemia is most often a clinically silent disease with few outward manifestations; however, these abnormalities, if severe enough, may lead to early clinical signs that depend on the particular lipid derangement.

The first type is the isolated hypercholesterolemia due to an isolated increase in LDL. This disorder is most often polygenic in origin, with total serum cholesterol between 250 and 350 mg per dL. At these concentrations, there are no obvious manifestations until the clinical effects of atherosclerosis are seen. Less common are the genetic disorders, such as familial hypercholesterolemia, that can lead to cholesterol levels of more than 500 mg per dL and accelerated atherosclerosis. At these concentrations, tendon xanthomas, tuberous xanthomas (soft nodules on the buttocks and elbows), and xanthelesmas (waxy cholesterol deposits over the eyelids) may form. A second type is hypertriglyceridemia. At triglyceride levels higher than 1,000 mg per dL, eruptive xanthomas (orange-red papules on the trunk and extremities) and lipemia retinalis (orange-red retinal vessels) may be seen. In addition, these levels of triglyceride are associated with an increased risk of pancreatitis. A third type of hyperlipidemia is the combined hypercholesterolemia and hypertriglyceridemia, seen in familial combined hyperlipidemia and dysbetalipoproteinemia. These disorders are usually clinically silent until vascular disease develops. In dysbetalipoproteinemia, deposits of cholesterol in the palmar creases (striae palmaris), which are specific for this disorder, and tuberous xanthomas may be seen.

DIAGNOSIS

As hyperlipidemia is most often clinically silent until the effects of vascular disease are present, it is most often a laboratory diagnosis. A lipid profile (total, HDL, and LDL cholesterol and triglycerides) should be performed after a 12-hour fast, as triglyceride levels rise after a fat-containing meal, and LDL levels are not measured but derived by using an equation incorporating triglycerides. Total and HDL cholesterol can be accurately measured in a nonfasting sample. Once hyperlipidemia is found, it is important to search for secondary causes including hypothyroidism, nephrotic syndrome, anorexia nervosa, and drugs, such as thiazides. Causes of hypertriglyceridemia include diabetes, chronic renal failure, alcoholism, pregnancy, and medications, such as estrogen, glucocorticoids, and beta-blockers.

The Framingham risk model is a helpful guide in identifying patients at the highest risk who would realize the greatest benefit from treatment. Red flags include known coronary heart disease (CHD) (angina or prior myocardial infarction) or CHD equivalents (diabetes, symptomatic carotid artery disease, peripheral arterial disease, or abdominal aortic aneurysm). Risk factors include smoking, hypertension, low HDL cholesterol (<40 mg/dL), first-degree relatives with CHD (<55 years old in men or <65 years old in women), or age over 45 in men and 55 in women. HDL cholesterol higher than 60 mg per dL removes one risk factor. Patients with CHD have a risk of subsequent myocardial infarction 20 times higher than do those without CHD. Patients with no known CHD and no or one risk factor have a low risk of developing CHD, less than 10% over 10 years. Total to HDL cholesterol ratio is another method of risk stratification. Men with a ratio of 6.4 or more had a 2% to 14% increased risk than predicted by LDL cholesterol alone. Women with a ratio of 5.6 or more had a 25% to 45% incrementally increased risk.

MANAGEMENT

Management is dependent on the risk factors present, as well as the specific lipid disorder (Table 27–1), and consists of lifestyle modification with or without medications. A metaanalysis of 38 primary and secondary prevention trials found that for every 10% reduction in serum cholesterol, CHD mortality was reduced by 15%. In addition to reduction in clinical events, reduction of LDL cholesterol below 100 mg per dL has been shown by serial angiographic studies to, in many cases, produce regression of coronary artery plaques.

Adult Treatment Pomel (ATP) III recommendations are based on the Framingham model. In patients with CHD or its equivalent, or without CHD but with two or more risk factors, lipid lowering should be initiated. Lifestyle modifications are an important part of treatment. Patients should be encouraged to increase physical activity and lose weight. Their diets should reduce saturated fats to less than 7% of caloric intake, limit trans-fatty acids, and reduce cholesterol intake to less than 200 mg per day. Instruction in reading nutrition labels on foods helps patients understand how to achieve this.

TABLE 27–1   Treatment Guidelines for Hyperlipidemia (LDL)

Risk Factors	Lifestyle Modification (mg/dL)	Drug Treatment (mg/dL)
0–1	>160	>190
2+	>130	>160
CHD or DM	>100	>130

CHD, coronary heart disease; DM, diabetes mellitus; LDL, low-density lipoprotein.

TABLE 27–2 Lipid-Lowering Agents

| Class | Drug Names | Effect on: | | | Adverse Reactions and Significant Drug Interactions |
		LDL	HDL	Triglycerides	
HMG-CoA reductase inhibitors	Atorvastatin Fluvastatin Lovastatin Pravastatin Simvastatin	Down 18–55%	Up 5–15%	Down 7–30%	Myopathy Increased LFTs
Bile acid binding resins	Cholestyramine Colestipol	Down 15–30%	Up 3–5%	May increase	GI upset Hyperchloremic acidosis in renal failure Decreased absorption of warfarin, digoxin, thiazides, and statins
Nicotinic acid	—	Down 5–25%	Up 15–35%	Down 20–50%	Hepatotoxicity Flushing Hyperglycemia Hyperuricemia GI distress
Fibrates	Gemfibrozil Fenofibrate	Down 5–20%	Up 10–20%	Down 20–50%	Dyspepsia Gallstones Myopathy Unexplained non-CHD deaths in WHO study

CHD, coronary heart disease; GI, gastrointestinal; HDL, high-density lipoprotein; HMG-CoA, 3-hydroxy-3-methylglutaryl coenzyme A; LDL, low-density lipoprotein; LFTs, liver function tests; WHO, World Health Organization.

Medications are often used in the treatment of hyperlipidemia. The goal of treatment is to bring the LDL below 100 mg per dL in patients with CHD or diabetes, below 130 mg per dL when two or more risks are present, and below 160 mg per dL in patients with less than two risk factors. Several classes of drugs are available and should be selected on the basis of the particular dyslipidemia present, as well as the side effect profile of each medication. Table 27–2 summarizes the various classes of medications, as well as their effects and adverse effects. Because of their effectiveness, statins are usually the first-line treatment of hypercholesterolemia, with the bile acid resins being added to them to improve control. In the case of severe hypertriglyceridemia, the fibrates are the drugs of choice in treatment. Because these drugs interact with one another, it is always important to keep their side effects and interaction profiles in mind. An important example is an increased incidence of severe rhabdomyolysis with the concurrent use of fibrates and statins.

Chapter 28

HYPERTENSIVE CRISIS

Jennifer L. Yeh

OVERVIEW

Approximately 20% to 30% of adults experience hypertension, and of these patients, less than 1% will have a hypertensive crisis, with a blood pressure (BP) elevation to above 120 diastolic and evidence of acute or ongoing end-organ damage. Because of the associated morbidity and mortality of potentially irreversible central nervous system, cardiac, or renal damage, it is essential to immediately recognize and manage hypertensive crisis, and tailor intensive intervention to the complications.

PATHOPHYSIOLOGY

At any given time, vascular tone reflects the balance between autocrine, paracrine, and neurohumoral factors that mediate relaxation and contraction. The acute BP elevation seen in hypertensive crisis is thought to be due to an abrupt increase in systemic vascular resistance secondary to both increased humoral vasoconstrictors (catecholamines, vasopressin, renin-angiotensin II, atrial natriuretic factor) and local mediators (prostaglandins and free radicals). Humoral vasoconstrictors result in a pressure-induced natriuresis, which causes a hypovolemic state. Volume depletion reinforces further release of humoral vasoconstrictors. Angiotensin II is thought to have a direct cytotoxic effect on the vessel wall. Local factors, such as inflammatory cytokines, monocyte chemotactic protein 1, endothelin 1, and vascular cell adhesion molecules, are up-regulated in the setting of mechanical stretch. The result is endothelial inflammation and progressive loss of endothelial function, evidenced as increased permeability, loss of local fibrinolysis, and activation of the clotting cascade, ultimately resulting in platelet deposition and aggregation. Their subsequent degranulation releases mitogenic and chemotactic factors that result in inflammation, thrombosis, fibrinoid necrosis, and myointimal proliferation. Furthermore, the endothelium, which normally releases relaxing factors, such as nitric oxide and prostacyclin, becomes overwhelmed and unable to compensate for this increased vascular tone. This cycle of vasoconstriction and myointimal proliferation with loss of compensatory mechanisms ultimately disrupts normal vascular autoregulatory function and homeostasis and manifests as tissue ischemia.

Underlying etiologies of hypertensive crises are multiple and include essential hypertension, withdrawal of or inadequate antihypertensive therapy, the postoperative state, intrinsic renal disease (acute glomerulonephritis, vasculitis, hemolytic uremic syndrome, thrombotic thrombocytopenic purpura), renovascular abnormalities (atheromatous or fibromuscular dysplasia, renal artery stenosis), eclampsia or preeclampsia, endocrine abnormalities (pheochromocytoma, Cushing's syndrome, renin or aldosterone-secreting tumors), collagen vascular diseases, drug ingestions (cocaine, sympathomimetics, erythropoietin, cyclosporine, amphetamines, lead poisoning, drugs that interact with monoamine oxidase inhibitors), autonomic hyperactivity syndromes (Guillain-Barré, spinal cord syndromes, acute intermittent porphyria), and central nervous system disturbances (head trauma, cerebrovascular accidents, malignancy).

CLINICAL PRESENTATION

Hypertensive crises typically occur in patients who have not only a preexisting diagnosis of hypertension, but also a history of its being poorly controlled, and are more common in the elderly and African-Americans. Chronic hypertensives may have no symptoms until diastolic BPs are in the mid-100s, whereas newly diagnosed hypertensives may be symptomatic with a diastolic BP as low as 100. Hypertensive encephalopathy may present with signs of cerebral edema, such as nausea, vomiting, headache, general or focal weakness, and confusion, whereas intracerebral and subarachnoid bleeds and stroke may present with focal neurologic findings. Chest pain or pressure may herald an acute myocardial infarction, whereas "tearing" or "searing" chest, back, and abdominal pain suggests aortic dissection. Left ventricular dysfunction may present with cough and dyspnea due to pulmonary edema. Renal insufficiency may manifest as decreased urinary output or hematuria. Retinal hemorrhages, exudates, and papilledema may be seen on funduscopic examination.

DIAGNOSIS

A diagnosis of hypertensive urgency is made when there is an acute, severe elevation in diastolic BP of greater than 120 to 130 without any evidence of end-organ damage, whereas hypertensive emergencies include the same degree of BP elevation but with evidence of end-organ damage. The history should ascertain the duration and severity of previously diagnosed hypertension, the antihypertensive medication regimen and compliance, previous history of hypertensive crises, previous underlying end-organ damage, and recent use of over-the-counter medications or illicit drugs. Symptoms and physical findings of end-organ damage should be sought. Orthostasis suggests volume depletion and is likely due to pressure-induced natriuresis. A significant difference in BP in both arms with pulse deficits, an aortic insufficiency murmur, or signs of limb or gut ischemia (or both) may indicate aortic dissection. Funduscopic evaluation may show acute retinal changes, such as flame or punctuate hemorrhages, hard or cotton-wool exudates, arteriolar spasm, or papilledema. The cardiovascular examination may reveal signs of congestive heart failure, such as jugular venous distention, a third heart sound (S_3), mitral regurgitation from increased afterload, or rales. A thorough neurologic evaluation should focus on evidence of depressed consciousness, delirium, and seizure associated with hypertensive encephalopathy.

Meningeal irritation, visual field deficits, or focal changes suggest an acute cerebrovascular accident from intracerebral bleeding or hypoperfusion-induced cerebral edema, because cerebral blood flow regulation is overwhelmed.

Helpful laboratory studies include serum electrolytes, blood urea nitrogen/creatinine, and urinalysis. Increased blood urea nitrogen/creatinine, metabolic acidosis, hypocalcemia, and hematuria or casts on urinalysis suggest renal insufficiency. A peripheral smear may show schistocytes as markers of microangiopathic hemolytic anemia. An electrocardiogram may demonstrate left ventricular hypertrophy or ST–T-wave changes consistent with ischemia or infarction, or both. A posteroanterior and lateral chest x-ray may demonstrate an enlarged heart, a widened mediastinum, or pulmonary edema. A head computed tomography scan may show evidence of a new stroke or a cerebral bleed. A transthoracic echocardiogram to assess left ventricular hypertrophy and to estimate ejection fraction is helpful but often not urgently available.

MANAGEMENT

Hypertensive urgencies require lowering of BP over 24 to 48 hours. The goal of therapy is to decrease the mean arterial pressure by 20% or achieve a diastolic BP of less than 120. Combinations of oral antihypertensives, such as angiotensin-converting enzyme inhibitors, calcium channel blockers, beta-blockers, and alpha-blockers may be used to achieve BP control. Monitoring for medication effects in the emergency department over several hours after the BP goal is achieved is typically sufficient if immediate outpatient follow-up can be arranged.

A hypertensive emergency mandates immediate BP control, given the presence of ongoing organ damage. Therapy should be initiated in an intensive care unit, and an arterial line should be placed for continuous hemodynamic monitoring. Because precipitous drops in BP may cause cerebral, myocardial, and renal hypoperfusion and subsequent ischemia or infarction (or both), the goal of therapy is to lower BP by 15% to 25% or to a diastolic BP of 100 to 110 (whichever value is higher) over 1 to 2 hours. Parenteral antihypertensive therapy is usually initiated by continuous infusion with such agents as sodium nitroprusside, nicardipine, fenoldopam, esmolol, or nitroglycerin, or by bolus injection of labetalol, diazoxide, phentolamine, hydralazine, or enalapril. In general, diuretics should be avoided in acute hypertensive situations, because patients are typically volume depleted in the setting of a pressure-induced natriuresis.

Therapy should be tailored to the specific end-organ complication. For patients with hypertensive encephalopathy, a 20% to 25% lowering or a diastolic BP of 100 within an hour is the goal of treatment, with special caution in elderly patients or those with chronically elevated BPs who are at risk for stroke. In addition to anticonvulsants (dilantin, benzodiazepines, or barbiturates), sodium nitroprusside is typically first-line treatment, but other appropriate agents include labetalol, enalapril, or hydralazine. In patients with cerebral ischemia, careful antihypertensive therapy is recommended, but abrupt decreases in BP may actually worsen hypoperfusion to an area where cerebral autoregulation is disrupted.

For patients with an acute myocardial infarction, intravenous nitrates decrease preload and afterload and improve coronary perfusion. Intravenous beta-blockers decrease myocardial work by decreasing heart rate and BP. Patients with congestive heart failure benefit from preload reduction with intravenous nitroglycerin, afterload reduction with sodium nitroprusside, volume removal with loop diuretics, and supplemental oxygen. Dosages are titrated to symptom relief. Aortic dissection requires very rapid diastolic BP lowering to a goal of 100 mm Hg over 10 minutes. A decrease in BP and heart rate reduce shear stress on the aortic wall. Agents of choice are therefore intravenous beta-blockers and sodium nitroprusside. In general, vasodilators, such as hydralazine and diazoxide, are avoided in cardiac complications of hypertensive emergencies because of their tendency to produce a reflex tachycardia and increase myocardial work.

The goal of therapy in patients with renal disease is to decrease systemic vascular resistance but to maintain renal perfusion and glomerular filtration rate. Labetalol, calcium channel blockers, and alpha-blockers are useful agents. Diuretics can worsen hypertension in patients who are already hypovolemic but may otherwise be beneficial. Angiotensin-converting enzyme inhibitors are contraindicated in patients with renal artery stenosis.

In patients with hypertension refractory to comprehensive medical management, secondary causes should be sought, as treating the underlying cause is the best way to treat the patient's hypertension.

Chapter 29

PERICARDIAL EFFUSION AND CARDIAC TAMPONADE

Seonaid F. Hay

OVERVIEW

Pericardial effusion refers to the accumulation of fluid within the pericardial space. Depending on the rapidity of accumulation (200 cc if rapid) and the amount of fluid (up to 2 L if more slowly), there can be serious hemodynamic compromise, a state known as *tamponade*. Tamponade is often fatal if not recognized and treated, and should be considered in patients who present with hypotension. The key to effective care is knowing in whom to suspect tamponade and monitoring for hemodynamic effect.

PATHOPHYSIOLOGY

Pericarditis, an inflammation of the pericardial sac, can lead to accumulation of pericardial fluid. Etiologies include infections, such as tuberculosis, and viruses (coxsackie, echo); uremia; cancer (usually metastatic); trauma; myocardial infarction; aortic dissection or aneurysm; collagen-vascular disease (rheumatic fever, systemic lupus erythematosus, rheumatoid arthritis, scleroderma); drug-induced (procainamide, hydralazine) causes; or idiopathic causes. The three most common causes of tamponade are neoplastic, idiopathic, and uremic pericarditis. Tamponade occurs when the pressure of the fluid causes constriction of the heart so that there is right heart collapse during diastole, interfering with diastolic filling and causing a decrease in cardiac output. Venous return to the right side of the heart is also compromised. In constrictive pericarditis, hemodynamic effect is due to an inelastic pericardium, and compression occurs in mid to late diastole, when ventricular volume is greatest. Constriction can be due to prior cardiac surgery or radiation therapy, collagen vascular disease, or neoplasm, and presents as a subacute process.

CLINICAL PRESENTATION

Patients with pericarditis may present with chest pain that is often relieved with sitting up and leaning forward. Tamponade can present with hypotension alone, which is why a high index of suspicion is necessary to make the diagnosis. Depending on the etiology, patients may also have fever or other systemic signs of the underlying disease. Tachycardia is a common finding, occurring to partly accommodate for the reduction in output.

Before a large amount of fluid accumulates, patients may have a pericardial friction rub. It may have three components per cardiac cycle, be high pitched and grating in quality, and be most evident with the patient sitting forward. With fluid between the inflamed pericardium and myocardium, however, the rub can disappear; the absence of a rub should not be used to rule out pericarditis or tamponade. Ewart's sign, dullness beneath the angle of the left scapula, is found when the left lung base is compressed by pericardial fluid.

With tamponade, hypotension and elevation of jugular pressure with a prominent x descent are seen. Distant heart sounds are heard. Symptoms of heart failure with dyspnea and orthopnea develop. Pulsus paradoxus, with more than a 10 mm Hg drop in systolic blood pressure from expiration to inspiration, is seen in tamponade and should be measured in every patient in whom tamponade is being considered. Kussmaul's sign, the absence of inspiratory decline in jugular pressure, is seen in constrictive pericarditis.

DIAGNOSIS

Chest x-ray can show a water bottle heart or be normal. Electrocardiography can show PR interval depression or diffuse ST segment elevation without reciprocal depressions, electrical alternans, or low QRS voltage, as well as sinus tachycardia. Echocardiography is a sensitive, specific, noninvasive way to diagnose pericardial fluid and tamponade. Pericardial fluid is easily seen by echocardiography, as are signs of right ventricular collapse during diastole. Right heart catheterization can make the diagnosis of tamponade by showing equalization of pressures, with the pulmonary capillary wedge pressure close to right atrial, right ventricular, and pulmonary artery diastolic pressures. Obtaining pericardial fluid samples for cell count, protein, cytology, culture, and acid-fast bacilli staining can help diagnose the underlying illness.

MANAGEMENT

Patients with pericarditis and pericardial fluid without tamponade should be treated according to the underlying disease and monitored for signs of tamponade. Volume depletion should be avoided. If tamponade is present or imminent, then pericardiocentesis should be performed emergently. A catheter can be placed in the pericardial space to continuously drain the fluid, and pericardial stripping or placement of a pericardial window can be performed to prevent the future accumulation of fluid. Constriction requires surgical removal of the pericardium.

Chapter 30

VALVULAR HEART DISEASE

James N. Kirkpatrick

OVERVIEW

An estimated 5 million Americans are afflicted with some form of valvular heart disease. The major forms include aortic stenosis (AS), aortic insufficiency (AI), mitral stenosis (MS), mitral regurgitation (MR), and tricuspid regurgitation (TR). Most of the morbidity and mortality arises from hemodynamic overload placed on the left ventricle (LV) or right ventricle (RV), or both ventricles, and subsequent myocardial dysfunction resulting in systolic and diastolic heart failure. The myocardial strain may also put valvular heart disease patients at increased risk of sudden death.

PATHOPHYSIOLOGY

AS usually arises from degeneration and calcification of the aortic valve leaflets, often arising in a bicuspid aortic valve. Afterload increases, leading to compensatory hypertrophy of the left ventricular myocardium. The increased oxygen requirements of the thickened LV are not well met by the reduced and fixed cardiac output through the stenotic valve, especially during exertion, leading to myocardial ischemia. Syncope results from the reduced cardiac output and a vasodepressor response in the carotid sinus that is not well understood. The hypertrophied ventricle has dysfunctional relaxation and compliance, leading to diastolic heart failure. Eventually, systolic heart failure occurs as the ventricle dilates. Once angina, syncope, or congestive heart failure (CHF) develops, survival is less than 5 years.

AI may result from leaflet dysfunction but also arises from dilatation of the aortic root. Damage to aortic leaflets is most often caused by endocarditis or rheumatic heart disease, or both. Root dilatation may be secondary to longstanding hypertension and age-related effects on the aorta, Marfan's syndrome, traumatic aortic dissection, collagen vascular disease, syphilitic aortitis, or annuloaortic ectasia (idiopathic). Although acute AI causes immediate volume overload and failure of the left ventricle, the much more common chronic aortic regurgitation leads to a compensatory hypertrophy and enlargement of the LV and increase in stroke volume. Pulse pressure is thereby widened, with development of systolic hypertension. Afterload values can reach as high as those found in AS.

MS is almost always a sequelae of rheumatic fever. Although not directly affecting the ventricle, the elevation of left atrial pressure leads to pulmonary edema and decreased cardiac output secondary to underfilling. Chronic backpressure in the pulmonary vascular circuit results in pulmonary hypertension and, eventually, right heart failure.

MR occurs acutely or chronically. Acute MR results most often from infective endocarditis, ruptured chordae, or papillary muscle dysfunction in the setting of inferior myocardial infarction. Early MR in myocardial infarction is a strong predictor of 1-year mortality (relative risk, 7.5). Chronic MR may result from the listed causes but also as a sequelae of rheumatic fever, collagen vascular diseases (systemic lupus erythematosus in particular), or myxomatous degeneration of the valve due to mitral valve (MV) prolapse. Acute MR causes immediate elevations in end-diastolic volume (preload) but reduces afterload as part of the stroke volume is ejected into the left atrium. Left atrial pressure and volume are elevated, leading to pulmonary hypertension. Acute MR may progress to chronic, compensated MR in which the LV eccentrically hypertrophies to accommodate the increased volume from the left atrium. The forward stroke volume normalizes owing to the increased volume handled by the LV. The LV hypertrophies, and ejection fraction remains normal. In chronic decompensated MR, the LV begins to fail, and the forward stroke volume drops off. The ejection fraction decreases. The end-diastolic volume increases and transmits increased pressure into the pulmonary circulation.

TR most often results from endocarditis secondary to intravenous drug use but can also result from dilatation of the RV secondary to chronic pulmonary hypertension, RV infarct, or biventricular dilated cardiomyopathy. The volume ejected backward into the right atrium returns to cause hypertrophy and eventual dilatation and failure of the RV, but is usually well tolerated in the absence of pulmonary hypertension. Back flow into the right atrium can cause edema and ascites.

CLINICAL PRESENTATION

AS usually presents in the sixth to eighth decades, but if accompanying a bicuspid aortic valve, it appears in the fourth to fifth decades. The classic historical progressive triad includes angina, exertional syncope, and symptoms of congestive failure. The harsh and often crescendo–decrescendo murmur of AS is best heard at the right sternal border, with radiation to the carotids. The murmur of mild AS usually peaks in early systole. In severe AS, the murmur peaks late. A_2 is decreased in intensity, and S_2 may become single. Peripheral manifestations include the traditional *parvus et tardus* (slow and late) carotid upstroke, but this sign lacks specificity in the elderly, who may have atherosclerotic vessels.

AI may present with congestive symptoms in acute or end-stage disease but is most often detected in chronic form from its blowing murmur in early diastole, heard best in full expiration with the patient leaning forward. Located at the left sternal border, it may radiate to the apex. The Austin Flint murmur, a diastolic rumble at the apex, results from the regurgitant aortic flow impinging on the anterior MV leaflet and causing physiologic MS. A host of systemic physical signs have been documented in association with AI, most of them arising from the increased stroke volume and widened pulse pressure. Two of the more reliable include Duroziez's sign, a to and fro murmur heard with the stethoscope compressing the femoral artery, and Hill's sign, systolic blood pressure differential of more than 30 mm Hg between leg and arm.

MS, found most often in developing nations and rarely in the United States and Europe because of the decline of rheumatic fever, occurs more often in women than in men. Patients present with symptoms of CHF and pulmonary hypertension, including hemoptysis, but may also have indications of systemic hypoperfusion, especially in advanced disease. Symptoms generally worsen with pregnancy secondary to hemodynamic alterations, and they are greatly exacerbated by the development of atrial fibrillation, because atrial systole provides much of ventricular filling through the stenotic valve. The MS murmur is an apical, low-pitched diastolic rumble preceded by an opening snap and followed by a loud S_1. It starts as a decrescendo that may die out in mid-diastole, only to reappear as a presystolic component that represents atrial systole. It may radiate to the left sternal border. P_2 may become accentuated and an RV heave develop secondary to pulmonary hypertension. Systemic signs include malar flush, prominent jugular *a* wave, jugular venous distention, peripheral edema, hepatomegaly, and ascites.

Acute MR presents with symptoms of CHF. Chronic compensated MR may be asymptomatic, but CHF returns with decompensation. Patients with MV prolapse have been noted to present with atypical chest pain, palpitations, light-headedness, and fatigue. The murmur of MR radiates from the apex to the axilla but may be heard over the entire precordium. It is often pansystolic and harsh in quality. In late states of chronic disease, an MS murmur may appear, indicating severely reduced excursion of the valve. The murmur of regurgitant MV prolapse follows a midsystolic click and is often described as a musical "whoop."

TR may present with symptoms of right-sided volume overload or failure, including lower extremity edema, congestive hepatopathy, and congestion of intestinal venous and lymphatic systems, leading to malabsorption. The murmur of TR is generally holosystolic, located at the left sternal border, and it may be differentiated from MR murmur by its lack of radiation to the axilla and accentuation in the left lateral decubitous position and with inspiration. It may be accompanied by an RV heave, jugular venous distention with increased *v* waves, and hepatomegaly.

DIAGNOSIS

Echocardiography is the test of choice for all valvular heart disease, although pressure measurements for gradients across stenotic valves may be more accurately elucidated by heart catheterization. Transthoracic echocardiography is generally indicated, but transesophageal echocardiography is more sensitive for lesions of endocarditis and for evaluating for dissection in AI. In advanced pathology in MR and TR, echocardiography may not be able to discern whether valvular disease produced dilated cardiomyopathy or vice versa, but otherwise echocardiography can accurately rule out valvular disease in the consideration of causes of cardiac dysfunction.

In AS, echocardiography can give a reasonable assessment of the valve area and gradient across the valve. Left heart catheterization is necessary before consideration of valve replacement, however, to investigate coronary arteries for possible concurrent bypass. An estimated 50% of AS patients also have significant coronary artery disease. In AI, an end-systolic volume higher than 60 mL per m^2 or an ejection fraction lower than 50% during exercise indicates decompensation. Echocardiography can provide planimetric calculation of the MV area and decay of the transvalvular gradient in MS. It also can give an estimate of pulmonary artery pressure. MR assessment by echocardiography includes semiquantitative severity of the regurgitant jet and presence of left atrial enlargement (>4 cm increases the risk of the development of atrial fibrillation). Assessment of ejection fraction and end-systolic diameter are crucial in the timing of surgery. Echocardiography can determine severity of the TR jet and development of right ventricular dysfunction.

MANAGEMENT

The main issues in management in valvular disease involve timing of surgery and endocarditis prophylaxis. Operative interventions include valve replacement, valve repair, and balloon valvulotomy. Mechanical prostheses are extremely durable and produce low transvalvular gradients. Anticoagulation is required. Bioprosthetic valves have reduced life expectancy, depending on age. In a 30-year-old, they may fail in an average of 10 years. In an 80-year-old, they may last 15 years. They do not require anticoagulation. There is less experience with human homografts, and they do not require anticoagulation.

The only definitive treatment for AS is valve replacement. It should be performed for any symptomatic patient, or when aortic valve area decreases to smaller than 0.8 cm and the valve gradient increases more than 50 mm Hg. Age is not a clear impediment to aortic valve replacement; octogenarians derive morbidity and mortality benefit. Without symptoms, a gradient less than 50 mm Hg or a valve area larger than 0.8 cm, the patient should receive yearly echocardiography. For a valve gradient greater than 50 mm Hg *or* valve area smaller than 0.8 cm, the follow-up is every 6 months. Balloon aortic valvulotomy has not proven beneficial. It has a higher than 10% mortality and shows no improvement in survival over the natural course. It may improve symptoms as a bridge to valve replacement in patients who cannot undergo surgery until a later date. Care must be exercised in the use of beta-blockers and angiotensin-converting enzyme inhibitors/angiotensin receptor blockers, as decompensated heart failure and hypotensive syncope can result.

AI patients should have the valve replaced when the left ventricular ejection fraction declines to below 50% or the end-systolic left ventricular dimension increases above 50 mm, or when symptoms of congestive failure develop, even if mild. In the meantime, vasodilators, such as dihydropyridine calcium channel blockers, and angiotensin-converting enzyme inhibitors/angiotensin receptor blockers can reduce systolic hypertension and keep patients asymptomatic for years. In the acute setting of AI secondary to endocarditis, the risk of death far outweighs the risk of prosthetic valve infection (which is <10%).

In mildly symptomatic MS, diuretics and sodium restriction may be beneficial to decrease CHF symptoms. Atrial fibrillation, if not causing acute decompensation, should prompt rate control measure and anticoagulation. If symptoms become more than mild, or if signs and symptoms of pulmonary hypertension develop, transatrial balloon mitral valvulotomy is the procedure of choice. MV repair or replacement, or open commisurotomy should be undertaken instead in the presence of heavy MV calcification, subvalvular distortion, or severe symptoms.

MR patients may benefit from afterload reduction, but repair or replacement should not be delayed if the ejection fraction decreases below normal (prognosis worsens with ejection fraction <60%). MV repair has lower mortality and better outcomes than does replacement, and it obviates the need for anticoagulation. Well-timed surgery for nonischemic MR leads to normal life expectancy, whereas operative mortality for ischemic MR is 10% to 20%.

Treatment of underlying pathology—usually endocarditis—is usually sufficient in TR. Diuretics are beneficial if dilated cardiomyopathy is the cause. TR patients without dilated cardiomyopathy are very preload sensitive and should not receive vasodilating agents. Tricuspid valve repair or replacement is rarely indicated.

Current recommendations for endocarditis prophylaxis in dental procedures are: by mouth (PO), within 1 hour of procedure: amoxicillin, 2 g, *or* clindamycin, 600 mg, *or* cephalexin/cefadroxil, 2 g, *or* azithromycin/clarithromycin, 500 mg. If unable to take PO, take intramuscularly or intravenously (IV) within 0.5 hour of procedure: ampicillin, 2 g, *or* clindamycin, 600 mg, *or* cefazolin, 1 g.

Endocarditis prophylaxis for gastrointestinal or genitourinary procedures: amoxicillin, 2 g PO 1 hour before the procedure, or ampicillin, 2 g intramuscularly or IV 30 minutes before. If penicillin-allergic, give vancomycin, 1 g IV, completed 30 minutes before the procedure.

Pulmonary and Critical Care

Chapter 31

ACUTE RESPIRATORY FAILURE

David Litvak

OVERVIEW

Acute respiratory failure is life threatening and demands immediate action. A wide variety of conditions can cause respiratory failure, and establishing a prompt and accurate diagnosis is crucial to guide treatment. An evaluation of underlying diseases and the respiratory pattern, lung examination, chest x-ray, and arterial blood gases is usually sufficient to uncover the mechanism for respiratory failure.

PATHOPHYSIOLOGY

Respiratory failure can be defined as the inability to maintain adequate gas exchange. Gas exchange can be subdivided into oxygenation and ventilation. Patients unable to oxygenate develop hypoxemic respiratory failure, and those unable to ventilate develop hypercarbic respiratory failure; however, patients frequently develop both conditions. Remember that in addition to oxygenation by the lungs, oxygen delivery depends on hemoglobin levels and cardiac output. Tissue hypoxia can occur owing to a low cardiac output or anemia.

Hypoxic respiratory failure can be divided into conditions with or without an increased alveolar-arterial (A-a) gradient. The causes of an increased A-a gradient are ventilation/perfusion ($\dot{V}/\dot{Q}$) mismatch, shunt, and abnormal diffusion. $\dot{V}/\dot{Q}$ mismatch is the most common cause for hypoxia. Alveolar filling is insufficient to meet the needs of the blood that continues to perfuse the alveolar capillary units owing to pus (pneumonia), water (edema), blood (alveolar hemorrhage), or collapse (atelectasis). The extreme of decreased ventilation is a "physiologic" shunt, when regions of the lungs continue to perfuse but have no ventilation at all. Causes include acute respiratory distress syndrome and lobar or whole-lung collapse. Another category of shunt is anatomic, when venous blood returns to the systemic circulation without ever passing through the pulmonary microcirculation. Examples include arteriovenous malformations and intracardiac right-to-left shunts. The difference between shunts and $\dot{V}/\dot{Q}$ mismatch is not simply semantic: Shunts do not respond to oxygen therapy, in contrast to $\dot{V}/\dot{Q}$ mismatch, which does. Last, abnormal diffusion of oxygen from the alveoli to the pulmonary capillaries (e.g., as occurs in interstitial lung disease) can limit oxygenation.

Hypoxic respiratory failure without an A-a gradient can be caused by hypoventilation or a decreased fraction of inspired oxygen, as in high altitudes or airplanes. Hypoventilation is frequently due to neurologic disease, including central respiratory drive depression (brainstem infarct), spinal cord disease (amyotrophic lateral sclerosis), or neuromuscular conditions (myasthenia gravis or Eaton-Lambert syndrome). These patients have a low PaO_2 and a high $PaCO_2$, but their degree of hypoxia is proportional to their degree of hypercarbia.

The most common causes of hypercapnia include excessive ventilation of dead space, hypoventilation (discussed previously) or overproduction of CO_2. Dead space includes the upper respiratory tract and alveolar units of the lung, which are not perfused. Thus, CO_2 carried in the blood does not reach sufficient alveoli involved in gas exchange. The three most common clinical conditions in which this problem occurs are chronic bronchitis, emphysema, and asthma. In chronic bronchitis, mucus obstructs upper airways. In emphysema, large air spaces are not perfused owing to alveolar capillary obstruction. In asthma, upper airways are obstructed by mucus, bronchospasm, and smooth muscle hypertrophy.

CLINICAL PRESENTATION

Acute respiratory failure is a syndrome based on the clinical picture. Laboratory results and imaging studies cannot rule in or rule out respiratory failure. Patients frequently have a history of pulmonary or cardiac disease. Their symptoms of dyspnea and tachypnea may be abrupt or subacute. On physical examination, hypotension should raise suspicion for a pneumothorax, pulmonary emboli, or heart failure. It is important to watch patients breathe to accurately assess respiratory rate and respiratory pattern (i.e., Cheyne-Stokes or Kussmaul's respiration). On lung examination, the focus should be on crackles, wheezes, and adequacy of air movement. Also, tracheal deviation, jugular venous distention, crepitus over the chest, and unilateral leg swelling should be sought. The chest x-ray is essential. Clues to the cause of the respiratory failure include flattening of diaphragms, infiltrates, atelectasis, vascular congestion, interstitial thickening, and pneumothorax. Often the chest x-ray is normal in pulmonary embolus, however. An arterial blood gas is important to assess for hypoxia, an A-a gradient, hypercarbia, and a coexisting metabolic disorder.

After gathering all of the data, the physician often finds that patients have mixed conditions. Conversely, patients with respiratory distress may have relatively preserved gas exchange. Their tachypnea may be due to a metabolic acidosis, anxiety, sepsis, or salicylates.

MANAGEMENT

The treatment of respiratory failure depends on making an accurate diagnosis and treating the underlying cause. The decision to intubate is based on the overall clinical assessment. In general, a PaO_2 lower than 60 mm Hg or an oxygen saturation of less than 90% on a 100% nonrebreather, a rising $PaCO_2$ with associated respiratory fatigue, or change in mental status are grounds for immediate intubation. Patients who appear likely to develop respiratory failure may warrant intubation, however, regardless of the results of blood gases. Noninvasive ventilation using continuous positive pressure ventilation or bimodal ventilation has been used with success in congestive heart failure and chronic obstructive pulmonary disease.

Chapter 32

ASTHMA

David Litvak

OVERVIEW

Asthma is a condition affecting all age groups, especially children and young adults. Despite extensive research, morbidity and mortality have risen since 1982. Asthma is characterized by hyperresponsiveness of bronchi to various stimuli causing airway obstruction due to bronchoconstriction. Episodes are at least partially reversible, producing a pattern of acute attacks interspersed with periods of diminished symptoms. This chapter focuses on the hospital management of an acute asthma attack.

PATHOPHYSIOLOGY

Many stimuli can lead to asthma exacerbations, including inhaled antigens (e.g., dust mites, cockroaches, animal dander, pollen), inhaled irritants (e.g., cigarette smoke, cocaine, crack, heroin, wood, metal, industrial chemical dust), infections, exercise, drugs, air pollution, and emotional stress. The mechanisms by which these stimulants cause asthma attacks vary, but the end pathologic response is the same: limitation of airflow secondary to smooth muscle cell constriction, mucus plug formation, and airway edema. In the most common example, inhaled antigens bind to immunoglobulin E antibody on the surface of mast cells, which release preformed substances, such as histamine. Immediately, bronchial smooth muscle cells contract, vascular permeability increases, and reflex vagal pathways are triggered, producing secondary bronchial constriction. Delayed responses, occurring up to 24 hours later, are characterized by the production of leukotrienes and recruitment of other inflammatory mediators and cells, such as eosinophils, polymorphonuclear cells, lymphocytes, and macrophages. Remodeling of the airway can eventually occur, calling into question the complete reversibility of asthma attacks.

CLINICAL PRESENTATION

Patients with acute asthma attacks typically present with shortness of breath and wheezing. It is imperative to assess the severity of the asthma attack. The history should focus on the severity of previous disease (prior intubations, frequency of hospitalizations, use of chronic steroids, baseline peak flow) and on features of the current attack (duration of symptoms, concurrent illness, use of beta-agonists and steroids). On physical examination, signs of severe asthma include a respiratory rate greater than 30, a heart rate greater than 120, a peak flow of less than 30% to 50% of a patient's personal best, an increased pulsus paradoxicus (>10 mm Hg), altered mental status, diaphoresis, subcutaneous emphysema, and use of accessory muscles.

DIAGNOSIS

An arterial blood gas usually shows a respiratory alkalosis, but in severe cases the PCO_2 may be normal or elevated, giving a respiratory acidosis. Lactic acid levels may rise, causing a metabolic acidosis, and the PaO_2 may fall. Chest radiography is not useful in ruling in the diagnosis of asthma, but it is helpful to exclude complications of asthma, such as barotrauma resulting in a pneumothorax, and to exclude other diseases that may mimic asthma, such as congestive heart failure and pneumonia. Laryngoscopy may be helpful to rule out vocal cord dysfunction in the subset of patients with stridor and concurrent psychiatric illness.

MANAGEMENT

The treatment of asthma exacerbations focuses on correcting hypoxemia with oxygen, relieving bronchospasm with beta$_2$ agonists, and reducing inflammation with corticosteroids. Second-line therapies include subcutaneous epinephrine, theophylline, and anticholinergics, particularly ipratropium. None of these second-line agents has proven benefit over beta$_2$ agonists alone, but their use may be warranted in patients who are not responding to continuous nebulizers and steroids. Other therapies, such as magnesium sulfate and heliox, are based on small studies and anecdotal evidence (Table 32–1).

The decision to intubate is primarily based on the patient's appearance and $PaCO_2$. Altered mental status, increasing fatigue, difficulty completing sentences, and a rising $PaCO_2$ usually warrant intubation. A large endotracheal tube (≥ 8 mm) should be used, if possible, to aid clearance of mucus secretions. Adequate sedation is crucial in preventing patient-ventilator dysynchrony. Neuromuscular blockers may be required to paralyze the patient. Ventilator settings should be adjusted to minimize auto–positive end-expiratory

TABLE 32–1   Treatments for Asthma

Drug	Dosage	Comment
Albuterol	2.5 mg in normal saline via nebulizer or 4 puffs by MDI with spacer	May increase dosage in severe attack. Can be given via an endotracheal tube.
Corticosteroids[a]	Methylprednisone, 40 mg q6h Prednisone, 50 mg t.i.d.	Many side effects, including hyperglycemia, hypokalemia, hypertension, and myopathy.
Theophylline	Load 5–6 mg/kg IV over 20–30 min (reduced if already on theophylline) Maintenance: 600 mg b.i.d.	Tachycardia and tremor common.
Ipratropium bromide	0.5 mg via nebulizer ×3	
Heliox	Mixture containing 60–80% helium	Enhances laminar flow; best for patients with sudden onset of severe asthma.

MDI, metered dose inhaler.
[a]All patients should receive, as is a crucial part of asthma treatment.

pressure (which occurs with inadequate expiratory ventilation) and keep plateau pressures less than 30 cm H_2O. This can be accomplished by permissive hypercapnia: setting a low respiratory rate and tidal volume to extend expiratory time, while allowing the CO_2 to rise, seeking to minimize dynamic hyperinflation. Permissive hypercapnea is safe as long as adequate oxygenation is ensured. On discharge, patient education is crucial to prevent subsequent hospitalizations.

Chapter 33

PNEUMOTHORAX

Daus Mahnke

OVERVIEW

Normally, the parietal and visceral pleura lie close together, separated only by a potential space. A *pneumothorax* is defined as air misplaced in that potential space. Pneumothoraces can be spontaneous and primary, spontaneous and secondary to underlying disease, traumatic, or iatrogenic. Spontaneous pneumothoraces occur in 2.5 to 18.0 per 100,000 people. They occur most commonly in 20- to 40-year-old (65%) men (85%) of taller than average stature. Smoking is a dose-dependent risk factor.

Secondary pneumothoraces (one-third of all cases) are more common in people older than age 50 years. Bullous pulmonary diseases [i.e., chronic obstructive pulmonary disease (COPD) or alpha$_1$-antitrypsin disease] are prevalent risk factors, implicated in up to 60% of cases. Acquired immunodeficiency disease with *Pneumocystis carinii*, inhaled drug use (drugs are often pulmonary toxins, and Valsalva maneuvers to increase drug effect increase risk of collapse), and tuberculosis and other infections are other important causes of pneumothorax. There are several rare diseases for which pneumothorax is a common event. Pneumothorax occurs in 25% of patients with Langerhans cell granulomatosis. Lymphangioleiomyomatosis is noted to have an 80% incidence of collapse. Patients with Marfan's syndrome also have a high risk of collapse. In addition, pneumothorax rarely can be associated with menses. Iatrogenic pneumothoraces are probably the most common form of pneumothorax. One-third of transthoracic needle aspirations generate one. Positive-pressure ventilation causes pneumothoraces in 5% of patients. Other procedures that incorporate risk of pneumothorax include central venous line placement using jugular or subclavian veins, nasogastric tube placement (or misplacement), pleural and lung biopsy, and cardiopulmonary resuscitation.

CLINICAL PRESENTATION

The symptoms associated with a pneumothorax usually correlate to its size. In spontaneous cases, symptoms occur at rest and can linger for hours to days before patients present for medical attention. Chest pain is the most common symptom (approximately 90%); it usually occurs suddenly and is pleuritic and associated with dyspnea (approximately 80%) and cough (approximately 10%). The most common sign of pneumothorax is tachycardia. If the pneumothorax is large enough (>20% lung volume) or is present in a patient with underlying disease, hypoxia and tachypnea may be present as well. Notable physical examination findings include decreased breath and voice sounds and normal or hyperresonance to percussion on the affected side. Subcutaneous air also may be present.

A tension pneumothorax is one in which sufficient air has entered the potential space to compromise the contralateral lung function and cardiac output. The presentation of tension pneumothorax is predictably more dramatic. Severe tachycardia, cyanosis, and hypotension should make one suspicious that a tension pneumothorax is present. In addition to these signs, tracheal deviation to the contralateral side and elevated jugular venous pressure (due to inhibited venous return) may be observed.

Of note, pneumothorax associated with COPD may present somewhat less dramatically. Pain is not as common, and dyspnea becomes more pronounced. The dyspnea may be out of proportion to the size of the collapse. Because the pneumothorax may be small, the classic physical examination findings may be absent or confused by the hyperresonance and decreased breath sounds that can accompany severe COPD. The differential diagnosis of pneumothorax includes those conditions that cause chest pain or dyspnea, or both, such as angina, heart failure, costochondritis, asthma, COPD exacerbation, aortic dissection, and pericarditis. The gold-standard diagnostic test—chest roentgenography—is easily available, painless, and generally fast.

DIAGNOSIS

Diagnosis is made with chest roentgenography. The roentgenographic findings may be subtle and missed if the collapse is small. Expiratory films may accentuate the findings if clinical suspicion is high and conventional inspiratory images reveal no collapse. Lateral decubitus views, with affected side up, are also useful. In the supine patient, a deep sulcus sign (deep lateral costophrenic angle) may be present on the affected side; other findings include a deep cardiophrenic sulcus and lucency at the bases. The size of a pneumothorax can be accurately assessed by a trained observer on a roentgenogram. Tension pneumothorax is a clinical diagnosis, as delaying diagnosis to obtain an x-ray can be fatal; however, x-ray findings can include shifting of the trachea and mediastinum to the contralateral side and flattening of the ipsilateral hemidiaphragm. Although not necessary for diagnosis, results of arterial blood gas measurements usually show an acute respiratory alkalosis and hypoxemia. Hypercapnea may occur in patients with significant underlying pulmonary disease.

MANAGEMENT

Treatment begins with assessing the patient's breathing and hemodynamics. The patient's clinical condition and the physician's clinical suspicion for tension physiology dictate the urgency of therapy. In all cases, therapy is aimed at both resolution of the acute condition (evacuation of the pleural space) and prevention of further pneumothoraces. The rate of recurrence is between

15% and 50% within 2 years, depending on the etiology. A reliable, otherwise healthy patient with mild symptoms who has a small (<15%) primary pneumothorax can be observed. A follow-up chest roentgenogram in 6 hours is necessary to confirm stability of lesion. After that, less frequent studies (one in 24 hours, and then weekly) can document resolution of the collapse. Administration of 100% oxygen may relieve symptoms and speed resolution. Roughly 1% to 2% of the intrapleural air volume can be reabsorbed each day. Progressing primary spontaneous pneumothoraces or those larger than 15% of hemithorax should be drained by simple aspiration with a thoracentesis catheter (7–14 French) or by insertion of a chest tube. Simple aspiration is the procedure of choice in patients younger than 50 years of age with less than 2.5 L of air. Successful aspiration requires close follow-up within days to assure reexpansion. If aspiration fails to reexpand the lung, a one-way valve (Heimlich) or water seal device can be attached to the catheter. Routine suction has not been shown to improve outcome. If these methods fail, chest tube insertion is indicated. The insertion of a chest tube (20–28 French) had been the traditional treatment for all pneumothoraces but is now more commonly reserved for failed simple aspiration or secondary pneumothoraces. Indications for chest tube are tension pneumothorax, significant underlying pulmonary disease, respiratory distress, persistent air leak or increase in pneumothorax size, more than 3 L air aspirated, positive pressure ventilation anticipated, bilateral pneumothoraces, and previous contralateral pneumothoraces.

Surgery is considered for patients with air leaks that persist beyond 4 to 7 days or for patients with secondary pneumothoraces. In the latter group, recurrent pneumothoraces are common enough to indicate surgery for prevention. The prevention of recurrence in resolved primary pneumothoraces is controversial. Some centers recommend interventions in all resolved pneumothoraces; others individualize the decision-making process. Younger patients have a greater lifetime risk of recurrence and better likelihood of benefiting from intervention. Procedures to prevent recurrence aim to fuse the pleural layers or remove bullae and include sclerosing agent instillation, thoracoscopic resection of bullae, thoracoscopic pleurodesis by mechanical abrasion, and talc insufflation, among others. Data comparing the efficacy of the various operative techniques are sparse.

Human immunodeficiency virus infection is a poor prognostic indicator. Most human immunodeficiency virus–positive patients die within 6 months of their pneumothorax. Therapy in these patients must be tailored to consider their overall prognosis. Pleural symphysis procedures are the choice to prevent recurrence in those patients who opt for intervention.

Chapter 34

HEMOPTYSIS

N. Christopher Kelley

OVERVIEW

Hemoptysis, or the expectoration of blood, can range from the streaking of sputum with blood to the presence of gross blood in the airways. Prompt diagnosis, especially in the setting of massive hemoptysis (generally defined as 600 mL of blood within a 24-hour period) is essential, as this disorder can be life threatening. As little as 400 mL of blood within the alveolar space can significantly hinder oxygen transfer without other signs associated with blood loss, such as orthostasis and tachycardia.

PATHOPHYSIOLOGY

The lungs receive blood from the systemic and pulmonary circulatory systems. The pulmonary arteries arise from the right ventricle and deliver unoxygenated blood to the pulmonary parenchyma. The bronchial arteries arise from the aorta (or, less commonly, the intercostal arteries) and are responsible for the delivery of nutrients and oxygen to the airways. Although the bronchial arteries account for 1% to 2% of the cardiac output, they are implicated in more than 90% of cases of hemoptysis. This is primarily because (i) the blood in the bronchial arteries traverses the circuit at systemic pressures, whereas the pulmonary arteries are part of a low-pressure circuit, and (ii) as the bronchial arteries supply the airways, they are more susceptible to disruption in the setting of anatomic abnormalities (as in neoplasm or bronchiectasis).

CLINICAL PRESENTATION

The presentation of hemoptysis can vary widely, from scant amounts of blood to frank hemorrhage. The duration of bleeding and estimated amount of blood loss are crucial data, as these facts can give clues to the underlying diagnosis and subsequently guide management. Massive hemoptysis accounts for only 1.5% of all cases of hemoptysis and should be treated as a medical emergency. When first interviewing and examining the patient, it is important to ascertain whether the bleeding site is truly located in the lower respiratory tract, as upper gastrointestinal bleeding and upper respiratory tract bleeding (e.g., epistaxis) can present in a similar fashion.

DIAGNOSIS

The history and physical examination can give important etiologic clues. The history should include questions pertaining to prior lung, cardiac, or renal disease; cigarette smoking; pulmonary infections; bleeding disorders; and the use of aspirin, nonsteroidal antiinflammatory drugs, and anticoagulants. The physical examination also can provide clues to the diagnosis. Skin rashes can suggest vasculitis, and telangiectasias on the skin may indicate the presence of arteriovenous malformations in patients with hereditary hemorrhagic telangiectasias. Wheezing or stridor should raise the suspicion of an obstructing endobronchial lesion. Hematuria is associated with both Wegener's granulomatosis and Goodpasture's syndrome.

In developed countries, bronchiectasis accounts for most cases of massive hemoptysis, whereas acute bronchitis is the cause of most cases of nonmassive hemoptysis. Other processes responsible for hemoptysis include malignant (both primary lung or metastatic), infectious (bronchitis, tuberculosis, aspergillosis and other fungal infections, necrotizing pneumonia, lung abscess), inflammatory (vasculitides, e.g., Wegener's, Behçet's, or Goodpasture's syndromes; collagen vascular diseases, e.g., systemic lupus erythematosus), hemodynamic (elevated pulmonary capillary wedge pressure, e.g., in congestive heart failure and mitral stenosis), hematologic (bleeding disorders), and vascular (arteriovenous malformations, bronchoarterial fistulas, pulmonary infarct) etiologies. Other miscellaneous causes include cocaine-induced hemorrhage ("crack lung"), pulmonary embolism, and iatrogenic causes (trauma from procedures, e.g., Swan-Ganz catheter placement). Up to 30% of patients with hemoptysis have no cause identified.

Diagnostic studies should start with a thorough history, standard laboratory tests (complete blood counts, chemistries, coagulation profiles), sputum examination (including Gram stain and cytology if malignancy suspected), and a chest x-ray (which gives clues as to the etiology of bleeding in more than 50% of cases). Fiberoptic bronchoscopy is often considered in patients with hemoptysis and a normal or nonlocalizing chest radiograph. High-resolution chest computed tomography has also recently become a useful diagnostic tool and is better than bronchoscopy at locating bronchiectasis. Although the relative utility of either study has yet to be determined, the current recommendations are to use bronchoscopy or computed tomography scan when suspicion of tumor is high (age >40 years, >40 pack-year history of smoking, duration of hemoptysis >1 week) and initial evaluation has not yielded an etiology.

MANAGEMENT

In most cases of nonmassive hemoptysis, medical therapy is supportive and should be geared toward treatment of the underlying process. Antitussives may be given, although their use may result in the accumulation of blood in the lower respiratory tract. Massive hemoptysis represents a medical emergency. Vital signs and oxygen saturation should be monitored closely. If the site of bleeding is known or suspected, the patient should be placed with the bleeding side in a dependent position to protect air exchange in the unaffected lung. The patient may require supplemental oxygen; in some cases, intubation and mechanical ventilation is necessary. An experienced anesthesiologist often can use a double-lumen endotracheal tube to further protect the nonbleeding lung from aspiration. Bedside fiberoptic bronchoscopy may allow for both visualization of the region of the lung that is bleeding and temporary hemostasis by balloon tamponade, iced saline lavage, or injection of the bleeding site with epinephrine or vasopressin; however, brisk bleeding often precludes adequate visualization of the bleeding site. In this case, rigid bronchoscopy (which requires an experienced operator in an operating room setting) is frequently preferred because of its superior suction capabilities. Arteriographic embolization of the bleeding bronchial artery has become the most effective nonsurgical treatment in massive hemoptysis. Bleeding is rarely seen on angiography, but abnormal vessels at the site may be visible. Emergent lung resection carries a high mortality (20% in some series) and should not be used in the acute setting unless it cannot be avoided. The major contraindications to surgery are an inability to localize a specific site, diffuse disease, and poor lung function.

Chapter 35

CHRONIC OBSTRUCTIVE PULMONARY DISEASE

Anya C. Harry

OVERVIEW

In the United States, chronic obstructive pulmonary disease (COPD) is the fourth leading cause of death, and it is the only common cause of death that is currently increasing in incidence worldwide. COPD is a condition characterized by progressive airflow obstruction. Most patients diagnosed with COPD have some varying combination of chronic bronchitis, emphysema, and asthma; however, each disease state manifests predominant clinical and histologic features. Chronic bronchitis is a clinical diagnosis characterized by a chronic cough with sputum production for most days of 3 months for 2 consecutive years. Emphysema is defined pathologically by the destructive changes of the alveolar walls, leading to permanent enlargement of the bronchiolar airspaces. Asthma is a generally reversible state with narrowing of the airways. Common use of the term COPD has excluded asthma, because it was originally thought to have a different cause, clinical course, response to therapy, and reversibility. This chapter focuses on chronic bronchitis and emphysema.

PATHOPHYSIOLOGY

Cigarette smoking is the most common risk factor, causing 80% to 90% of COPD. Other factors include airway irritants, such as environmental exposures to pollution, passive smoke, acute respiratory illnesses, occupational exposures to dusts, noxious gases, and a genetic predisposition as seen in alpha$_1$-antitrypsin (AAT) deficiency.

In the healthy lung, maximal expiratory flow rates are achieved through a dynamic interaction between the airways caliber, elastic recoil pressures, and collapsibility of the airways. In COPD, this interplay is lost, mainly as a result of airways remodeling. The earliest pathologic finding is an inflammatory reaction in the respiratory bronchioles and mucus gland hyperplasia in the large and central airways. In the relatively mild airflow obstruction typical of chronic bronchitis, the obstruction is primarily irreversible and occurs at the level of the small airways, the bronchioles. Compromise of the airway caliber develops in response to intraluminal secretions, bronchospasm, thickening of the airway wall by edema, inflammatory cells, fibrosis, and enlargement of the mucus-secreting apparatus.

In severe obstructive disease, there is destruction of the alveolar walls with enlargement of terminal air spaces typical of emphysema. Alveolar wall breakdown diminishes the elastic recoil property and airway support, resulting in a more compliant or less stiff lung. Airways collapse during forced expiration, which causes air trapping. The three recognized types of emphysema are distinguished based on localization of the lesion: (i) centrilobular is most often associated with cigarette smoking and selectively affects the respiratory bronchioles in an irregular pattern and affects the upper portions of the lung. (ii) Panlobular is found in AAT deficiency with the proteinase inhibitor phenotype, PiZZ, and AAT levels below 10% of normal values. The panlobular subtype mainly involves the entire alveolus in a characteristically uniform pattern predominantly in the lower lobe. (iii) Distal acinar emphysema involves distal alveolar sacs and alveolar ducts, resulting in subpleural blebs or bullae.

CLINICAL PRESENTATION

Historically, patients with COPD have been categorized as "blue bloaters" or "pink puffers." These oversimplifications are useful in describing the clinical features salient to each disease. The patients with predominant chronic bronchitis exhibit problems with gas exchange. They are usually hypoxemic, hypercapnic, and overweight, and often present with cyanosis, thus the descriptor blue bloater. Morning headaches and hypersomnolence may indicate CO_2 retention. On physical examination, peripheral edema with distended neck veins corresponds to right ventricular failure, cor pulmonale. Chest auscultation may reveal slowed expiration, wheezing, or coarse crackles, and percussion is usually resonant with hyperinflation. The patient with predominant emphysema is usually thin and has a tendency to maintain near-normal PaO_2 by increasing the work of breathing; this patient looks adequately oxygenated, thus the pink puffer descriptor.

The disease course is punctuated by periods of exacerbation defined by increased symptoms associated with worsening lung function. They are often secondary to respiratory tract infections, mainly viral (e.g., influenza, rhinovirus, and parainfluenza); however, common bacterial pathogens include *Haemophilus influenzae*, *Streptococcus pneumoniae*, and *Moraxella catarrhalis*.

DIAGNOSIS

Spirometry reveals an obstructive pattern with characteristic patterns of lung volumes consistent with obstructive airways disease. A low forced expiratory volume in 1 second (FEV_1); moderate increase in total lung capacity, functional residual capacity, and residual volume; decreased diffusing capacity of lung from carbon monoxide ($DLCO$) and a ratio of FEV_1 to forced vital capacity of less than 70% is the typical pattern. The chest radiograph may reveal a barrel chest, hyperinflation, and flattened diaphragm. Electrocardiographic changes most commonly include P-wave abnormalities, such as a negative P wave in aVL or P pulmonale with peaked P waves in II, III, and aVF. Predictors of mortality in patients with COPD include advancing age; severity of airflow obstruction, as indicated by a low FEV_1; severity of hypoxemia; and the presence of hypercapnia.

MANAGEMENT

Smoking cessation is the only proven intervention that slows the progression of COPD. Abstinence rates appear to be more successful with pharmacologic intervention, such as bupropion and nicotine replacement, combined with counseling.

Outpatient management of stable COPD should be approached according to the level of pulmonary dysfunction and tolerance of side effects of each intervention. The classes of bronchodilators include anticholinergics (ipratropium), beta$_2$ adrenergic agonists (e.g., albuterol), phosphodiesterase inhibitors (theophylline), antiinflammatory agents (corticosteroids), and others, such as mast cell inhibitors (cromolyn) and leukotriene receptor antagonists.

For mild, varying symptoms, a selective beta$_2$ agonist as an inhaler on an as-needed basis leads to rapid symptomatic relief in many patients. For mild to moderate ongoing symptoms, ipratropium bromide or the longer-acting tiotropium can enhance and prolong bronchodilation when added to beta$_2$ agonists. The combination of a beta$_2$ agonist with an anticholinergic drug appears to provide more bronchodilation than either drug alone. As a third-line agent, theophylline may be added if response to previous intervention is unsatisfactory or for patients less compliant with aerosol therapy. Greater monitoring is required, however, when achieving therapeutic levels owing to side effects. A course of steroids (e.g., prednisone) can be added if symptoms are ongoing. They may be abruptly discontinued if no improvement is seen or may be tapered and subsequent aerosol form used if steroids appear to be beneficial.

Oxygen is the only documented therapy to reduce mortality and improve quality of life in patients with severe COPD and chronic hypoxemia. Supplemental oxygen is indicated in patients who are medically stable with a PaO$_2$ <55 mm Hg or patients with PaO$_2$ between 55 and 59 mm Hg who have tissue hypoxia manifest by cor pulmonale or reactive erythrocytosis.

In the acute decompensation period, hospitalization may be indicated. Aerosolized beta$_2$ agonists and anticholinergics may be given more frequently in the acute setting. An intravenous form of theophylline can be added if response is inadequate. Systemic corticosteroids have been shown to provide a beneficial effect in acute exacerbations, with improved clinical outcome and reduced length of hospitalization. Antibiotics are recommended in patients with severe exacerbation and evidence of infection, such as fever, leukocytosis, or a change in chest radiograph. The antibiotic choice should be selected based on common pathogens, local hospital patterns, and sputum culture and sensitivities. Noninvasive positive-pressure ventilation may reduce the need for mechanical ventilation in acute exacerbations. AAT augmentation is indicated in those with severe AAT deficiency. Pulmonary rehabilitation can improve exercise tolerance and quality of life for those with severe COPD. Lung reduction surgery has shown improvements in lung function, exercise capacity, and quality of life for patients with severe disease.

Chapter 36

PULMONARY EMBOLISM

David S. Smith

OVERVIEW

Pulmonary embolism (PE) is an acute clinical syndrome usually characterized by sudden shortness of breath, pleuritic chest pain, hypotension, or some combination of these. It is caused by obstruction of a pulmonary artery on migration of a venous thrombus originating in the legs or pelvis. Accurate diagnosis of PE is critical, because prompt treatment with anticoagulants reduces mortality from 30% to 2% to 8%. In the United States, it is estimated to cause 50,000 deaths per year and two-thirds of these cases are undiagnosed before the terminal event. Diagnosis is an art, as clinical recognition is difficult, the noninvasive lung scan and helical computed tomography scan have false-positives and false-negatives, and the gold standard pulmonary angiogram is resource intensive and has inherent risk of morbidity.

PATHOPHYSIOLOGY

A venous thrombus usually begins as a platelet nidus at a damaged venous valve. It propagates within the venous lumen by accretion of platelets, fibrin, fibrinogen, and adhesive proteins, such as von Willebrand's factor. Risk factors identified by the Prospective Investigation of Pulmonary Embolism Diagnosis (PIOPED) study were immobilization, surgery within 3 months, stroke, history of venous thromboembolism, and malignancy. Patients with a PE without risk factors may have an underlying "hypercoagulable state" due to deficiencies of protein C or S, antithrombin III, factor V Leiden mutation, or dysfibrinogeninemia. When the embolic thrombus lodges in the pulmonary vascular bed, lung is ventilated and not perfused. Inflammatory mediators are released, increasing gas exchange abnormalities due to surfactant dysfunction and causing changes in vascular permeability and functional intrapulmonary shunting, which leads to hypoxia. Right heart failure may also result from a massive pulmonary embolus, particularly in patients with preexisting cardiopulmonary disease.

CLINICAL PRESENTATION

The hallmark of PE is the sudden onset of symptoms of pleuritic chest pain and dyspnea. Hemoptysis, when present, is an important diagnostic clue. In the PIOPED study, the most common presenting symptoms were dyspnea (73%), pleuritic chest pain (66%), cough (37%), and hemoptysis (13%). Physical findings included tachypnea (70%), rales (51%), tachycardia (30%), a fourth heart sound (S_4) (4%), and accentuated pulmonic component of the second heart sound (S_2) (23%). Pleuritic pain or hemoptysis without hypotension was found in 65%, and isolated dyspnea in another 22%.

DIAGNOSIS

PE most commonly leads to a sinus tachycardia, although transient atrial fibrillation can be seen. A classic large S wave in I, a Q wave in III, and an inverted T wave in III ($S_1Q_3T_3$) indicate right heart strain from a massive PE. Electrocardiography is also useful in ruling out myocardial infarction, an important alternative diagnosis. Chest x-ray shows atelectasis or a parenchymal abnormality in 69% and excludes pneumonia and pneumothorax. Infrequently, peripheral radiolucency due to oligemia (Westermark's sign) or a wedge-shaped pleural-based density (Hampton's hump) are seen. Arterial blood gas measurement usually shows a reduced PaO_2, but a PaO_2 higher than 90 does not exclude the diagnosis (normal PaO_2 may be found in up to 15%).

Ventilation/perfusion lung scan is performed by injecting isotopically labeled protein microspheres into a vein. When they are transiently held up in the capillaries of the lung vasculature, they can be imaged with a gamma camera. Absence of tracer infers absence of flow. These images can be complemented with those made by inhalation of radioactive xenon gas. A peripheral wedge-shaped defect on the perfusion scan with preservation of ventilation is a classic finding in PE. There are many causes of false-positive and false-negative readings, however. The most helpful findings are a normal scan, which virtually rules out a PE, and a "high-probability" scan [large mismatched defect(s) with a normal chest x-ray, seen in 42% of patients with PE], which is reasonably diagnostic of a PE. A helical computed tomography scan with intravenous contrast has a sensitivity of 53% to 87% and a specificity of more than 90%, which is slightly better than the lung scan, especially for larger thrombi. It can also provide information about competing diagnoses.

Pulmonary angiography remains the gold standard of diagnosis and should be done when the clinical suspicion of PE remains moderate to high, despite results of noninvasive testing. A PE should never be ruled out based on a negative ventilation/perfusion or computed tomography scan alone when there remains significant clinical suspicion. Because it is personnel-intensive and time-intensive, and carries a risk of morbidity and mortality, pulmonary angiography should be used judiciously, but definitively.

The serum marker D-dimer has a high negative predictive value but a low specificity, so it is helpful in ruling out PE if negative. A D-dimer level below 500 ng per mL by enzyme-linked immunosorbent assay or a negative SimpliRED assay in conjunction with a low clinical probability or other negative noninvasive tests is effective in excluding significant PE (negative predictive value, 99.5%). Duplex ultrasound of the legs can accurately detect proximal deep vein thrombosis. If thrombosis is found, PE is implied, and anticoagulation is justified. If the ultrasound is negative, one must be concerned that the reason is that the thrombus is already in the lung, as is found in one-third of patients with PE.

MANAGEMENT

Intravenous (IV) heparin is given promptly and dosed according to the patient's weight, starting with an IV bolus at 80 U per kg and followed with a continuous infusion of 18 U per kg per hour. The partial thromboplastin time should be rechecked in 4 to 6 hours, and heparin adjusted to prolong the partial thromboplastin time to twice control. An alternative gaining wider acceptance is low-molecular-weight heparin (enoxaparin), 1 mg per kg SC q12h. Monitoring is not needed. These treatments are intended to prevent fresh thrombus from forming at the source, with a potential for another, possibly fatal, embolism. The patient should remain at reduced activity, and IV or subcutaneous treatment continued for 1 week to allow the thrombus to organize while oral warfarin (Coumadin) is instituted. The patient's international normalized ration should be adjusted to 2 to 3 and maintained there for 6 months. Oxygen should be given if the PaO_2 is low and IV fluids given if indicated for hypotension. An inferior vena caval filter is indicated when anticoagulation is contraindicated (e.g., recent intracranial surgery or gastrointestinal bleeding) and in selected patients with large or recurrent PEs while anticoagulation is continued. In patients with massive PE with cardiopulmonary compromise, IV thrombolysis or embolectomy can be lifesaving.

Chapter 37

PLEURAL EFFUSION

David N. Smith

OVERVIEW

Despite making approximately 2.5 L of fluid per day, the pleural cavity normally contains only 7 mL of transudative fluid. Generally, an effusion is classified as primary or secondary based on the origin of the pathology (inside vs. outside the lung). Increased pleural space fluid to the point of clinical illness (progressive dyspnea, cough, or pleurisy) warrants an evaluation to define the etiology, treatment, and, often, prognosis.

PATHOPHYSIOLOGY

Starling's equation dictates three causes of pleural effusions: increased hydrostatic pressure [congestive heart failure (CHF)]; decreased oncotic pressure, generally in the setting of volume overload (nephrosis, liver failure); or decreased clearance of the fluid by increased lymphatic pressure (tumor, obstructing mass) in the pleural space. Other important causes may not be related to Starling's forces; these include chylous effusion, empyema, and malignant effusion. Cirrhosis as well can cause a right-sided effusion by ascitic fluid's crossing the diaphragm. Simply, "effusion" develops from overproduction or low drainage of pleural fluid. The fluid is either dilute and consistent with plasma (transudate) or concentrated with proteins, inflammatory cells, or both (exudate). The natural history of serous drainage is that it evolves into fibrinous deposition. Because the pleura covers the lung viscera as well as the chest wall and pericardium, the sources of increased fluid are broad.

CLINICAL PRESENTATION

Patients may be asymptomatic from the effusion until it grows to limit lung compliance. Then, patients report progressive shortness of breath, cough, or chest pain, which is often pleuritic in inflammatory conditions. Chronically debilitated patients may never express symptoms. Breath sounds are reduced over the area of the effusion, and percussion produces a dull note compared with aerated zones. Whisper pectoriloquy and fremitus are dampened. At least 200 mL of fluid must be present to see costophrenic angle blunting on the chest x-ray (meniscus sign). If present, a lateral decubitus film should show layering of the fluid to the dependent side if it is free flowing and not loculated. Ultrasonography can be used to prove fluid consistency.

DIAGNOSIS

The differential diagnosis can be limited by dividing the causes of pleural effusion into transudative versus exudative types. Transudative effusions are of low (<3.0 g/dL) protein content and usually associated with CHF (right sided more than left), liver cirrhosis (hepatic hydrothorax), nephrotic syndrome, protein-losing enteropathy, and Meig's syndrome. The etiologies of exudative effusions are much more diverse. Inflammatory conditions may be intrapulmonary, such as tuberculosis or other pneumonia; aspiration; abscess; pulmonary embolism; collagen-vascular disease; pancreatitis; or bronchitis. Malignancy is the most common cause of exudative effusion in those older than 60 years of age and is usually associated with primary breast, lymphoma, lung, and metastatic tumors. Esophageal rupture (Boerhaave's syndrome) may result in orogastric fluid in the pleural cavity with chemical inflammation. Chylothorax, usually from trauma, tumor, or yellow-nail syndrome, may also cause exudate. Blood in the pleural cavity usually results from trauma, cancer, ruptured aortic aneurysm, or bleeding diathesis. Human immunodeficiency virus–associated effusions are usually infectious (tuberculosis, *Pneumocystis carinii* pneumonia) or malignant. Left-sided effusions are more common with pancreatitis, post–coronary artery bypass graft sternotomy, and aortic dissection; CHF may rarely present with a predominantly right-sided effusion. Empyema or pus in the pleural space results from trauma, malignancy, or anaerobic bacterial infections.

Realizing the potential sources of effusion, the physician should send obtained fluid for biochemistry (serum and fluid lactate dehydrogenase, total protein, pH, and glucose). Depending on the suspected causes, other tests may be done, including amylase, lipase, and lipids; microbiology (Gram stain and routine culture ± fungal or acid-fast bacteria smear and stains if indicated); and cytology examinations (cell count with differential; three samples to pathology if suspected malignancy). A closed-needle pleural biopsy can be done in conjunction with thoracentesis for suspected tuberculosis or pleural-based tumor.

MANAGEMENT

Most small effusions have low risk of adverse events and need not be completely drained; however, a diagnostic tap of the fluid is sufficient in an asymptomatic patient. Large (>25% of lung field), acidic (pH <7.2), or infected (positive culture or Gram stain) effusions require complete drainage. A bedside thoracentesis is performed by inserting a 14-gauge to 21-gauge needle in the midscapular line one interspace level below the upper level of the effusion. The patient sits upright, similar to lumbar puncture. Alternatively, an ultrasound-guided thoracentesis could be performed by an experienced radiologist.

After drainage of the fluid, repeat chest imaging should be used to evaluate progress and search for pleural-based nodules, masses, lymphadenopathy, or plaques that may have caused the effusion.

If the effusion is a transudate, treat the underlying cause and follow the patient's symptoms and oxygen saturation. Therapeutic thoracentesis may be required periodically.

Recurrent exudates, acidic (<7.2) effusions, effusion with low glucose in the setting of infection, and empyema require chest tube insertion for complete evacuation of the fluid. Low, continuous suction helps mobilize the fluid. When the underlying condition is treated and less than 100 mL per 24 hours is draining via the chest tube, it can be removed and a surveillance chest x-ray obtained. If the fluid is loculated, a 2-day to 3-day trial of fibrinolytic (e.g., urokinase) infusion may help mobilize loculated fluid. Video-assisted thoracic surgery may be effective for limited decortication and débridement during the fibropurulent phase.

For malignant or recurrent transudative effusions, sclerotherapy or pleurodesis is performed. Usual agents include talc, tetracycline, bleomycin, or radioisotopes. In prolonged cases, ambulatory sclerotherapy through small-bore tubes is an attractive, cost-effective approach. Periodic chest x-rays should look for lung reexpansion within a few weeks. Surgical placement of a pleuroperitoneal shunt should be considered in large effusions in which a large amount of fluid is continuously being made.

Chapter 38

INTERSTITIAL LUNG DISEASE

David J. Horne

OVERVIEW

More than 150 acute and chronic clinical conditions are associated with interstitial lung disease (ILD) (diffuse parenchymal lung disease). Many have a similar course involving alveolar and perialveolar injury's leading to inflammation with either resolution or scarring (fibrosis). In general, ILD is characterized by progressive dyspnea, an abnormal chest x-ray, and restrictive ventilatory defect on pulmonary function tests.

As the causes are myriad, it is helpful to break them down into broad categories by etiology:

1. Occupational/environmental exposures and medications (e.g., asbestosis, inhalational injury, radiation, aspiration, crack cocaine, antibiotics, anticancer drugs)
2. Systemic diseases (e.g., systemic lupus erythematosus, rheumatoid arthritis, ankylosing spondylitis, anti–glomerular basement membrane)
3. Granulomatous diseases (e.g., sarcoidosis, Langerhans cell histiocytosis, Wegener's, hypersensitivity pneumonitis)
4. Idiopathic pulmonary disease [e.g., idiopathic pulmonary fibrosis (IPF), bronchiolitis obliterans organizing pneumonia (BOOP), Hamman-Rich syndrome, chronic eosinophilic pneumonia]

IPF (also known as cryptogenic fibrosing alveolitis) is the most common ILD, accounting for approximately 30% of cases; sarcoidosis is the second most common, at 19%. The prevalence of IPF ranges from 6 to 15 per 100,000, increasing with age to a prevalence of 250 per 100,000 among those 75 years of age and older. IPF is a serious illness with mean survival from time of diagnosis of 2 to 4 years.

PATHOPHYSIOLOGY

ILD may involve an acute inflammatory phase, although often only a chronic fibrotic phase is seen. Features of acute inflammation include the expression of inflammatory cytokines and migration of inflammatory cells into the alveolar structures, leading to tissue injury. The chronic phase involves parenchymal remodeling with myofibroblast proliferation, collagen deposition, and fibrosis. Depending on the underlying process, inflammation may be present diffusely or only in peribronchiolar tissue. At least seven different histologic categories of ILD exist. Different clinical entities may produce the same histopathologic picture and, conversely, a single disease may be associated with different histologic categories.

Usual interstitial pneumonia is the pattern seen in IPF and must be present to make this diagnosis pathologically. Usual interstitial pneumonia features patchy, subpleural interstitial fibrosis and honeycombing interspersed with interstitial inflammation and normal lung. The interstitial inflammation consists of alveolar septal infiltrate, mainly composed of lymphocytes and plasma cells. Acute interstitial pneumonia (Hamman-Rich syndrome) consists of diffuse alveolar damage with epithelial injury and intraalveolar hyaline membranes initially, leading to fibrosis as the disease progresses. Acute interstitial pneumonia is often considered to be acute respiratory distress syndrome without an underlying precipitating injury.

CLINICAL PRESENTATION

ILD is usually chronic and insidious and may present at any time, although the average age is in the fifties; patients with IPF are usual older than 60 years of age. Patients usually present with a dry, nonproductive cough or progressive dyspnea, or both. Depending on the etiology, there may or may not have been an acute phase illness. Nonspecific symptoms, such as weight loss, anorexia, and arthralgias, may also be present.

Signs may include tachypnea, cyanosis, and clubbing. Patients may have a normal physical examination, although bibasilar end-inspiratory rales are common. In advanced disease, signs and symptoms of right heart failure (due to pulmonary hypertension) may be present. Although most ILDs are a subacute to chronic process, a number of disorders may present acutely over 1 to 14 days. The presentation may resemble a viral or mycoplasma pneumonia with dyspnea, fever, nonproductive cough, and malaise. These acute ILDs (e.g., Hamman-Rich, acute eosinophilic pneumonia, acute BOOP) may progress rapidly to respiratory failure.

DIAGNOSIS

A thorough medical and occupational history is of greatest importance in working up an ILD and identifying the likely etiology, especially because environmental exposures may be subtle. The patient's medication regimen must be reviewed, as certain drugs (e.g., nitrofurantoin, amiodarone, tricyclic antidepressants, gold) may cause ILD. Old chest x-rays should be sought to assess for the presence of subtle changes in the past and thus indicate a chronic process. Laboratory studies can aid in the diagnosis, especially if it is related to a systemic process (antineutrophil cytoplasmic antibodies, connective tissue serologies, urinalysis, complete blood cell count with differential, human immunodeficiency virus antibody). Arterial blood gases may show hypoxemia and a respiratory alkalosis.

Pulmonary function tests most commonly show a restrictive pattern (decreased lung volumes) and reduced diffusion, although a mixed picture with obstructive disease may be present with coexisting chronic obstructive pulmonary disease and certain interstitial diseases, such as Langerhans cell histiocytosis. Chest x-ray can show many patterns: reticular, nodular, reticulonodular, and alveolar filling. The first three patterns are interstitial patterns; the latter is an alveolar pattern. Chest x-ray may be normal in 10% of patients with ILD.

Definitive diagnosis, after infection has been ruled out, is necessary for direct treatment and to establish a prognosis, and is based on one or more of the following tests: (i) high-resolution computed tomography (HRCT), (ii) bronchoscopy, and (iii) lung biopsy with either video-assisted thoracic surgery or open-lung biopsy. Bronchoscopy with bronchoalveolar lavage may be indicated in an acute process to rule out infection, and bronchoalveolar lavage fluid cellular profile may assist in making the diagnosis in certain cases of ILD (sarcoidosis, hypersensitivity). Transbronchial biopsy is generally not recommended, as the small tissue yield rarely provides diagnosis (except in sarcoidosis). HRCT is approximately 90% sensitive in making the diagnosis but is not very specific. It shows an abnormality but only occasionally yields a specific diagnosis by itself. Typical findings are "ground glass," correlating with cellular inflammation, or a reticular pattern, connoting fibrosis. HRCT may aid in targeting lung biopsy sites or even avoiding biopsy; if IPF is suspected and HRCT shows more than 25% pulmonary fibrosis in an elderly patient, biopsy would be unlikely to change management. Lung biopsy, whether video-assisted thoracic surgery or open-lung biopsy, remains the gold standard and is indicated when diagnosis remains in question or infection has not been ruled out. Surgical lung biopsy is recommended in most patients with suspected IPF, and no contraindications to surgery; surgical lung biopsy is especially important if clinical or radiologic features that are not typical of IPF are present.

MANAGEMENT

Treatment is targeted at preventing tissue damage related to inflammation and progressive scarring. The traditional treatment involves combined therapy of prednisone with either azathioprine or cyclophosphamide; colchicine is an alternative in patients who do not respond to or cannot tolerate steroids. The most promising area of research in this area is the use of gamma interferon. Antiinflammatory therapies work poorly, in part because the predominant process is progressive scarring that is not closely tied to the degree of inflammation.

As only 20% to 30% of patients have an objective response (improvement or stabilization of disease) and treatment-associated morbidities are high, a treatment trial may not be appropriate for all patients. A more aggressive treatment approach should be taken in younger patients (<70 years) and treatment stopped if no response is observed within 3 to 6 months based on pulmonary function tests and cardiopulmonary exercise testing. In addition to improving pulmonary function, successful treatment has been shown to increase survival by a mean of 3 years. ILD due to other etiologies generally has higher rates of response to steroids alone (e.g., sarcoidosis 50%, BOOP 70–80%, eosinophilic pneumonia >90%).

Single-lung transplantation is an option for IPF patients who continue to progress in their disease despite medical management. Although transplantation improves function, it has no apparent effect on survival. Treatments involving antioxidants and antibodies to leukocyte adhesion molecules are also being examined.

Chapter 39

SARCOIDOSIS

Henry Klar Yaggi

OVERVIEW

Sarcoidosis is a multisystem inflammatory disease characterized pathologically by the presence of noncaseating granulomas. The granulomas can occur in any organ system but most commonly occur in the lung, lymph nodes, skin, or eyes, or some combination of these. The disease has an estimated prevalence of 10 to

20 per 100,000 and affects people throughout the world of all races and ages; however, in the United States, the highest incidence is observed in blacks (particularly black females), who tend to be affected more acutely and with more severe disease than do whites, who tend to present with asymptomatic and chronic disease. The etiology of sarcoidosis remains unknown.

PRESENTATION

Sarcoidosis presents between ages 10 and 40 years in 70% to 90% of patients. The most common presenting symptoms are those of pulmonary sarcoidosis, including cough, dyspnea, and chest pain. The most prominent areas and symptoms of extrapulmonary sarcoidosis include the skin (erythema nodosum, papules, nodules, and plaques), eyes (pain, visual changes), and reticular endothelial system (fever, night sweats, fatigue, malaise). Findings of neurologic or cardiac dysfunction may signify life-threatening disease.

DIAGNOSIS

Establishing the diagnosis of sarcoidosis depends on the clinical correlation of these nonspecific symptoms with supportive radiographic and histologic findings, as well as the exclusion of other known causes of granulomatous disease, such as Wegener's granulomatosis, fungal disease, and particularly mycobacterial infection. Lung involvement occurs in more than 90% of patients with sarcoidosis, and the classic chest x-ray reveals bilateral hilar adenopathy, which may occur in combination with parenchymal infiltrates depending on the stage of the disease. Stage I is defined as the presence of bilateral hilar adenopathy. Stage II consists of bilateral hilar adenopathy and interstitial infiltrates, which usually occur in the upper more than the lower lung zones. Stage III disease consists of interstitial disease with shrinking hilar nodes, and stage IV disease is defined by advanced fibrosis. The granulomas of sarcoidosis typically do not contain focal areas of necrosis (caseation) and tend to occur in lymph nodes, perivascular sheaths, and connective tissue spaces. Serum angiotensin-converting enzyme levels have not consistently been associated with disease activity. The American Thoracic Society recommends a comprehensive initial evaluation that focuses on determining the extent and severity of individual organ system involvement. This initial evaluation should include (i) a complete neurologic examination, electrocardiogram, and complete ophthalmologic examination to exclude critical organ involvement; (ii) chest radiographs, pulmonary function tests, liver function tests, blood urea nitrogen levels, creatinine levels, urine analysis, complete blood counts, and serum calcium levels to determine the extent and severity of disease; and (iii) occupational and environmental exposure history and tuberculin skin test to exclude other diseases.

MANAGEMENT

With respect to the natural history and prognosis of sarcoidosis, spontaneous complete remission occurs in a significant number of patients who do not receive treatment, but fatalities occur usually as a result of progressive respiratory, central nervous system, or cardiac involvement. Negative prognostic indicators include lupus pernio (a chronic rash of papules and plaques, usually on the face), nasal mucosal involvement, chronic uveitis, hypercalcemia, progressive pulmonary decline, neurosarcoidosis, and cardiac involvement. Löfgren syndrome, the acute onset of erythema nodosum, or periarticular ankle inflammation together with bilateral hilar or right paratracheal lymphadenopathy is typically associated with a benign course.

Treatment decisions in sarcoidosis are based on the presence of symptoms and the extent and severity of organ involvement. Patients who are asymptomatic or who are at low risk for disease progression (Löfgren syndrome) can be observed without treatment with close follow-up. Patients with severe symptoms, vital organ involvement, or progressive organ dysfunction require corticosteroid therapy. The optimal dose of corticosteroids is not known, so choosing a dose requires balancing the risk of side effects with the likelihood of response. In practice, relatively high doses of oral prednisone (1 mg/kg) are used initially, followed by a slow taper to the lowest effective dose for a total duration of therapy between 6 and 12 months. Patients who cannot tolerate or do not respond to corticosteroids may benefit from immunosuppressive, cytotoxic, or antimalarial drugs, such as azathioprine, infliximab, methotrexate, or hydroxychloroquine.

Section 4

Gastroenterology

Chapter 40

ACUTE ABDOMINAL PAIN

David S. Smith

OVERVIEW

Acute abdominal pain is a classic symptom that can herald conditions ranging from the trivial to the life threatening. The accurate diagnosis and timely management of abdominal pain require an understanding of the mechanisms of pain, recognition of typical patterns of clinical presentation, a broad differential of common causes, and an index of suspicion for variant presentations and unusual causes.

PATHOPHYSIOLOGY

Parietal pain, caused by inflammation of the parietal peritoneum, is a sharp, steady, aching pain, well localized over the inflamed area and accentuated by pressure. Tonic reflex spasm of the abdominal musculature is present. *Visceral pain*, caused by obstruction of a hollow viscera, is classically intermittent and cramping, but distention may produce dull, steady pain. The patient with visceral pain writhes incessantly, whereas the patient with parietal pain lies still in bed. *Referred pain* is aching and perceived to be near the surface, often accompanied by skin hyperalgesia and increased tone of the abdominal wall. *Vascular occlusion* can be recognized by severe pain out of proportion to physical findings in a patient with vascular disease or atrial fibrillation.

Visceral pain is perceived at the level the nerves enter the spinal cord. An example is gallbladder pain, which first may be perceived at the scapula, then later in the right upper quadrant (RUQ), when the somatically innervated overlying parietal peritoneum is inflamed.

CLINICAL PRESENTATION

Upper Abdominal Pain Syndromes

Biliary colic begins with sudden onset of severe, steady pain or crescendo pain lasting 15 minutes to hours. Cystic duct obstruction causes RUQ pain, whereas common duct obstruction causes epigastric pain, early jaundice, and prominent emesis. The pain may radiate to the scapula. *Acute cholecystitis*, in contrast, has RUQ pain that radiates to the scapula and is accompanied by nausea, vomiting, and fever. Murphy's sign (inspiratory arrest with palpation over the gallbladder) is present, and a distended gallbladder is palpable in 30%. There is often a background history of biliary colic. Fever and rigors herald a suppurative cholangitis. *Hepatitis* occurs after a prodromal phase of anorexia and malaise. The icteric phase is dominated by RUQ pain and tenderness, fever, jaundice, nausea, dark urine, and light stool. *Pancreatitis* has left upper quadrant pain boring through to the back, prominent nausea, and vomiting. A history of heavy alcohol use or gallstones are important clues. The patient sits up and leans forward, or lies on the side in a knee-chest position. Hiccups may be present. *Peptic ulcer disease* produces a gnawing, aching, burning, or hunger pain in the epigastrium, relieved temporarily by food or antacids. Radiation into the back suggests perforation into the pancreas. Duodenal ulcer pain may occur 1 to 2 hours after meals and at night. *Pyelonephritis* is typically accompanied by dysuria, fever, prominent nausea, and costovertebral angle tenderness, although it may present with poorly localized abdominal pain.

Lower Abdominal Pain Sydromes

Appendicitis classically begins as poorly localized pain in the periumbilical region and moves to the right lower quadrant, where the pain is progressive and focal. There is tenderness over McBurney's point, with or without rebound. Anorexia or nausea and low-grade fever are usually present. In *diverticulitis,* the presentation is subacute, with low-grade fever and left lower quadrant abdominal pain. There may be constipation or diarrhea. A tender mass with indistinct borders may be palpable on abdominal or rectal examination. *Ovarian torsion* is seen in a young woman with acute onset of pain and a tender adnexal mass but no fever. *Ruptured ectopic pregnancy* should be suspected when there is a missed or late period (although this history is presented in only 85% of cases) with an adnexal mass. Rupture is accompanied by acute pain that may project to the shoulder, cervical bleeding, shock and a full, boggy cul-de-sac. There is a history of pelvic inflammatory disease in 25%. *Ruptured corpus luteum cyst* occurs midway between menses, causing transient (hours) unilateral lower abdominal pain of sudden onset. The patient does not look ill and has moderate adnexal tenderness. *Salpingitis* should be considered in a sexually active woman who presents with lower abdominal pain. Pelvic examination reveals a yellow discharge from the cervix, cervical motion tenderness ("chandelier sign") or a tender adnexa, or both. An exquisitely tender adnexal mass indicates a tubo-ovarian abscess. *Ureteral calculus* causes severe, cramping flank pain that radiates to the groin. The patient is pale and restless. The urine dipstick is positive for blood. In *inflammatory bowel disease,* pain, fever, and diarrhea with blood or mucus accompany flares. Crohn's disease may be recognized by systemic signs, such as arthritis. Terminal ileal involvement may simulate acute appendicitis.

Diffuse Abdominal Pain Syndromes

Gastroenteritis causes diffuse, crampy abdominal pain; fever; and nausea, with hyperactive bowel sounds and mild diffuse abdominal tenderness. Bacterial infections cause higher fever; frequent, watery diarrhea; and foul-smelling, often bloody, stools. *Mesenteric ischemia* due to acute vascular occlusion presents with severe midabdominal pain out of proportion to the physical findings. The pain begins as colicky, then progresses. In later stages, fever and hypotension occur. An embolic source is the key clue. The stool is hemoccult positive. *Intestinal angina* presents with recurrent colicky abdominal pain and distention 20 to 30 minutes after a meal and lasting 2 to 3 hours. It may be manifest as food aversion or a malabsorptive diarrhea (steatorrhea) with prominent weight loss. There is often a bruit in the upper abdomen. *Abdominal aortic dissection* produces a migrating, severe, tearing back pain. The patient is often in early shock: hypotensive and restless. There may be a pulsating, enlarged, tender aorta palpable through the abdomen. A femoral pulse may be absent. Loss of motor function and sensation in a leg suggests dissection with spinal artery compromise. With *small bowel obstruction,* the pain is colicky, severe, and poorly localized, coming in intense waves, with short pain-free intervals in proximal small bowel obstruction, and longer ones in distal obstruction. Vomiting, which may become feculent, is common in proximal obstruction. The abdomen is distended in distal obstruction, and the rectum has an empty, "ballooned" feel. Tenderness to palpation is not impressive unless perforation has occurred. High-pitched, hyperactive bowel sounds are characteristic, but they may be hypoactive or absent in 25%. Most patients (80%) have a history of prior abdominal surgery. *Large bowel obstruction* is accompanied by constipation or a change in bowel habits that often precedes complete obstruction. Pain is felt below the umbilicus. Distention is prominent, but pain is less than with small bowel obstruction. With *obstipation,* the patient is distended, with stool palpable through the abdominal wall, and only mild abdominal tenderness. There is usually a history of absence of bowel movements for several days, although a small amount of diarrhea may appear around the fecal obstruction. *Peritonitis* characteristically has early vomiting, boardlike abdominal rigidity, rebound tenderness, fever, and a silent abdomen. The patient lies absolutely still. The pain is often localized (e.g., appendicitis) before becoming generalized. In *rectus abdominis muscle strain,* the history suggests strain or overuse. The pain is constant, aching, and exacerbated by movement. There is superficial tenderness over the muscle, and spasm may mimic guarding. A hematoma may simulate an abdominal mass.

DIAGNOSIS

History indicates the diagnosis in 85% to 90% of cases. Consider the organs located in the region of maximum pain, and the time course of onset. Features such as quality, severity, aggravating and alleviating factors, and associated symptoms help narrow the differential diagnosis. The ultimate decision may require repeated history and physical examination over several hours. Narcotic analgesics should be withheld until a diagnosis is established, because they can mask the expression of diagnostic characteristics of the disease. An intrathoracic source must always be considered with upper abdominal pain.

On physical examination, peritoneal signs can be elicited with gentle percussion of the abdomen, as opposed to sharply releasing the depressed hand (rebound tenderness). Muscular rigidity or "guarding" is an early sign of peritoneal inflammation. Pelvic and rectal examinations are mandatory in every patient with abdominal pain. Auscultation may reveal silence, consistent with ileus or advanced peritonitis, hyperactive high-pitched sounds with early bowel obstruction, or a friction rub with splenic infarct or hepatic metastases.

Pregnancy should be ruled out by urine pregnancy test in every young woman with abdominal pain. The white blood cell count is usually elevated but may be normal early in the course of infection or in noninfectious causes, such as renal colic. The urinalysis can help in assessing hydration state, urinary tract infection, renal stone, and diabetes. The amylase may be elevated in pancreatitis, perforated ulcer, acute cholecystitis, and intestinal obstruction. Plain and upright abdominal films may show air-fluid levels suggesting ileus, dilated small intestine suggesting obstruction, or a crescent of free air under the diaphragm, suggesting perforated viscus. Ultrasound can detect gallstones, an enlarged pancreas or ovary, ureteral obstruction, or a tubal pregnancy. Computed tomography (CT) scan is useful for specific questions, such as a ruptured spleen or intraabdominal abscess, and used when the differential is broad. CT has a sensitivity of 96% to 98% and specificity of 83% to 89% for diagnosing appendicitis. Helical CT is becoming the imaging modality of choice for evaluating nephrolithiasis and vascular structures.

MANAGEMENT

Begin with a rapid initial survey. Obtain vital signs (including orthostatics), assess perfusion (alertness, cool extremities), gently examine for peritoneal signs, and perform a rectal examination, looking for blood or tenderness. Treat shock immediately if present (large-bore intravenous access with 1 L normal saline over 15 minutes, O_2, catheter to monitor output, nasogastric tube if ileus or vomiting, triple antibiotics (cefoxitin, gentamicin, and clindamycin). Medical or surgical therapy is determined by the specific diagnosis.

Chapter 41

ACUTE GASTROINTESTINAL BLEEDING

Lynn E. Sullivan

OVERVIEW

Upper gastrointestinal bleeding (UGIB) is considered bleeding from a source originating above the ligament of Treitz, whereas lower GI bleeding (LGIB) is from a source distal to the ileocecal valve. "Middle" GI bleeding is between upper and lower GI bleeding. Bleeding can range from occult amounts to frank hemorrhage. Initial management of a patient with an upper or lower GI bleed is essentially the same, whereas the diagnostic measures and long-term management can be very different. In either case, one should have a low threshold for treating the patient as a medical emergency and potentially monitoring him or her in an intensive care setting.

PATHOPHYSIOLOGY

In looking for the etiology of a GI bleed, it is important to look at the patient's presentation, age, and concurrent medical conditions. A UGIB typically presents with hematemesis (vomiting blood) or melena (black, tarry stools), whereas an LGIB typically presents with hematochezia (bright red blood from the rectum) or maroon-colored stools. More than 50% of UGIBs are from peptic ulcer disease, either from *Helicobacter pylori* infection, nonsteroidal antiinflammatory medications (NSAIDs), stress, or gastric acid reflux. Other causes include varices, Mallory-Weiss tears, esophagitis, duodenitis, erosion, and tumors. More than 50% of young patients presenting with LGIB are found to have hemorrhoids as the cause of their bleeding. In older patients, 30% to 50% have bleeding secondary to diverticulosis. Although tics are more commonly found in the left colon, they more commonly bleed if they are in the right colon. Other causes of LGIB are angiodysplasia, colitis (ischemic, infectious, or inflammatory), and malignancy, or from sites in the small bowel.

DIAGNOSIS

It is crucial to take a thorough history from the patient, including duration of bleeding; presence of abdominal pain, nausea, or vomiting; quality of stools; presence of dizziness or lightheadedness; and use of aspirin, NSAIDs, or anti-coagulating medicines. On physical examination, checking vital signs is of paramount importance. Having the patient remain supine for 2 minutes and checking the vital signs and then having the patient stand for a full minute and again checking vital signs gives important information regarding volume status. The most sensitive indicators for orthostatic changes are a postural change in heart rate of more than 30 mm Hg and the inability of the patient to stand secondary to severe dizziness. Supine tachycardia is also a specific indicator of blood loss. Other important aspects of the physical examination include looking for pallor, the abdominal examination, the rectal examination, and looking for evidence of concurrent liver disease. In obtaining blood work, the hematocrit should be checked and monitored, although it correlates poorly with the degree of blood loss and one may not see a decrease in its value for up to 4 to 6 hours. Other important laboratory tests include prothrombin time, partial thromboplastin time, a platelet count, liver function tests, electrolytes, and a blood urea nitrogen and creatinine, as an increased blood urea nitrogen with a normal creatinine is consistent with UGIB.

To diagnose the location of the bleeding, certain investigative tools can be used. If the suspected source is in the upper tract, upper endoscopy, which is very sensitive and specific, should be performed. If the source is thought to be in the lower tract, colonoscopy has an accuracy level of 70% to 85%. If these procedures yield normal results, radionuclide scans should be used. The most accurate but invasive study is angiography, which requires large amounts of active blood loss, at a rate of at least 1.0 to 1.5 mL per minute.

MANAGEMENT

The initial management of GI bleeding from any source focuses on stabilization of the patient. The patient needs adequate intravenous (IV) access, including at least two large-bore IVs of 16 gauge or larger, and should receive IV hydration with normal saline. The patient's blood should be typed and crossed, and the patient should be transfused packed red blood cells, if necessary. If the patient has an elevated prothrombin time, other blood products, including platelets and fresh-frozen plasma, should be transfused. A nasogastric tube should be inserted to prevent the patient from aspirating, and the patient should be restricted from any oral intake. H_2 blockers or proton pump inhibitors should be administered; any medicines exacerbating bleeding, such as aspirin, NSAIDs, heparin, and warfarin (Coumadin), should be discontinued; and beta-blockers should be discontinued, as they can mask a symptomatic tachycardia. Conjugated estrogens can be used in the treatment of arterio-venous malformations, antibiotics should be administered if an infectious coli-tis is diagnosed, and antiinflammatory or immunosuppressant medications can be used in the case of inflammatory colitis. The GI and surgical services should be contacted immediately, because the patient may require endoscopic therapy with banding, sclerotherapy, or laser treatment, or surgical intervention.

Chapter 42

ACUTE MESENTERIC ISCHEMIA

Caroline Loeser

OVERVIEW

Patients with acute mesenteric ischemia (AMI) have mortality rates exceeding 60%. Risk factors include advanced age, cardiac diseases, generalized atherosclerosis, and intraabdominal malignancy. Cardiac risk factors include arrhythmias, recent myocardial infarctions, low cardiac output, congestive heart failure, and severe valvular disease. The incidence of AMI is increasing, owing to increasing recognition of the disease, an aging population with morbidities that place them at risk for AMI, and advancing medical care that prevents previously fatal events, which cause subsequent secondary ischemia as a consequence.

PATHOPHYSIOLOGY

AMI can be classified into four major etiologies: acute mesenteric arterial embolism, acute mesenteric arterial thrombosis, nonocclusive ischemia, and acute mesenteric venous thrombosis (MVT). The development of ischemia depends on systemic perfusion, collateral circulation, the number and caliber of vessels affected, and the duration of the insult. Three major vessels providing blood to the bowel are the celiac axis, the superior mesenteric artery (SMA), and the inferior mesenteric artery (IMA). The celiac axis and SMA supply the duodenum. The SMA supplies the jejunum, ileum, cecum, appendix, and ascending colon, and the proximal one-third of the transverse colon. The IMA supplies the distal one-third of the transverse colon, the descending colon, and the sigmoid colon. Ischemia and distention are the two basic stimuli that produce pain in the gastrointestinal tract. Typically, AMI produces diffuse abdominal pain. Ischemia causes the bowel to spasm, which contributes to "gut emptying" in the form of emesis or diarrhea. The bowel wall is pale, hypertonic, and contracted secondary to spasm. The spasm subsides, and the bowel wall becomes engorged with blood. The visceral veins become thrombosed, and the bowel becomes inert and cyanotic. The mucosa may slough and cause gastrointestinal bleeding. Each of the etiologies of the AMI has a different mechanism leading to bowel ischemia. Embolic events cause initial spasm and then thrombosis of a distal artery. Arterial thrombosis often occurs in vessels with underlying atherosclerotic disease, and thromboses of these vessels lead to vasospasm. The pathogenesis of nonocclusive mesenteric ischemia involves vasospasm of the mesenteric vessels to maintain cardiac and cerebral blood flow. It occurs in the setting of cardiac failure, sepsis, alpha-adrenergic agents, diuretics, and digitalis. MVT causes bowel wall outflow resistance, causing edema of the bowel wall. This phenomenon results in systemic hypotension and increased blood viscosity. The arterial flow is diminished, causing submucosal hemorrhage and subsequent bowel infarction.

CLINICAL PRESENTATION

The hallmark of AMI is pain out of proportion to physical findings. The pain may be sudden or more insidious, depending on the mechanism of AMI. Patients may have gut emptying and hypoactive bowel sounds. They may have bloody diarrhea as a consequence of mucosal sloughing. As the ischemia progresses to transmural necrosis, the bowel wall becomes cyanotic and weeps serosanguineous fluid into the peritoneal cavity, causing the physical signs of peritonitis. Bowel sounds are absent, and the abdomen may become distended. The patient becomes febrile and hypotensive. The prognosis is worse when physical signs are present. Patients may also present with minimal pain but with diarrhea with or without bleeding.

Acute mesenteric arterial embolism accounts for 50% of AMI. Of all the syndromes of AMI, embolic events manifest the most intense abdominal pain. The patients typically do not have a history of peripheral vascular disease, although they do have coronary artery disease. The source of emboli is from the left atrium, ventricular thrombi, or cardiac valvular lesions. Because of its anatomic location and size, the SMA and its branches are the sites of the majority of emboli. Of the emboli to the SMA, 15% are found at the origin, with the majority just past the origin of the middle colic artery. Emboli to the IMA are rare. Arterial thrombosis makes up 15% to 25% of all cases of AMI. Patients with arterial thrombosis often have diffuse peripheral vascular disease and typically have aortoiliac disease that is often associated with visceral atherosclerosis of the mesenteric arteries. Thrombosis occurs typically at the origin of the celiac axis or SMA and involves two major splanchnic arteries. Patients may have a history of chronic mesenteric ischemia. Patients with arterial thrombosis do not have the dramatic presentations as do patients with embolic events. Owing to their underlying atherosclerotic disease, they typically have developed more collateral circulation, so their presentation is more insidious, with symptom progression over a longer period of time. The event may occur in the setting of an intercurrent illness that causes emesis and diarrhea. Patient's complaints are out of proportion to their physical examination and may be attributed to the other illness. Nonocclusive mesenteric ischemia accounts for 20% to 30% of AMI, but the severity and location are more variable. Patients are often elderly, with a history of atherosclerotic disease. The patient is often hospitalized in the setting of cardiogenic or septic shock. Patients may have received digoxin that can cause vasoconstriction, even at nontoxic levels, or they may have received vasopressors to support their blood pressure. Other causes include ergot medications and cocaine. Only 5% of AMI are caused by MVT. MVT is more difficult to diagnose and may occur in young adults, which is rare in the other syndromes. Almost all of the patients have fever and abdominal pain, whereas only two-thirds of them have peritonitis. Risks for developing acute MVT include a hypercoagulable state, portal hypertension, pancreatitis, visceral infections, a perforated viscus, blunt abdominal trauma, and malignancy in the portal region. Reportedly, 40% to 50% of cases are due to inherited thrombotic disorders.

DIAGNOSIS

Early diagnosis is difficult owing to the lack of early signs and indicators of ischemia. Blood work may reveal a leukocytosis with a left shift and an increased hematocrit due to hemoconcentration. Other laboratory tests that may be elevated include creatine phosphokinase, alkaline phosphatase, lactic dehydrogenase, and amylase. Patients often have a metabolic acidosis. In certain cases, the recommendation is to treat a patient with acute abdominal pain and a metabolic acidosis as having AMI. There is no serum marker that is sensitive or specific enough to establish or exclude the diagnosis. Often, the laboratory tests are elevated late in the disease, when transmural necrosis is already present. A radiograph of the abdomen should be performed to rule out other causes of abdominal pain. Early in AMI, the radiograph has no abnormalities, whereas late in the disease, the radiograph shows signs of bowel wall edema. Barium contrast evaluation is contraindicated. Doppler ultrasonography is highly specific, 92% to 100% for identification of occlusions or stenoses, whereas the sensitivity is only 70% to 89%. Asymptomatic patients may have occlusion of splanchnic vessels; therefore, identifying a stenosis does not establish the diagnosis of AMI. It is also limited in that it cannot detect emboli beyond the proximal main vessel and has no role in diagnosing nonocclusive mesenteric ischemia. Computed axial tomography (CAT) is valuable in the diagnosis of MVT. CAT is the recommended initial imaging study for patients presenting with abdominal pain and a history of deep venous thrombosis or thrombophlebitis, or a family history of hypercoagulability. In other causes of AMI, CAT is similar to plain radiograph in that abnormalities can be detected late in the course of the disease. CAT can demonstrate pneumatosis or portal vein gas indicating AMI. Similar to Doppler ultrasound, magnetic resonance angiograms have high sensitivity and specificity for severe stenosis or occlusions at the celiac axis and SMA; however, it is limited in the diagnosis of peripheral occlusions and nonocclusive mesenteric ischemia and is often not readily available. Angiography is the gold standard for the diagnosis of AMI, as only angiography, along with surgery, allows for early diagnosis of AMI. The sensitivity of angiography is 74% to 100%, and the specificity is 100%. In the appropriate clinical setting, angiography is indicated in a patient with a normal radiograph, abdominal pain, and an unimpressive examination. The limitations of angiography include that it cannot be performed in a hypotensive patient, and it actually may delay surgery. Colonoscopy is also useful for colonic ischemia and is being used more and more for its diagnosis.

MANAGEMENT

If AMI is suspected, immediate surgical consultation should be obtained. Surgical intervention may be required, depending on the clinical presentation of the patient. Patients with peritoneal findings typically go to surgery immediately; however, in certain cases, it is recommended that angiography be performed before surgery to identify the mechanism of AMI and to administer intraarterial vasodilators, if needed. The management of AMI includes volume resuscitation, correcting acidosis, and administration of antibiotics. Patients should have hemodynamic monitoring with a peripheral arterial catheter. A nasogastric tube and Foley catheter should be placed. Depending on the clinical setting, immediate angiography or surgery should be performed. Angiography is diagnostic but can be therapeutic as well. Embolectomy with thrombolytic agents, infusion of papaverine, and angioplasty with stent placement may all be performed during angiography. Systemic thrombolytics are indicated in certain patients with embolic AMI. The use of immediate anticoagulation is controversial and depends on the mechanism of AMI. If the patient has MVT, anticoagulation should be started immediately, although the duration of anticoagulation has not been established. Patients with the other etiologies of AMI should receive heparin. There is no consensus on when to start anticoagulation. Although there are some recommendations to wait 48 hours owing to the risk of gastrointestinal bleeding, there are theories that the benefits of heparin actually reduce this risk. Other recommendations include starting heparin if there is no evidence of infarction, but this practice is also debatable. Despite the course of treatment, the patient requires close monitoring in an intensive care setting.

Chapter 43

ACUTE PANCREATITIS

Xinqi Dong

OVERVIEW

The incidence of acute pancreatitis ranges between 70 and 700 per million populations but is substantially higher among the human immunodeficiency virus population. The rate of mortality of acute pancreatitis is 5% to 10% and may increase to as high as 35% if certain complications develop, such as organ failure or local complications of pancreatic necrosis, pseudocyst, or fistula. In acute pancreatitis, there is an absence of continuing inflammation and the process is reversible, whereas in chronic pancreatitis, there are irreversible structural changes and permanent impairment of exocrine and endocrine pancreatic function.

The severity and mortality of acute pancreatitis may be determined using Ranson's criteria:

- On admission:
  - Age older than 55 years
  - White blood count higher than 16,000 per mm^3
  - Glucose higher than 11 mmol per L
  - Lactate dehydrogenase higher than 350 IU per L
  - Aspartate aminotransferase higher than 250 U per L
- During the initial 48 hours:
  - Packed cell volume decrease higher than 10%
  - Blood urea nitrogen increase higher than 1.8 mmol per L
  - Calcium less than 2 mmol per L
  - Partial pressure of oxygen lower than 60 mm Hg
  - Base deficit higher than 4 mmol per L
  - Fluid sequestration higher than 6 L
- Mortality with numbers of criteria:
  - Two or fewer: less than 1%
  - Between three and four: 16%
  - Five or more: higher than 40%

PATHOPHYSIOLOGY

Pathologic changes found in acute pancreatitis are primarily due to the activation of trypsin, causing autodigestion of the pancreas. Pancreatic proteases, such as trypsin, chymotrypsin, phospholipase A, carboxypeptidase, and elastase, are secreted as proenzymes requiring activation for catalytic activity. Trypsin is essential to this role and is activated by enterokinase, a duodenal brush border enzyme. Activated trypsin not only digests pancreatic and peripancreatic tissues, but also can trigger other proteolytic enzymes. Phospholipase A may be responsible for the pulmonary manifestations of acute pancreatitis, such as acute respiratory distress syndrome. Elastase causes vascular damage and hemorrhage by a direct effect on the elastic fibers of blood vessels. Fat necrosis occurs as a result of the action of lipase. Chymotrypsin causes edema and vascular injury.

The two most common causes of acute pancreatitis are alcohol use and gallstones. Other causes include obstruction secondary to pancreatic tumors, pancreatic divisum, and foreign bodies obstructing the papilla; trauma to abdomen and iatrogenic causes, such as secondary to endoscopic retrograde cholangiopancreatography or endoscopic sphincterotomy; metabolic abnormalities of hypertriglyceridemia and hypercalcemia; infections, such as ascariasis, mumps, rubella, coxsackie, cytomegalovirus, the viral hepatitides, mycoplasma, and human immunodeficiency virus; idiopathic causes; toxins or drugs, such as alcohol, azathioprine, mercaptopurine, valproic acid, pentamidine, didanosine, asparaginase, furosemide, estrogens, and scorpion bite venom.

CLINICAL PRESENTATION

Classically, acute pancreatitis presents with poorly localized, continuous epigastric pain that is often worse in the supine position and radiates to the back in 50% of patients. Signs of peritoneal irritation, such as rebound tenderness, are often absent on initial presentation. Most patients have vomiting and nausea that can lead to rapid depletion of intravascular volume. Abdominal distention and ileus are common. Evidence of retroperitoneal hemorrhage, specifically periumbilical bruising (Cullen's sign) and flank bruising (Grey Turner's sign), is rare but should be considered as a prognostic indicator. Pleural effusion and atelectasis can worsen the hypoventilation associated with acute pancreatitis. Acute respiratory distress syndrome is a rare complication of acute pancreatitis but can be potentially fatal. The differential diagnosis for acute pancreatitis includes cholecystitis, hepatitis, pyelonephritis, renal calculi, ovarian cysts, ovarian torsion, diverticulitis, appendicitis, constipation, bowel obstruction, gastroenteritis, esophageal reflux, hiatal hernia, ulcer disease, tubal pregnancy, ischemic bowel, and chronic pancreatitis.

DIAGNOSIS

An elevated amylase level is 70% specific and can be seen in other conditions, such as salivary gland inflammation, ischemic bowel, renal insufficiency, and a perforated viscus. Simultaneous determination of amylase and lipase offers a sensitivity and specificity of 90% to 95%. Elevated alanine aminotransferase and bilirubins may indicate gallstone pancreatitis. Ultrasound and endoscopic retrograde cholangiopancreatography are used to diagnose intraductal stones and other forms of obstruction. Contrast-enhanced computed tomography is the most useful imaging study in moderate and severe pancreatitis. This study may show pancreatic necrosis, pseudocysts, and intraabdominal fluid.

MANAGEMENT

The mainstay of therapy includes supportive measures, such as aggressive intravenous hydration, placement of a nasogastric tube for symptomatic relief, parenteral analgesia, total parenteral nutrition correction of electrolytes, and appropriate pulmonary, vascular, and renal support. Patients should be restricted from any oral intake. Diet should be advanced slowly from clear liquids to low-protein and low-fat diets as the patient's clinical presentation improves. Urgent endoscopic retrograde cholangiopancreatography is indicated in severe pancreatitis with impacted stones. A pancreatic pseudocyst is a localized collection of pancreatic secretions that lacks an epithelial lining and persists for more than 4 weeks. It is a potentially dangerous complication, and drainage should be considered if a pseudocyst enlarges beyond 5 to 6 cm in diameter or causes pain or gastric outlet obstruction. There are no uniform recommendations for the use of antibiotics for prophylaxis. If patients have pancreatic necrosis or signs of systemic collapse in the setting of fever, use of antibiotics, such as imipenem or combined ciprofloxacin and metronidazole, is indicated and may reduce mortality. The benefit of surgical débridement of necrotic tissues and use of jejunal tube feeding are areas of controversy.

Chapter 44

CHOLELITHIASIS AND CHOLECYSTITIS

Haider A. Akmal

OVERVIEW

Gallstones are a major cause of morbidity worldwide, and it is estimated that approximately 1 million new cases of cholelithiasis develop in the United States each year.

PATHOPHYSIOLOGY

Gallstones are classified into three major types: cholesterol, pigmented, and mixed. Up to 80% of gallstones are made of cholesterol or are mixed (usually containing more than 70% cholesterol). The remaining 20% are pigment stones containing primarily calcium bilirubinate and less than 10% cholesterol. The mechanism of gallstone formation is supersaturation with an excess of biliary cholesterol in relation to bile acids and phospholipids. Additional factors contributing to gallstone formation are nucleation of cholesterol monohydrate with subsequent crystal formation, biliary stasis, and increased calcium in bile. Cholelithiasis is most common in obese, middle-aged females with a family history of gallstones. Other risk factors include pregnancy, total parenteral nutrition or prolonged fasting, ileal disease (Crohn's disease), resection, or bypass. Cholelithiasis is also associated with certain drugs, including oral contraceptive agents, fibrates, octreotide, and ceftriaxone. In addition to these risk factors, pigment stones are much more prevalent in Asians and are associated with biliary tract infections, chronic hemolysis, and alcoholic cirrhosis. The most common etiologic organisms are *Escherichia coli*, *Klebsiella*, enterococci, and pseudomonads. Rarely, cytomegalovirus and cryptosporidia can cause cholecystitis and cholangitis in immunocompromised patients. Infection with salmonellae can result in gallbladder colonization without inflammation, resulting in a carrier state.

CLINICAL PRESENTATION

Gallstones cause symptoms by inflammation or obstruction of the cystic or common bile duct. The pain of biliary colic is of sudden onset and is severe, steady epigastric or right upper quadrant pain, rapidly increasing in intensity, frequently radiating to the right scapula or shoulder, and lasting 1 to 4 hours. It is thought to be secondary to spasm of the cystic or common bile duct when obstructed by stones. *Cholecystitis* refers to inflammation of the gallbladder wall and presents as either an acute or chronic condition. Unlike the pain of chronic cholecystitis, which lasts 1 to 4 hours before resolving spontaneously, acute cholecystitis typically lasts more than 6 hours and is associated with fever and rigors. In 30% to 40% of patients with acute cholecystitis, the gallbladder is palpable, and jaundice is noted in approximately 15% of patients. Cholangitis is an infection of the biliary tract and is a common complication of choledocholithiasis, presenting with right upper quadrant pain, jaundice, and chills (Charcot's triad). It can progress to sepsis, characterized by the addition of hypotension and altered mentation (Reynold's pentad). Elderly patients can have a much more subtle presentation. In 5% to 10% of patients, acute cholecystitis may present as an acalculous disorder, typically affecting older patients in the setting of critical illness or total parenteral nutrition.

DIAGNOSIS

In uncomplicated cases of biliary colic, hematologic and biochemical tests are usually unrevealing; however, in acute cholecystitis, leukocytosis with a "left shift" is usually observed. Alkaline phosphatase, serum aminotransferase levels, and bilirubin may also be mildly elevated. Elevation in serum amylase usually suggests the diagnosis of gallstone pancreatitis. Ultrasonography provides more than 95% sensitivity and specificity for the diagnosis of gallstones larger than 2 mm in diameter. Ultrasonographic findings suggestive of acute cholecystitis include pericholecystic fluid, gallbladder wall thickening, and sonographic Murphy's sign. Nuclear medicine tests, such as an iminodiacetic acid scan, can help confirm or exclude the diagnosis of acute cholecystitis. A normal hepatobiliary scan virtually rules out acute cholecystitis, but the lack of specificity in fasting, critically ill patients limits the use of the hepatobiliary scan to exclusion of acute acalculous cholecystitis rather than confirmation of the diagnosis. Endoscopic retrograde cholangiopancreatography provides diagnostic and therapeutic options, and has a sensitivity and specificity of 95% for the detection of common bile duct stones.

MANAGEMENT

The treatment of choice for symptomatic patients with cholelithiasis is surgical removal of the gallbladder. Elective cholecystectomy is not recommended for patients with asymptomatic gallstones. The decision to pursue prophylactic cholecystectomy in patients should be based on assessment of three factors: (i) frequency and severity of symptoms; (ii) prior complication of gallstone disease, such as a history of acute cholecystitis, pancreatitis, or gallstone fistula; and (iii) presence of an underlying condition predisposing the patient to increased risk of cholangiocarcinoma or gallstone complications, such as a calcified or porcelain gallbladder, polyps larger than 10 mm, gallstones larger than 2 cm, congenitally anomalous gallbladder, and carrying salmonellae. Nonoperative therapies, such as gallstone dissolution with ursodeoxycholic acid and lithotripsy, are rarely used owing to high rates of recurrence and low effectiveness.

Patients with acute cholecystitis often require medical stabilization in the hospital before cholecystectomy. Analgesia is best provided with meperidine, because it may produce less spasm of the sphincter of Oddi than would morphine. Oral intake is discontinued, and emesis is managed with nasogastric suction and antiemetics. Volume depletion and electrolyte abnormalities require correction before surgical intervention. Intravenous antibiotics, such as a second-generation or third-generation cephalosporin, are usually indicated in patients with acute cholecystitis. Broad-spectrum antibiotic treatment is indicated in diabetic or debilitated patients, and in patients with gram-negative sepsis. Early cholecystectomy (within 24–48 hours) is preferred once the diagnosis of acute cholecystitis is made and if the patient is hemodynamically stable. Delayed surgical intervention is reserved for patients whose medical conditions constitute an unacceptable risk for early surgery.

Chapter 45

CIRRHOSIS AND PORTAL HYPERTENSION

E. Scott Swenson

OVERVIEW

Cirrhosis is associated with significant morbidity and mortality, and is currently the tenth leading cause of death in the United States. Complications of liver disease can be broadly categorized in terms of liver insufficiency or portal hypertension. Liver insufficiency causes impairment of protein synthesis, metabolite and drug catabolism, and glycogen storage. Portal hypertension (HTN) commonly presents with ascites, splenomegaly, and excessive venous collateralization with potentially catastrophic gastrointestinal (GI) bleeding. Hepatocellular carcinoma (HCC) usually occurs in the setting of cirrhosis.

PATHOPHYSIOLOGY

Cirrhosis is the end result of chronic hepatocellular injury, resulting in hepatic fibrosis and nodular regeneration that is irreversible. Common causes of cirrhosis include alcohol abuse and chronic viral infection. Less commonly, cirrhosis results from hemochromatosis; nonalcoholic steatohepatitis; Wilson's disease; alpha$_1$-antitrypsin deficiency; chronic biliary obstruction secondary to stones, stricture, or malignancy; primary sclerosing cholangitis; primary biliary cirrhosis; or idiopathic causes. Histologically, there is extensive hepatic fibrosis with multiple regenerating nodules. Features of chronic alcohol abuse or chronic viral infection may also be present. Portal HTN is defined as a pressure gradient (wedged minus free hepatic vein pressure) of greater than 6 mm Hg. Clinically significant complications of portal hypertension typically do not arise until the pressure gradient exceeds 10 to 12 mm Hg, however. Obstruction to portal flow may arise before, within, or beyond the liver. The most common form of portal HTN is intrahepatic sinusoidal portal HTN due to alcoholic or viral cirrhosis, in which structural and hemodynamic changes in the hepatic sinusoidal endothelium lead to increased resistance to blood flow. Less commonly, portal HTN may arise independent of cirrhosis. Presinusoidal (intrahepatic) portal HTN is exemplified by schistosomiasis or sarcoidosis, whereas veno-occlusive disease is an example of postsinusoidal (intrahepatic) portal HTN. Portal HTN can also be caused by prehepatic obstruction (e.g., portal vein thrombosis) or posthepatic obstruction (e.g., hepatic vein thrombosis, inferior vena cava web, constrictive pericarditis, or tricuspid regurgitation). Doppler ultrasound is a useful tool for making this important distinction. Sinusoidal, postsinusoidal, or posthepatic portal HTN favor formation of ascites, whereas portal HTN of any etiology can cause splenomegaly with thrombocytopenia and abnormally large venous collaterals (varices) throughout the abdomen and pelvis.

CLINICAL PRESENTATION

Signs and symptoms of liver insufficiency include jaundice, fatigue, muscle wasting, ecchymoses, spider angiomas, and encephalopathy. Mild portosystemic encephalopathy (PSE) manifests with sleep-wake disturbance and the flapping tremor of asterixis. More severe PSE is characterized by frank delirium followed by coma. Although PSE is typically associated with a high blood ammonia level, ammonia alone does not account for the encephalopathy, and serum ammonia levels are less useful to follow than the clinical examination. Other findings of liver insufficiency in men include gynecomastia, testicular atrophy, and impotence.

Signs and symptoms of portal HTN include ascites, splenomegaly, and dilated abdominal wall veins termed *caput medusa*; upper GI bleeding due to spontaneous hemorrhage from gastroesophageal varices may be dramatic and life-threatening. The modified Childs-Pugh classification is a widely used scoring system to assess the severity of liver disease (Table 45-1).

Cirrhotic patients are particularly susceptible to bacterial and fungal infections owing to impairment of the reticuloendothelial system and decreased synthesis of opsonic proteins. SBP is a life-threatening complication that may be subtle in its presentation. The absence of abdominal pain or fever in a cirrhotic with ascites is *not* reassuring, and a high index of suspicion should be maintained.

Hepatorenal syndrome is an ominous development associated with advanced cirrhosis, characterized by hypotension, azotemia, oliguria, hyponatremia, and a urine sodium less than 10. It is a diagnosis of exclusion. Histo-

TABLE 45-1 Modified Childs-Pugh Classification

	Points Assigned		
Parameter	1	2	3
Ascites	None	Slight	Moderate or more
Bilirubin (mg/dL)	≤2	2–3	≥3
Albumin (g/dL)	≥3.5	2.8–3.5	≤2.8
PT (sec over control)	1–3	4–6	≥6
Encephalopathy	None	Gr 1–2	Gr 3–4

Gr, grade; PT, prothrombin time.
Total score of 1–6 is considered grade A, or well compensated. Total score of 7–9 is considered grade B, or significantly compromised. Total score of 10–15 is considered grade C, or decompensated cirrhosis.

logically, the kidneys are normal, and the pathogenesis of renal failure involves disturbances of local and circulating mediators of renal blood flow. Renal function can return to normal after liver transplantation. Pulmonary HTN may be associated with cirrhosis and portal HTN. The pathogenesis is unknown, and the prognosis generally poor. The hepatopulmonary syndrome (not to be confused with portopulmonary HTN) is associated with hypoxia and an abnormal alveolar-arterial gradient, likely due to failure of the liver to clear venodilatory substances, resulting in intrapulmonary vascular dilation and right-to-left shunt. HCC is almost always associated with cirrhosis (any cause) or chronic hepatitis B infection (even without cirrhosis).

DIAGNOSIS

Typical end-stage physical findings are described in Clinical Presentation, but well-compensated disease can be very subtle. Blood chemistries may reveal elevated transaminases, but in advanced disease, the transaminases can be normal. There may be a moderately elevated alkaline phosphatase or bilirubin, with hypoalbuminemia and hypergammaglobulinemia. The most sensitive indices of liver *synthetic* function are prothrombin time and albumin. Hyponatremia and metabolic alkalosis are late manifestations. Hematologic abnormalities of macrocytosis, anemia, thrombocytopenia, and coagulopathy are common.

Diagnostic paracentesis of approximately 20 cc fluid is a safe procedure that should be performed in the setting of new-onset ascites, or with the development of fever, leukocytosis, upper GI bleed, hepatorenal syndrome, or encephalopathy in a patient with ascites (essentially any cirrhotic being admitted to a hospital). Mild or moderate coagulopathy and thrombocytopenia are not contraindications to diagnostic paracentesis. At minimum, samples should be sent for cell count, culture, and sensitivity; total protein; and albumin, but consider also requesting acid-fast staining and cytology. Although a positive Gram stain or culture is obviously diagnostic of SBP, an absolute neutrophil count greater than 250 is also diagnostic of SBP, even in the absence of a documented organism. A serum-ascites albumin gradient (serum albumin minus ascites albumin) of greater than 1.1 g per dL is consistent with, but not diagnostic of, ascites due to portal HTN.

Direct visualization of the esophagus and stomach by esophagogastroduodenoscopy provides sensitive detection of varices. Ultrasound has limited sensitivity for evaluating hepatic nodularity and the presence of ascites or masses, but Doppler techniques may be helpful to assess portal and hepatic vein flow. Computed axial tomography and magnetic resonance imaging are more sensitive than ultrasound for assessing hepatic contour and masses. Serum alpha-fetoprotein may be elevated in both cirrhosis and HCC.

MANAGEMENT

Preventive action and proactive investigation of potential complications are essential. Patients with cirrhosis must abstain from alcohol and other hepatotoxins (do not use aminoglycosides). All cirrhotic patients who have not been immunized should receive hepatitis A and B immunization. Selection of well-compensated cirrhotic patients for treatment of chronic viral hepatitis should be made in consultation with a hepatologist, based on the age of the patient, duration of infection, severity of disease, viral genotype, and other medical issues (e.g., renal disease, human immunodeficiency virus co-infection, psychiatric disease). Decompensated cirrhosis (PSE, large varices, ascites) is, in most cases, a contraindication to antiviral therapy with interferon or ribavirin, or both.

Upper GI bleeding is a major cause of morbidity and mortality due to varices, peptic ulcer disease, or portal hypertensive gastropathy. Clinically, it is most important to distinguish variceal from nonvariceal upper GI bleeding. Active bleeding from known or suspected varices should be managed with red blood cell and plasma transfusion and fluid resuscitation in an intensive care setting; however, excessive transfusion (hematocrit >30) should be avoided because it can cause ongoing or recurrent variceal bleeding by elevating portal venous pressure. Endoscopic band ligation or injection sclerotherapy of actively bleeding varices are the mainstays of treatment. Although somatostatin analogs, such as octreotide, are often used in the management of acute variceal hemorrhage, their value is controversial. For variceal hemorrhage refractory to endoscopic treatment (typically after two failed endoscopic attempts), sustained reduction of portal pressure may be achieved by placement of a TIPS in carefully selected patients. This procedure reduces portal pressure by creating a direct connection between the portal and hepatic veins by placement of a stent through the liver parenchyma under fluoroscopic guidance. Complications of TIPS include exacerbation of encephalopathy and shunt thrombosis.

Preferably, elective esophagogastroduodenoscopy should be performed if cirrhosis is suspected (thrombocytopenia <100,000/mm^3 correlates with portal HTN and predicts presence of varices). If medium or large varices are present, prophylactic therapy with a nonselective beta-blocker (propranolol or nadolol) to reduce portal pressure decreases the incidence of variceal bleeding. Beta-blocker should be titrated to a target heart rate of 55 to 60 as tolerated. Elective endoscopic obliteration of varices can be considered in patients with contraindication or intolerance to beta-blockers. Patients should be advised to avoid aspirin or other anticoagulants and instructed to seek immediate attention for symptoms of GI bleeding.

Common SBP pathogens include *Escherichia coli, Streptococcus pneumoniae, Enterococcus* species, and *Klebsiella pneumoniae*. Third-generation cephalosporin or fluoroquinolone is the agent of choice. Upper GI bleeding in the cirrhotic patient with ascites is associated with increased risk of SBP, so these patients should have an early diagnostic paracentesis and be treated prophylactically with fluoroquinolone. Patients with history of SBP are at risk for recurrence and should receive indefinite prophylaxis with norfloxacin or trimethoprim-sulfamethoxazole.

The presence of new or worse PSE, even in a chronically decompensated cirrhotic, should prompt an aggressive search for a precipitating cause, such as upper GI bleed, SBP, dietary indiscretion, or medication side effect. Treatment of hepatic encephalopathy includes dietary protein restriction and administration of lactulose to reduce ammonia production by enteric flora and trap ammonia intraluminally to reduce its absorption. Lactulose should be titrated to produce two to three soft bowel movements daily. Unconscious or uncooperative patients can be given lactulose by enema. Encephalopathy often complicates acute upper GI bleeding owing to the protein load from blood in the GI tract and may resolve promptly with cessation of bleeding.

Peripheral edema and refractory ascites may be particularly difficult to treat in advanced cirrhosis. If the patient is hyponatremic, sodium should be restricted to 2 g daily, and water to 2 L or less. Nonsteroidals promote sodium retention and should be avoided. If these measures fail to improve ascites and peripheral edema, diuretics can be added cautiously. Spironolactone is started at 100 mg daily and gradually increased to 400 mg daily. Furosemide can be added cautiously after maximizing spironolactone, but it usually does not work alone. Volume status should be monitored by daily body weight. Renal function and electrolytes must be monitored closely. Refractory ascites may be managed by large-volume paracentesis, but reaccumulation is common. If more than 5 L is removed, give 6 to 8 g intravenous albumin per liter removed to support the effective circulatory volume. Large-volume paracentesis should not be performed in patients with active upper GI bleed, SBP, or hepatorenal syndrome (although *diagnostic* paracentesis may be appropriate).

Anemia is often present and may be associated with GI bleeding, iron deficiency, or folic acid deficiency. Thrombocytopenia may be severe enough to require platelet transfusion if there is active bleeding. Coagulopathy manifesting as elevation in the prothrombin time is multifactorial in origin and usually does not respond to vitamin K supplementation, in which case fresh-frozen plasma provides at least transient benefit for the actively bleeding patient.

In the hepatorenal and hepatopulmonary syndromes, medical management options are limited, but the syndromes may reverse with liver transplantation. Advanced pulmonary HTN is generally irreversible and is a contraindication to liver transplantation. Echocardiography is a sensitive means of ruling out pulmonary HTN in the liver transplant candidate.

Early diagnosis of HCC is essential. All cirrhotic patients should be screened every 6 months for HCC using serum alpha-fetoprotein and imaging with ultrasound or computed tomography. In HCC, if the tumor is unresectable but solitary and smaller than 5 cm, or there are no more than three lesions, each smaller than 3 cm in diameter, transplantation may be considered. Radiofrequency ablation and alcohol injection are useful treatment measures for unresectable small tumors, regardless of whether the patient is a candidate for transplant. Palliative surgery and chemotherapy for HCC may provide some benefit, although the overall prognosis is poor. For additional reading, see Garcia-Tsao G. Current management of the complications of cirrhosis and portal hypertension; variceal hemorrhage, ascites, and spontaneous bacterial peritonitis. *Gastroenterology* 1999;120(3):726–748.

Chapter 46

DIVERTICULAR DISEASE

John Toksoy

OVERVIEW

Diverticula may be congenital or acquired and occur in the small or large intestine. Congenital diverticula of the colon are rare and solitary, and involve the full thickness of the bowel wall ("true" diverticula). Acquired diverticula are common and usually multiple and involve mucosal herniations through the muscular wall ("false" diverticula). *Diverticulosis* refers to the presence of multiple false diverticula in the colon. In Western societies, diverticulosis occurs most commonly in the distal colon, with 90% of patients having involvement of the sigmoid colon. In contrast, in Asian countries, diverticula occur predominantly in the proximal colon. The prevalence of diverticulosis increases with age, ranging from less than 10% in those younger than 40 years to between 20% and 50% in those older than 50 years of age. The size of each diverticulum is typically 5 to 10 mm but can exceed 2 cm. They are thought to result from the higher intraluminal pressures that are required to move the small fecal bulk in those with decreased intake of dietary fiber. Approximately 20% of patients may manifest symptoms. Symptomatic, uncomplicated diverticular disease refers to recurrent abdominal pain, often in the left lower quadrant, as well as constipation or diarrhea, or alternating constipation and diarrhea. These patients do not manifest signs of inflammation or bleeding. Complicated diverticular disease refers to either diverticulitis (with its potential complications of perforation, obstruction, abscess formation, and fistula development) or lower intestinal hemorrhage. Diverticulitis affects 10% to 25% of the patients and occurs three times as often in the left as in the right colon. Bleeding diverticula, on the other hand, occur more often in the right colon. The remainder of this chapter focuses on diverticulitis.

PATHOPHYSIOLOGY

Diverticulitis refers to the inflammation or infection, or both, associated with one or more diverticula and is the most common complication of diverticulosis. The development of diverticulitis begins with the obstruction of the neck of a diverticulum by a hard mass, called a *fecalith*, consisting of undigested food residues and bacteria. This mass causes local abrasion and inflammation of the sac that further impair drainage, diminish blood flow, and thereby allow the growth of bacteria. Decreased venous and arterial flow cause the mucosa of the sac to be susceptible to invasion by the expanding colonic flora. After invasion, the bacteria may then extend through the full wall, ultimately leading to a microperforation or macroperforation. The clinical presentation depends on the progression of infection after the perforation. Microperforations may spontaneously regress or lead to a small abscess contained by the pericolic fat and mesentery. Macroperforations can extend longitudinally along the colon or extend to other hollow organs, resulting in fistula formation. Uncommonly, a diverticulum may rupture freely into the peritoneum and cause a life-threatening bacterial peritonitis.

CLINICAL PRESENTATION

In Western societies, patients with acute diverticulitis usually present with left lower quadrant abdominal pain, fever, and change in bowel habits (either diarrhea or, more commonly, constipation). They may experience anorexia, nausea, and vomiting. Urinary frequency and dysuria may also occur secondary to local irritation of the bladder by the adjacent inflamed diverticulum. Physical examination usually reveals tenderness in the left lower quadrant that may be accompanied by guarding and rebound tenderness. There may be a palpable, tender mass on abdominal or rectal examination. Stool has microscopic blood in 25% of patients. Bowel sounds are usually decreased but could be normal in mild cases or increased in obstruction. The most common laboratory abnormality is a polymorphonuclear leukocytosis.

DIAGNOSIS

The signs and symptoms of acute diverticulitis are usually sufficient for confirming the diagnosis. Other disorders to consider in the differential diagnosis include Crohn's disease, colon cancer, and ischemic colitis. In female patients, ruptured ovarian cysts, ovarian torsion, ectopic pregnancy, and pelvic inflammatory disease should be considered and excluded. In most patients with abdominal pain, an upright chest radiograph, as well as upright and supine abdominal radiographs, should be obtained. The chest film is used to detect pneumoperitoneum, whereas the abdominal films are used to detect bowel dilation, obstruction, or soft tissue densities. If the diagnosis is in doubt, a complication is suspected, or the patient is seriously ill, a computed tomography scan is generally performed. It has a sensitivity of 69% to 98% and a specificity of 75% to 100%. In addition, computed tomography may be used therapeutically in guiding percutaneous drainage of abscesses. A second-line tool is ultrasonography, which has a sensitivity of 84% and a specificity of 93%. It is lower in cost and noninvasive, and may be useful in female patients when a gynecologic pathology is suspected. Single-contrast enema examinations are a third-line tool. Barium is less expensive than water-soluble contrasts and provides better detail, but its use is contraindicated because of the risk of barium peritonitis if perforation occurs. Air contrast studies and endoscopies are contraindicated in diverticulitis for fear of perforation. A colonoscopy should be done 6 to 8 weeks after resolution of a presumptive case of diverticulitis to exclude colon cancer, especially in the elderly.

MANAGEMENT

When a patient presents with diverticulitis, the first decision is whether he or she requires outpatient or inpatient treatment. Patients who are elderly or immunocompromised, or who have significant comorbidities, high fevers, marked leukocytosis, or poor home support, should be hospitalized. In all patients, bowel rest should be assured with clear liquids or nothing by mouth. For hospitalized patients, intravenous fluids are generally used to maintain adequate intravascular volume. Antibiotics should be initiated and selected to cover both gram-negative aerobic and gram-negative anaerobic bacteria, such as *Enterobacteriaceae* and *Bacteroides* species. Clinical improvement is expected within 2 to 4 days, at which time the diet could be advanced. Patients should complete a 7-day to 10-day course of antibiotics. Most patients respond to medical therapy alone.

Approximately 30% of the patients need surgical intervention during an initial presentation. Complications that require prompt surgical intervention include perforation, obstruction, abscess formation, and fistula development.

For perforation, obstruction, and abscess formation, resection of the involved segment (usually the sigmoid colon) is required with a diverting colostomy and closure of the rectal stump (Hartmann's procedure). In several weeks, a second stage is performed with colostomy takedown and anastomosis to the rectal stump. Colovesicle fistula is the most common type of fistula formation and occurs in approximately 4% of cases. Patients may have no symptoms or present with refractory urinary tract infections, fecaluria, and pneumaturia. Treatment involves primary closure of the bladder and resection of the sigmoid colon with primary anastomosis. Patients with diverticulitis have an approximate risk of recurrence of 30%. Patients who have had two episodes of severe diverticulitis should be considered for elective sigmoid colectomy, because recurrent attacks increase the risk of complications and are less likely to respond to medical therapy.

Chapter 47

DYSPHAGIA AND GASTROESOPHAGEAL REFLUX DISEASE

Mark Nyce

OVERVIEW

Normal swallowing requires a complex series of closely coordinated neuromuscular contractions, commonly divided into oropharyngeal and esophageal stages. *Dysphagia* is the subjective sensation of difficulty in swallowing. It suggests an obstruction or a functional disturbance with the movement of food along the pathway from the mouth and pharynx through the esophagus and into the stomach. Dysphagia is a common symptom affecting as many as 12% of hospitalized patients and 50% of those in extended care facilities. It is considered an alarm symptom requiring immediate evaluation to determine etiology and direct treatment. A careful medical history correctly discerns between oropharyngeal or esophageal dysphagia and identifies the likely etiology in approximately 80% of patients.

PATHOPHYSIOLOGY

Oropharyngeal dysphagia involves difficulty with preparing and transferring a food bolus to the hypopharyngeal area through the upper esophageal sphincter into the proximal esophagus. It is usually the result of a functional problem rather than an obstruction and manifests as a systemic disease rather than a disease specific to the oropharynx. Most frequently, oropharyngeal dysphagia has a neuromuscular etiology. Esophageal dysphagia involves difficulty passing a food bolus down the esophageal body, through the lower esophageal sphincter (LES) and into the stomach. The etiologies involve disorders affecting esophageal muscle peristalsis or conditions that obstruct flow toward the stomach. Common causes of functional disorders are scleroderma, diffuse esophageal spasm, and achalasia, whereas carcinoma, peptic strictures, and Schatski's rings are common obstructive disorders.

CLINICAL PRESENTATION

Clinical assessment should distinguish between oropharyngeal and esophageal dysphagias; determine whether solid, liquid, or both types of food are causing the problem; specify the temporal progression as intermittent or progressive; and identify any associated symptoms, such as heartburn. Symptoms of oropharyngeal dysphagia typically include difficulty transferring food or liquid from the mouth into the esophagus, the sensation of food sticking in the throat during swallowing, and the necessity for repeated swallows to pass food into the esophagus. Patients with pharyngeal dysfunction often localize their symptoms to the cervical region immediately after swallowing and may have associated dysarthria, coughing, choking, or nasal regurgitation. A sudden onset associated with cranial nerve or cerebellar dysfunction suggests a cerebrovascular cause, such as stroke. A subacute onset may present with extrapyramidal movement disorders, such as Parkinson's, whereas muscle weakness, fasciculation, and atrophy with signs of pharyngeal dysfunction suggest an inflammatory myopathy, myasthenia, or motor neuron disease. Oropharyngeal dysphagia to solids often indicates an obstruction, such as strictures, webs, diverticuli, thyroid masses, and oropharyngeal tumors. Zenker's diverticulum, a mucosal outpouching located in the distal pharynx, is typically associated with an underlying upper esophageal sphincter motility dysfunction and a history of regurgitating undigested food, halitosis, and pulmonary aspiration. Odynophagia or pain on swallowing indicates a mucosal problem. Potential etiologies include infection, malignancy or inflammation from a corrosive agent, radiation treatment, or medication.

Symptoms of esophageal dysphagia typically include difficulty moving food down the esophagus, localizing the problem behind the sternum several seconds after initiating the swallow, and the absence of oropharyngeal symptoms, such as difficulty initiating swallowing, swallowing accompanied by nasopharyngeal regurgitation, pulmonary aspiration, and sensation that residual material remains in the pharynx. Patients who report dysphagia with both solids and liquids usually have an esophageal motility disorder. In achalasia, persistent contraction of the LES causes complete obstruction of the esophagus that lasts until the sphincter relaxes or hydrostatic pressure of the retained material exceeds the LES tone. Symptoms are progressive over time and are sometimes relieved with various maneuvers, such as throwing the shoulders back. Other symptoms include weight loss and regurgitation of undigested food, particularly at night. In contrast, spastic motility disorders are typically intermittent, associated with chest pain (nutcracker esophagus), and exacerbated by hot or cold foods.

Patients who report dysphagia only after swallowing solid but not liquid foods usually have an obstruction. The esophageal lumen may narrow secondary to intrinsic causes, such as mucosal inflammation, fibrosis, or neoplasm, or extrinsic causes, such as mediastinal disease that encases and obstructs by direct invasion, lymphadenopathy, or vessel enlargement. Intermittent and nonprogressive dysphagia without weight loss is characteristic of an esophageal web or ring. Webs generally occur in the upper and mid esophagus, whereas rings, such as a Schatzki's ring, occur at the gastroesophageal junction. Patients may present with acute dysphagia after swallowing a large piece of meat (termed "steak house syndrome"), requiring emergent endoscopic intervention to remove the food bolus. Solid food dysphagia that is progressive is usually a peptic esophageal stricture or carcinoma. Neoplasms of the esophagus or gastric cardia tend to present in older patients with associated anorexia, weight loss, and rapidly progressive dysphagia to solids. High-grade obstruction of the esophageal lumen, however, may involve dysphagia to both liquids and solids. The two major neoplasms are squamous cell carcinoma, usually associated with a history of alcohol and tobacco use, and adenocarcinoma, usually in the setting of long-standing heartburn with Barrett's esophagus. Benign peptic strictures are a complication in approximately 10% of patients with gastroesophageal reflux disease (GERD). Most patients have slowly progressive dysphagia to solids, chronic heartburn, and acid regurgitation without significant weight loss or anorexia. In addition to GERD, peptic strictures occur in other disorders that lead to increased esophageal acid exposure, such as scleroderma or Heller myotomy for achalasia. Esophageal dysphagia may also occur from radiation, caustic, pill, and infectious esophagitis. These injuries are usually acute and present predominantly with odynophagia. Radiation esophagitis may be acute or chronic, lasting more than 2 months, and may involve ulceration and strictures and localize to the area of maximal radiotherapy. Medications likely to cause esophagitis include antibiotics, such as doxycycline, potassium chloride, nonsteroidal antiinflammatory drugs, quinidine, and alendronate. Infectious esophagitis from candida, cytomegalovirus, and herpes are frequently seen in immunocompromised patients, as seen in 30% to 40% of patients with acquired immunodeficiency syndrome. Extrinsic causes of esophageal dysphagia include vascular compression, such as from a thoracic aortic aneurysm (dysphagia aortica) or an enlarged left atrium in patients with mitral valve disease, and mediastinal masses.

DIAGNOSIS

The choice of specific testing for esophageal or oropharyngeal dysphagia should be based on the history and physical examination. In oropharyngeal dysphagia, testing by barium swallow, videofluoroscopy, upper endoscopy, fiberoptic nasopharyngeal laryngoscopy, and esophageal manometry is used to confirm the diagnosis. Videofluoroscopy or nasopharyngeal laryngoscopy is commonly used to assess a patient's risk for aspiration. In cases of esophageal dysphagia, a barium swallow is useful before endoscopy if the clinical suspicion is high for achalasia or a lesion that may pose a hazard to endoscopy, such as a proximal esophageal lesion. Endoscopy is recommended for most patients with dysphagia of esophageal origin to confirm a diagnosis, establish the presence of esophagitis, exclude malignancy, and implement therapy when appropriate. Esophageal manometry is used when barium swallow and endoscopy are unremarkable, and is the gold standard for esophageal motility disorders, such as achalasia, diffuse esophageal spasm, and disorders associated with collagen vascular diseases. Ambulatory esophageal pH monitoring is useful in patients with atypical reflux symptoms or equivocal endoscopic findings, or those refractory to antireflux therapy.

MANAGEMENT

Therapy for oropharyngeal dysphagia includes swallowing rehabilitation and dietary modifications in the case of patients with strokes, therapeutic endoscopy for webs and strictures, and surgery for neoplasms. These treatments are intended to improve food transfer and prevent aspiration. The choice of treatment of esophageal dysphagia is determined by the underlying cause. Achalasia treatment options include pneumatic dilatation, botulinum toxin injections, and surgical myotomy. Medical therapies such as nitrates and calcium channel blockers for documented achalasia and esophageal spasm are usually ineffective. Patients with persistent dysphagia and no definable cause may benefit from treatment with an anxiolytic or antidepressant. Esophageal webs, rings, and strictures are generally treated with progressive dilatation using bougies or balloons. Disorders associated with GERD, such as peptic strictures, esophageal spasm, and esophageal carcinoma arising within Barrett's esophagus, require aggressive antireflux therapy. Mild symptomatic GERD can be managed with lifestyle and dietary modifications, along with nonprescription H_2-receptor antagonists, but more severe symptoms are better treated with proton pump inhibitors. GERD refractory to medical management should be evaluated with endoscopy, ambulatory pH testing, and esophageal manometry before referral for antireflux surgery.

Chapter 48

INFLAMMATORY BOWEL DISEASE

Jeffrey D. Kravetz

OVERVIEW

Inflammatory bowel disease (IBD) is the second most common chronic inflammatory disorder, after rheumatoid arthritis, and causes substantial morbidity and mortality worldwide. IBD affects all age groups, with peak incidence between the ages of 15 and 35 years, and a second peak in the eighth decade. IBD is comprised of two related syndromes with overlapping and distinct clinical features: Crohn's disease (CD) and ulcerative colitis (UC). There is no pathognomonic presentation of IBD, and awareness of its prevalence in all age groups facilitates obtaining the diagnostic studies necessary to establish the diagnosis.

PATHOPHYSIOLOGY

Both CD and UC are idiopathic, chronic inflammatory disorders that affect and involve different parts of the gastrointestinal (GI) tract. The hallmark of CD is transmural inflammation of any portion of the GI tract, from the mouth to the anus, with segmental involvement and corresponding inflammation in the mesenteric fat and lymph nodes. More than 75% of cases of CD involve the small intestine, usually terminal ileum, and one-half of patients with CD have small and large bowel involvement. Full-thickness specimens (surgical or autopsy specimens) reveal noncaseating granulomas in 50% of specimens. Chronic transmural inflammation leads to fibrosis, bowel wall thickening, and ulceration, leading to such dreaded complications as intestinal obstruction and fissure or fistula formation.

UC is predominantly defined by mucosal inflammation beginning in the rectum and extending proximally, without skip lesions, through the colon with occasional, minimal involvement of the terminal ileum termed *backwash ileitis*. Biopsies rarely reveal granulomas but commonly contain crypt abscesses. Long-standing inflammation can lead to atrophy and fibrosis, causing shortening of the colon with a "lead pipe" appearance.

CLINICAL PRESENTATION

The clinical features of IBD are varied and nonspecific and a result of idiopathic inflammation of the entire wall (CD) of the GI tract or just the mucosa (UC). Symptoms depend on the extent of the inflammation, location of disease activity, and extraintestinal manifestations. Because the majority of CD involves the terminal ileum, its major clinical features are fever, right lower quadrant abdominal pain, bloody or nonbloody diarrhea, and weight loss from malabsorption and steatorrhea. Crohn's colitis can also present with abdominal pain and bloody diarrhea. Perineal disease, consisting of perianal fistulas or abscesses, is seen in one-third of patients with CD. Longstanding CD can be complicated by fistula formation, bowel obstruction, perforation, abscess formation, toxic megacolon, colon cancer, and small or large bowel adenocarcinoma.

UC classically presents with bloody diarrhea and less severe abdominal pain than does CD. Patients complain of tenesmus, mucus in stool, weight loss, and fever. Perineal disease is rare in UC. Complications of UC include massive hemorrhage, perforation, toxic megacolon, large bowel strictures, and colon cancer.

Extraintestinal manifestations of IBD are thought to be a result of immune-mediated mechanisms secondary to chronic inflammation and can be classified into those associated with intestinal inflammation and those unrelated to inflammation. Peripheral, usually migratory, arthritis; erythema nodosum; pyoderma gangrenosum; episcleritis; anterior uveitis; and aphthous ulcers tend to correlate with intestinal disease activity. Sacroiliitis, ankylosing spondylitis, and primary sclerosing cholangitis can progress independent of underlying GI inflammation.

DIAGNOSIS

IBD is diagnosed based on the clinical picture, stool examination, radiologic or endoscopic appearance, and histologic specimen. Either CD or UC can be mistaken for ischemic colitis, especially in the late peak of IBD; collagenous or microscopic colitis; infective colitis (*Yersinia, Campylobacter, Shigella, Salmonella, Escherichia coli* O157:H7); amebiasis; pseudomembranous colitis; tuberculosis with ileal involvement; gonorrhea with proctitis; appendicitis; or diverticulitis. Obtaining stool culture is imperative to rule out infective colitis before initiating immunosuppressive therapy. Laboratory tests are nonspecific and can reveal evidence of malabsorption or leukocytosis. Diagnosis depends primarily on evaluation of the bowel wall and biopsy specimen. Endoscopic evaluation is essential and can reveal mucosal edema, erythema, and exudate seen in UC; evaluate for skip lesions and reveal cobblestoning in CD; and be a tool to obtain tissue biopsy. If features of UC are present on sigmoidoscopy, colonoscopy is not necessary acutely. In cases of CD not involving the distal colon, colonoscopy or upper endoscopy may be indicated with small bowel biopsy. Radiologic evaluation with barium enema or small bowel series, or both, can aid in the diagnosis of IBD and its complications, allowing visualization of fistulas or strictures not seen on endoscopy.

MANAGEMENT

Treatment of IBD can be surgical or medical, inpatient or outpatient, depending on associated complications and severity of disease. Medical management of IBD consists of antiinflammatory and immunomodulatory medications. Steroids, either oral or intravenous, are effective in inducing remission in UC and are often required in acute exacerbations, depending on disease severity. 5-Aminosalicylates have topical antiinflammatory activity and can be used to treat mild UC exacerbations. Mild distal UC can also be treated with 5-aminosalicylate or steroid enemas, including budesonide, which may produce less systemic complications. Severe cases of UC, which fail to respond to intravenous steroids, may be treated with cyclosporine or may ultimately require total colectomy. Maintenance therapy with 5-aminosalicylates, azathioprine, or 6-mercaptopurine is often required to maintain remission in UC. Long-term steroids should never be used to maintain remission. Mild CD exacerbations can be treated with 5-aminosalicylates, which are available in different formulations to allow for delivery to the small or large bowel. Metronidazole and ciprofloxacin may be effective in treating perianal disease in CD and may also be useful for mild exacerbations. Moderate to severe CD is best treated with oral or intravenous steroids. Budesonide can be used as a topical steroid to the bowel with fewer systemic side effects. As in UC, maintenance of remission should be accomplished without the use of steroids. Immunomodulatory agents, such as azathioprine and 6-mercaptopurine, are effective in the maintenance of remission in CD. Methotrexate, especially when given parenterally, has been shown to be effective in steroid withdrawal and maintenance of remission in CD. Infliximab, an antibody to tumor necrosis factor-α, is effective in inducing remission, healing fistulas, and maintaining remission in CD.

Surgical management is required for perforation, toxic megacolon, fistulas, obstruction, abscesses, and poor response to medical treatment. Colectomy is necessary for management of diffuse colonic dysplasia to prevent colon cancer. Seventy percent of patients with CD will require surgery during the course of their disease, usually for management of complications. Disease tends to recur at surgical margins in CD, making surgery a last resort. Approximately one-quarter of patients with UC will require colectomy, which can be performed with maintenance of continence, after rectal mucosal stripping.

UC or CD involving the colon can lead to dysplasia of the mucosa secondary to chronic inflammation. True polyps are difficult to distinguish from pseudopolyps; thus, surveillance biopsies throughout the colon are recommended in patients with IBD involving the colon every 1 to 3 years beginning 10 years after disease onset.

Chapter 49

MALABSORPTION

Joseph K. Lim

OVERVIEW

Malabsorption represents a clinical syndrome in which there is impairment of the ability of the gastrointestinal tract to digest or absorb nutrients. This phenomenon may involve specific macronutrients (carbohydrates, proteins, and fat) or micronutrients (vitamins and trace elements). It may be global, in the case of a diffuse mucosal defect, or partial, in the case of malabsorption of a specific nutrient. Patients may present with symptoms of specific nutritional deficiencies, such as pernicious anemia and vitamin B_{12} deficiency, but more commonly report nonspecific findings of diarrhea or weight loss. The focus of evaluation should be placed on identifying the underlying etiology, which is often revealed by a careful history and examination, and a series of basic, directed diagnostic studies.

PATHOPHYSIOLOGY

Defects may occur at any of the several steps of normal nutrient digestion and absorption, including (i) controlled release of food bolus; (ii) primary digestion by salivary and gastric enzymes, pancreatic juice, and bile; (iii) terminal digestion by brush border enzymes; (iv) luminal processing within small intestinal enterocytes; (v) mucosal absorption; and (vi) nutrient transport. Fats are typically ingested as triglycerides that are solubilized and hydrolyzed into emulsions. These emulsions are broken down by pancreatic lipase and colipase into monoglycerides and fatty acids that form micelles with bile salts, allowing absorption of fats and fat-soluble vitamins (A, D, E, K) within the proximal two-thirds of the jejunum. Disordered or diminished pancreatic function, bile acid metabolism, absorptive surface, or lymphatic flow may result in fat malabsorption. Gastric pepsins in the acidic stomach environment initially digest proteins where amino acid products stimulate cholecystokinin-mediated release of pancreatic proteases, such as trypsinogen and chymotrypsinogen. Enterokinases within the duodenum convert pancreatic proenzymes to their active form, allowing for digestion of proteins into amino acids or dipeptides/tripeptides, which are efficiently absorbed via sodium-dependent transporters in the jejunum. Abnormal or decreased gastric acid production, gastric emptying, pancreatic function, or absorptive surface may lead to protein malabsorption. Carbohydrates, usually starch or the disaccharides sucrose and lactose, are broken down into monosaccharides by salivary and pancreatic amylases and brush border disaccharidases before their absorption via facilitated diffusion and active or passive transport processes. Disordered or diminished saliva production, disaccharidase activity, pancreatic function, or absorptive surface may lead to carbohydrate malabsorption. The most common example seen in clinical practice is lactase deficiency. Although most micronutrients are absorbed in the proximal half of the small intestine, vitamin B_{12} is absorbed in the distal jejunum and ileum via specific interactions between an ileal receptor and the B_{12}-intrinsic factor complex.

Any disease or resection of distal small bowel may cause vitamin B_{12} malabsorption. Bile acids are also absorbed in the ileum and are similarly affected by disease of the distal small bowel.

CLINICAL PRESENTATION

Clinical manifestations are dependent on the specific underlying etiology of malabsorption. Fat malabsorption is characterized by pale, voluminous, greasy, foul-smelling stools and weight loss. Protein malabsorption is often associated with wasting, edema, and muscle atrophy. Carbohydrate malabsorption may present with watery diarrhea, abdominal distention, borborygmi, and flatulence 1 to 2 hours after ingestion. Patients may present with symptoms related to secondary micronutrient deficiencies. Folate deficiency may present with macrocytic anemia and glossitis; vitamin B_{12} deficiency is associated with similar findings but may also present with signs of subacute combined degeneration, including paresthesias, ataxia, and impaired vibration and position sense. Malabsorption of fat-soluble vitamins leads to characteristic findings, including hypocalcemic paresthesias and tetany (vitamin D), ecchymoses and petechiae (vitamin K), and follicular hyperkeratosis and night blindness (vitamin A).

DIAGNOSIS

Patients should be specifically asked about prior medical conditions that may lead to an underlying cause, including prior surgeries (i.e., intestinal resection), alcohol use, and chronic pancreatitis, and recurrent or refractory peptic ulcer disease, seen in the setting of a gastrinoma. Basic laboratory and radiographic studies focused on likely etiologies for the individual patient should be obtained. Initial testing should include a complete blood count, iron, vitamin B_{12}, folate, calcium, albumin, and coagulation parameters. Further serologic studies can evaluate for specific causes of global malabsorption, such as antigliadin or antiendomysial antibodies for celiac sprue.

Fat malabsorption may be detected by a simple serum carotene assay, although more definitive diagnosis is achieved by direct analysis of fecal fat from collected stool specimens. Sudan III–stained stool smear is a simple, timely, qualitative test that may detect more than 90% of clinically significant steatorrhea. Significant variability in performance and interpretation of this test, however, limits its reliability and utility. The gold standard remains a quantitative fecal fat analysis in a 3-day stool collection, during which the patient ingests 80 to 100 g fat per day. Healthy individuals absorb more than 94% dietary fat, and therefore a fecal fat excretion of more than 6 g per day is diagnostic of fat malabsorption. Although normal fat excretion may be up to 6 g per day, most healthy individuals excrete less than 2.5 g per day. Notably, most patients with clinically significant steatorrhea may dramatically exceed diagnostic limits, often excreting more than 20 to 25 g per day. Additional precision is achieved by maintaining an accurate record of dietary fat intake in grams per day, allowing for the calculation of the fractional fat absorption that is the percentage of actual dietary fat intake that is absorbed.

Tests evaluating carbohydrate malabsorption rely on the fermentation of maldigested carbohydrates by intestinal bacteria after administration of a test dose. The most commonly used instrument is the xylose absorption-excretion test, which measures the capacity of the intestinal mucosa to absorb D-xylose. After a test dose of 25 g D-xylose, urine is collected for 5 hours, and serum is collected at 1 hour. Serum xylose of less than 20 mg per dL or urine xylose of less than 6 g is diagnostic for abnormal carbohydrate absorption, usually suggesting diffuse mucosal disease, such as in celiac sprue. This test is limited by frequent false-positive results caused by renal insufficiency, ascites, edema, disordered gastric emptying, medications, and bacterial overgrowth. The lactose tolerance test specifically evaluates for malabsorption of the sugar lactose. After a test dose of 50 g lactose, blood glucose is measured at 0, 60, and 120 minutes. An inappropriate increase in blood glucose of less than 20 mg per dL in the presence of typical symptoms is diagnostic. This test is often inaccurate in the setting of disordered gastric emptying, bacterial overgrowth, or diabetes mellitus. Several breath tests measuring excreted H_2 and $14CO_2/13CO_2$ from bacterial fermentation of ingested carbohydrates have been used to diagnose specific forms of malabsorption, but variations in performance and interpretation limit their reliability and utility.

No tests are routinely used to evaluate for protein malabsorption, which is most commonly the result of intestinal protein loss secondary to bacterial overgrowth or a protein-losing enteropathy. Specific studies evaluating for the site of protein loss, such as technetium 99m-albumin scintigraphy, or the degree of intestinal injury, such as plasma citrulline determination, have been helpful.

Pancreatic insufficiency may be diagnosed through invasive or noninvasive approaches. The secretin stimulation test is an invasive study that evaluates the ability of the pancreas to release bicarbonate and amylase in response to secretin administration. This study involves duodenal intubation with a Dreiling tube, which allows sampling of duodenal contents after administration of intravenous secretin (1 U/kg). A peak HCO_3 level of less than 80 mEq per L is diagnostic of pancreatic exocrine insufficiency. Loss of pancreatic function may also be seen with the excessive release of fluorescein on the pancreolauryl test that evaluates the function of pancreatic esterase, or by the presence of pancreatic calcifications on radiographic imaging. Endoscopic ultrasound may be a helpful adjunct in the diagnosis of chronic pancreatitis.

Although frequently diagnosed by decreased serum levels (<100 pg/mL), elevated serum levels of methylmalonic acid (>500 nmol/L) and homocysteine more accurately detect clinically significant vitamin B_{12} deficiency. Once a diagnosis is made, the underlying etiology can be determined by performing a Schilling test. After saturation of tissue receptors in the terminal ileum with a large intramuscular dose of vitamin B_{12}, oral radiolabeled vitamin B_{12} is administered, followed by a 24-hour urine collection (stage I). Normal patients excrete more than 7% of the test dose in their urine; excretion of less than 3% confirms vitamin B_{12} malabsorption. Correction of the deficiency when this test is repeated with radiolabeled vitamin B_{12} and intrinsic factor (stage 2) suggests a diagnosis of pernicious anemia. Normalization of vitamin B_{12} excretion with the administration of vitamin B_{12} and antibiotics (stage 3) suggests a diagnosis of bacterial overgrowth. Similar examinations with the addition of pancreatic enzymes or a gluten-free diet can lead to the diagnosis of pancreatic insufficiency and celiac disease, respectively.

MANAGEMENT

Treatment must be aimed at the underlying etiology, as well as at control of symptoms, maintenance of fluid and electrolyte homeostasis, and correction of vitamin and mineral deficiencies. Special dietary modifications may be required in cases of celiac sprue (gluten-free diet), lactose intolerance (lactose-free diet or lactase supplementation), and pancreatic insufficiency (pancreatic enzyme supplementation and low-fat diet). Surgery or long-term antibiotics may be required for bacterial overgrowth syndromes once an underlying etiology has been determined, such as diverticuli, blind loop syndrome, impaired motility due to amyloidosis, or hypogammaglobulinemia. Nonspecific antidiarrheal agents, such as loperamide, diphenoxylate, and tincture of opium, may be helpful for symptomatic relief in cases in which the underlying disease process cannot be corrected. In cases of severe malabsorption, consideration must be given for enteral or parenteral nutrition.

Chapter 50

PEPTIC ULCER DISEASE

Daus Mahnke

OVERVIEW

Peptic ulcer disease is a chronic ulcerative disorder of the upper gastrointestinal (GI) tract. The most common sites of involvement are the stomach and proximal duodenum. The development of an ulcer in these locations is dependent on the balance between mucosal defense mechanisms and acid secretion. It is a common and chronic problem with potentially life-threatening consequences if the ulcer progresses to perforation or hemorrhage.

PATHOPHYSIOLOGY

The secretion of acid by parietal cells is tightly regulated by humoral, chemical, and neural factors. The sight, smell, taste, and anticipation of food begin the cascade of acid production. The hormone gastrin is the most potent stimulator of parietal cell hydrogen ion secretion. Under vagal stimulation, gastrin is secreted by G cells, which are located in the antrum and proximal duodenum. In addition to gastrin, vagal nerve input and histamine act directly on parietal cells to stimulate hydrogen ion secretion. The inhibition of acid production occurs through several mechanisms. As the luminal pH of the stomach and duodenum decreases, the release of gastrin slows. At a pH below 1.5, gastrin production is nearly halted. Other peptides and hormones, such as somatostatin, secretin, vasoactive intestinal peptide, peptide YY, and urogastrone, play a role in acid suppression. In addition to the neurohormonal defenses against acid, the gastric lining has some mechanical defenses. Mucus secreted by the gastric epithelium protects the stomach lining. Epithelial cells can also secrete bicarbonate in response to increasing hydrogen ion concentrations. With these protective mechanisms, the pH at the face of the gastric epithelium is close to 6 or 7, whereas the pH on the other side of the protective mucus layer can be as low as 1 or 2. The balance between acid production and suppression, and the health of the epithelial cells lining the upper GI tract are what determine a patient's susceptibility to peptic ulcer disease.

The most important risk factors for the development of peptic ulcer disease are nonsteroidal antiinflammatory drug (NSAID) use and *Helicobacter pylori* infection. The risk of significant GI toxicity from NSAID use is 2% to 5% per year. This risk can be lowered by using cyclooxygenase-2 selective agents or by concomitant therapy with acid-suppressive agents. Nonselective agents appear to contribute to ulcer formation through breakdown of mucosal defense mechanisms. There is significant evidence to suggest that *H. pylori* infection is a major etiologic factor in the development of duodenal and gastric ulcers (GUs). Eighty percent to 95% of duodenal ulcers (DUs) are caused by *H. pylori*, and elimination of the infection hastens ulcer regression. *H. pylori* infection is also highly associated with dyspepsia, GUs, and gastric cancer. There is a high prevalence of infection among asymptomatic people, with as many as 50% of Americans older than 60 years of age being colonized. An even higher rate of colonization exists in developing nations. Only 10% to 15% of colonized people ultimately develop ulcers. *H. pylori* infection appears to contribute to ulcer formation by increasing gastric acid secretion, causing gastric metaplasia of duodenal mucosa, and decreasing mucosal defenses by instigating an inflammatory response.

CLINICAL PRESENTATION

DUs are present in 5% to 10% of the U.S. population, and approximately 10% of men and women will be affected in their lifetime. The natural history of a DU is one of relapse and recurrence, with more than 80% recurring within 2 years. Several factors increase the risk of developing a DU, including tobacco use; increased acid production, as in the case of Zollinger-Ellison syndrome; NSAID use; and *H. pylori* infection. The most common presenting complaint in a DU is epigastric pain. Characteristically, the pain occurs 60 to 180 minutes after a meal and is improved by eating food or taking antacids. Nighttime and early morning pain is rare. When pain becomes constant or involves radiation, especially to the back, penetration of the ulcer to the extraluminal space must be considered. Notably, many patients with active ulcer disease may have no symptoms. GI hemorrhage is a worrisome complication of a DU, but DUs typically have more subtle occult blood loss. Ninety-five percent of DUs occur in the duodenal bulb. If ulcers are detected beyond the bulb, secondary diagnoses, such as Zollinger-Ellison syndrome, should be considered.

The incidence of GUs peaks in the sixth decade, approximately 10 years after the peak in incidence of DUs. Men are slightly more affected than are women, and in contrast to DU disease, the incidence of GU has been increasing. Although DU patients typically have increased acid secretion, GUs usually occur in patients with normal to slightly reduced secretion of acid. It is thought the primary process in the development of GUs is the loss of the mucosal surface. The most important risk factor for the development of a GU is *H. pylori* infection, with 75% of GUs being caused by *H. pylori*. NSAID use is another important risk factor, with approximately 15% of chronic NSAID users developing a GU. Concomitant steroid use increases this risk even further, and as opposed to overall GU rates, the rate of GUs secondary to NSAID use appears to be slightly higher in women. As in DUs, epigastric pain is the most common symptom. With GUs, however, symptoms are brought on by eating and are not as responsive to antacids. Weight loss and anorexia may be present, and nausea and vomiting occur more frequently in GUs than in DUs. The most dangerous complication of a GU is bleeding, which occurs in 25% of patients. A bleeding GU has a threefold higher mortality than does a bleeding DU.

DIAGNOSIS

Radiography and endoscopy are the diagnostic modalities that are most help-ful in peptic ulcer disease. Selective serum markers may also be of assistance if alarm signs or symptoms are present. Barium examination of the upper GI tract is the most common technique used to identify DUs or GUs. The radio-graphic hallmark of an ulcer is barium visualized in an "ulcer niche." Other secondary findings of luminal deformities or flattened fornices can be sugges-tive as well. The sensitivity of barium examination approaches 80% to 90% in the hands of an experienced radiologist. Esophagogastroduodenoscopy (EGD) is the gold standard for diagnosis, with a higher than 90% sensitivity. In addition to identifying the shallow ulcers that barium may miss, EGD offers the ability to biopsy an ulcer to rule out *H. pylori* infection and malignancy.

Testing for *H. pylori* is indicated if the patient has active peptic ulcer dis-ease with radiographic or EGD evidence of ulcer, history of peptic ulcer dis-ease, or history of gastric mucosa–associated lymphoid tissue. There is a high incidence of *H. pylori* infection in GU and DU, and it is recommended that patients with DU be checked for *H. pylori* and treated based on a positive test result. Asymptomatic patients without a history of peptic ulcer disease should not be tested unless gastric cancer is suspected. The recommendations for testing and treatment in nonulcer dyspepsia are currently controversial. The diagnosis of *H. pylori* infection can be made at endoscopy by biopsy, urease testing (90–95% sensitive and specific), or histology of a biopsy specimen. Noninvasive testing also exists for making the diagnosis of *H. pylori* infection. Measurement of serum antibody markers (85–95% sensitive and 75–85% spe-cific), urease breath testing (90–96% sensitive and 88–98% specific), and serum enzyme-linked immunosorbent assay techniques (85–95% sensitive and 75–95% specific) are available to clinicians.

MANAGEMENT

The goals of therapy in peptic ulcer disease are to provide pain relief, acceler-ate ulcer healing, prevent ulcer relapse, and, if appropriate, eliminate *H. pylori* infection. Management begins with eliminating peptic ulcer disease risk factors, such as tobacco use, NSAIDs, and alcohol. Of note, diet, caffeine, and psychodynamic factors do not appear to be risks for peptic ulcer disease. Once risks have been modified, pharmacotherapy is recommended. Antacids speed ulcer healing and offer symptomatic relief. These medicines have sig-nificant side effects, such as constipation and diarrhea, and they frequently have high electrolyte content and may not be suitable for chronic use in many patients, such as those with renal insufficiency.

H_2 receptor antagonists are potent medications with few recorded seri-ous side effects. They slow the parietal cell secretion of acid stimulated by H_2 receptor activation. Healing rates with these medications are comparable to those of antacids, but compliance is much greater with these drugs. Healing rates approach 92% after 8 weeks for DUs, and for uncomplicated ulcers, therapy can be withdrawn after 8 weeks.

Coating agents, sucralfate being the most common of these agents, act by binding to the bed of an ulcer where the pH is the lowest, adding extra defense against the caustic acid environment. Sucralfate has been shown to be almost as effective as H_2 receptor blockade or antacids for DU and GU but is U.S. Food and Drug Administration approved only for use in DUs. Bismuth compounds have the unique feature of being able to eradicate *H. pylori* infec-tion when used in combination with other drugs. Coating agents are less well tolerated than are H_2 receptor antagonists, but they may be well suited to intensive care unit patients with nasogastric tubes in place. Oral medicines must be dosed on a schedule compatible with the chosen coating agent. The ultimate step in acid production is accomplished by an H^+K^+-adenosine triphosphatase on the apical membrane of the parietal cell. Proton pump inhibitors inhibit this enzyme and are extremely potent suppressors of acid production. These agents act more quickly than do H_2 blockers and provide greater than 90% healing rates after 4 weeks of therapy for GU and DU. They are, however, more expensive than H_2 blockers and available only by prescription. For uncomplicated ulcers, therapy can be withdrawn after 6 weeks.

Treatment of *H. pylori* has led to an increased ability to cure peptic ulcer disease through *H. pylori* eradication. Sensitive biopsy and serum tests allow clinicians to accurately identify patients with *H. pylori* infection, and, in the setting of known ulcer disease, eradication of *H. pylori* is indicated. In populations where *H. pylori* prevalence is higher than 90%, empiric therapy is indicated. The role of *H. pylori* eradication in nonulcer dyspepsia is less clear.

Several effective drug regimens for the eradication of *H. pylori* exist and usually involve one or two antimicrobial agents, an acid suppressant, and a bismuth compound. Ninety-five percent eradication rates are common. Complicated ulcers or patients with persistent symptoms may benefit from a post-treatment confirmation of *H. pylori* eradication. Surgery is reserved for complicated peptic ulcer disease refractory to medical therapy. The notable indications for operative resection of ulcer are hemorrhage, obstruction, and perforation.

Section 5

Hematology and Oncology

Chapter 51

ANEMIA

Holly Craig

OVERVIEW

Anemia is defined as the reduction in hemoglobin (HGB) level or number of circulating red blood cells (RBCs). By numbers, this reduction translates to less than two standard deviations below the mean HGB (<13.5 g/dL in men, <12.0 g/dL in women) or below the mean hematocrit (HCT) (<41% in men, <36% in women). The World Health Organization criteria for anemia is defined as an HGB less than 13 g per dL in men and less than 12 g per dL in women. More important than strict numeric definitions is whether the effect of decreased oxygen delivery to tissues has any clinical effect. Symptoms of anemia can range from barely detectable to very severe, depending on the cause and rate of onset of anemia, and may exacerbate symptoms of other comorbid illnesses. Notably, anemia in the elderly is frequently overlooked and erroneously attributed to the normal consequence of aging. Correction of the underlying cause, found in as many as 80% of elderly patients, can significantly improve quality of life. The causes of anemia are numerous but relatively straightforward to categorize, and therefore treatment is tailored to the cause.

PATHOPHYSIOLOGY

RBCs carry oxygen from the lung to tissues via an iron-containing heme moiety in HGB. Normally, RBC production equals RBC destruction. Erythropoietin is a hormone produced by peritubular interstitial cells in the kidney in response to tissue oxygenation. It enhances the growth and differentiation of erythroid precursors in the bone marrow. When the progenitor cells extrude the nucleus, they become reticulocytes, which are larger than the mature RBC and still contain some of the ribosomal network capable of HGB synthesis, seen as blue on hematoxylin and eosin staining. Reticulocytes constitute approximately 1% of the circulating blood cells, but this number increases as erythropoietin levels increase and the bone marrow becomes stimulated to increase production. A reticulocyte normally spends approximately 3 days in the bone marrow and 1 day in the periphery before maturing to an RBC, whose life span is approximately 120 days before being destroyed by circulating macrophages. The life cycle of an RBC is dependent on normal renal function, bone marrow, HGB synthesis, and an adequate supply of iron and other nutrients required for cell division and RBC production. A disruption in any one of these steps can result in anemia. Functionally, anemia can be caused by increased RBC destruction or loss, or by decreased RBC production.

CLINICAL PRESENTATION

Clinical symptoms are related to the cause, degree, and rate of decrease in tissue oxygen delivery. A mild anemia can be compensated by a shift in the HGB-oxygen dissociation curve to maintain oxygen delivery at rest, but vague symptoms of fatigue and dyspnea may be present with minimal exertion. Iron-deficient patients may report a sore mouth or a craving for ice and dirt known as *pica*. Individuals with anemia may also experience worsening symptoms of comorbid illnesses, such as angina and claudication. Severe anemia, rapid in onset, such as caused by hemorrhage, may present with signs and symptoms of hypoxia and hypovolemia, such as tachycardia, postural hypotension, and even vascular collapse. Key in the physical examination is to look for clues to hematologic disorders that are associated with anemia, such as lymphadenopathy, bone pain, and petechiae. Signs of pallor in the palmar creases, conjunctivae, and nail beds may be present, and jaundice may be seen in cases of severe hemolysis.

DIAGNOSIS

Although the clinical presentation may vary widely, certain simple laboratory tests can quickly lead to a diagnosis. In the setting of an acute decrease in the HCT, blood loss from certain areas, such as the gastrointestinal tract, must be investigated immediately. In these cases, patients need a focused physical examination and appropriate imaging studies to locate the site of acute bleeding. In the case of chronic anemia, initial studies should include a complete blood count, peripheral blood smear, and reticulocyte count. The white blood cell and platelet counts are important in determining whether other cell lines are involved. The reticulocyte count provides a reliable measure of the bone marrow's response to anemia, and can therefore distinguish between increased RBC destruction or loss and decreased production.

The best measure of the bone marrow function is the reticulocyte production index (RPI), which corrects for changes in a patient's HCT and for the effect of erythropoietin on the early release of marrow reticulocytes, called a "shift factor."

$$RPI = \% \text{ reticulocyte count} \times HCT/45\% \times 1/\text{shift factor}$$
(Where shift factor = 1 for HCT = 45%, add 0.5 for every 10% decrease in HCT.)

A normal RPI is 1. Anything over 2 is considered an adequate marrow response, and anything less points to decreased production. An increased RPI indicates the cause of anemia is related to blood loss or hemolysis. Laboratory results such as an increased lactate dehydrogenase, indirect bilirubin, or decreased haptoglobin suggest hemolysis, a diagnosis that can be further supported by the peripheral blood smear.

The mean corpuscular volume can also help determine the etiology of the anemia. Macrocytosis is seen in vitamin B_{12} or folate deficiencies, myelodysplastic syndromes, alcohol abuse, liver disease, and hypothyroidism. Normocytic anemias can result from hypoproliferative disorders, renal disease, or chronic disease, or may represent a mixed disorder, which the peripheral blood smear helps to clarify. Microcytosis is seen in iron deficiency, chronic disease, lead poisoning, and genetic reductions in heme or globin production, as in the thalassemias. A low iron, high iron-binding capacity, and low serum ferritin characterizes iron deficiency, whereas anemia of chronic disease is characterized by low serum iron, low iron-binding capacity, and a normal or elevated ferritin.

MANAGEMENT

In the setting of acute blood and volume loss, a patient must be aggressively resuscitated with fluids and colloids to ensure tissue oxygen delivery. In less severe cases, one has time to make the diagnosis and therefore can tailor appropriate therapy. Iron deficiency requires identification and correction of iron loss as well as the addition of iron to the diet. Similarly, vitamin B_{12} and folate deficiencies can be corrected with supplementation. Erythropoietin is used in cases of anemia associated with renal disease. Treatment of chronic infections, inflammatory disorders, and malignancies can correct anemia of chronic disease. Frequently anemia, especially in the elderly, is multifactorial, which may complicate the diagnosis and management and therefore require careful delineation between RBC loss or destruction versus decreased production.

Chapter 52

EOSINOPHILIA

Devan L. Kansagara

OVERVIEW

Eosinophilia refers to the accumulation of excess eosinophils, which normally comprise only a small percentage of leukocytes, in blood or tissue. It is seen in diverse settings and may be a benign, clinically unimportant finding or may provide the initial clue to allergic disorders, helminthic infections, and potentially devastating conditions, such as malignancy and the hypereosinophilic syndrome. The differential diagnosis is broad, so obtaining a complete history is necessary to evaluate the protean clinical manifestations.

PATHOPHYSIOLOGY

Peripheral eosinophilia is defined as the presence of more than 450 eosinophils per µL of blood. Infection with helminthic parasites (*Ascaris, Schistosoma, Strongyloides, Trichinella,* and others) is the most common cause of eosinophilia in developing nations. Allergic and atopic diseases, including asthma, allergic rhinitis, and drug allergies, account for the majority of cases in developed countries. These causes account for more than 90% of all cases of eosinophilia. Other important causes are leukemia, lymphoma (seen in 15% of Hodgkin's cases and 5% of non-Hodgkin's lymphoma), solid organ cancers (lung, stomach, colon, uterus, and others), fungal infections (*Aspergillus*), the eosinophilic pneumonias (Löffler's syndrome), vasculitis (Churg-Strauss syndrome), cholesterol embolization, and adrenal insufficiency. The major cytokines regulating eosinophil production are granulocyte-macrophage colony-stimulating factor, interleukin-3, and interleukin-5. Conditions associated with an overproduction of these molecules, linked to the T-helper cell type 2 immune response seen in asthma, or the malignant production of cytokines in some lymphomas, can result in eosinophilia. Eosinophils can serve an adaptive function in some instances, whereas they may contribute to the pathogenesis of disease in others. Eosinophils play a role in host defense in helminthic infections. They are recruited as part of the T-helper cell type 2 immune response to the multicellular parasites and are capable of secreting toxic cationic proteins. In other disease states, the presence of excess eosinophils may actually play a role in the disease process. They may be proinflammatory in asthma and can directly cause tissue damage, as in the case of the hypereosinophilic syndrome.

CLINICAL PRESENTATION

The clinical presentation varies markedly, depending on the cause of the eosinophilia. A travel and dietary history is important to look for a source of helminthic infection. Patients may be asymptomatic or may present with gastrointestinal or respiratory symptoms. The presence of transient pulmonary infiltrates with a peripheral eosinophilia is characteristic of Löffler's syndrome. People with pet dogs may be at risk for *Toxocara* infection. Patients with atopic disease present with wheezing, cough, allergic rhinitis, or eczema. Patients with drug allergies as the cause of eosinophilia are often asymptomatic, although some medications cause organ-specific symptomatology, such as in the case of nonsteroidal antiinflammatory medication and pulmonary infiltrates. Eosinophiluria and renal failure can be seen in allergic interstitial nephritis. Constitutional symptoms suggestive of malignancy, such as weight loss and night sweats, may be present. Anemia, thrombocytopenia, and marked eosinophilia may be seen in eosinophilic leukemia. Sustained marked eosinophilia with no identifiable cause associated with dyspnea, chest pain, cough, or heart failure is suggestive of the potentially fatal hypereosinophilic syndrome. Tissue-specific eosinophilia can present as cellulitis (Wells' syndrome) or fasciitis (Shulman's syndrome). Symptoms of asthma, pulmonary infiltrates, and bronchiectasis are seen in allergic bronchopulmonary aspergillosis. Asthma associated with vasculitis, neuropathy, and pulmonary infiltrates is seen in Churg-Strauss syndrome.

DIAGNOSIS

The discovery of a mild eosinophilia alone on routine blood smear is relatively common, as high as 10%, in the general population and may not warrant an extensive workup. The diagnosis is often apparent on history. The workup for moderate to severe eosinophilia or persistent mild eosinophilia with no known cause should include serial stool examinations for ova and parasites, a peripheral blood smear, and urinalysis. When there is a suspicion of helminthic infection, serologic testing is also indicated. Serologic testing for *Strongyloides* is especially important, because a potentially fatal hyperinfection syndrome can develop in people unwittingly treated with glucocorticoids. People with long-standing eosinophilia of unknown cause should also have periodic echocardiograms to search for end-organ damage suggestive of hypereosinophilic syndrome. In specific circumstances, tissue or bone marrow biopsy may be indicated.

MANAGEMENT

Perhaps the most important part of the management of eosinophilia is making the correct diagnosis of the underlying cause and treating accordingly. Certain drugs used in asthma, such as the leukotriene inhibitors and cromolyn, interfere with eosinophil-mediated inflammation. In the case of a drug allergy, discontinuation of the medication is not necessary if there is no evidence of organ involvement. For patients with eosinophilia and end-organ damage, therapy directed at lowering the eosinophil count is indicated. Glucocorticoids are the first-line treatment. For glucocorticoid-resistant eosinophilia, hydroxyurea or interferon-alpha may be useful. Future treatments may include antibodies to interleukin-5 and an eosinophil chemokine receptor.

Chapter 53

LYMPHADENOPATHY AND SPLENOMEGALY

Caroline Loeser

OVERVIEW

The list of diseases that may present with lymphadenopathy (LA) is extensive. The most common disease categories presenting with LA include malignancies, infections, connective tissue diseases, granulomatous disorders, and hypersensitivity syndromes. Factors such as patient characteristics, associated signs and symptoms, and lymph node location should be considered to narrow the differential diagnosis.

PATHOPHYSIOLOGY

The lymphatic system provides defense against microorganisms and foreign antigens and drains excess fluid from the body. It includes circulating lymphocytes; lymph plexuses; lymph nodes; aggregations of lymphoid tissue in the walls of the digestive system, such as the tonsils; and the spleen and thymus. Lymphatic fluid flows through the afferent vessel to the subcapsular sinus and exits via the single efferent lymphatic vessel. Through this process, lymph is exposed to B and T lymphocytes, macrophages, and dendritic cells. These cells act together to process foreign antigen and ultimately to proliferate, leading to lymph node enlargement. Lymph nodes larger than 1 to 2 cm are considered abnormal in an adult. The larger the lymph node, the more likely a serious underlying cause exists. Lymph nodes are normally freely movable. Nodes can become fixed to one another or to adjacent tissues by invading cancers or by inflammation surrounding the nodes. The consistency of nodes may provide clues regarding the etiology of their enlargement. Nodes become hard owing to fibrosis, which may be found secondary to cancer, or previous inflammation that has led to scarring. Lymphomas and chronic leukemia often cause firm, rubbery nodes. A tender node may suggest the stretching of pain receptors in the capsule from rapid enlargement. The formation of a sinus tract to the skin is usually due to infection but may also be caused by aggressive malignancy.

The spleen has multiple roles: cellular and humoral immunity; removal of bacteria, senescent (old) red blood cells, cell fragments, and foreign particles from the circulation; and extramedullary hematopoiesis if the marrow is damaged. If the spleen enlarges rapidly, as in viral infections, it may become tender. If the process develops slowly, as in the case of polycythemia vera, the patient may not experience any tenderness. The pain or discomfort may be felt in the left upper quadrant or referred to the left shoulder. A patient may also experience early satiety due to encroachment on the stomach. If the patient experiences acute left upper quadrant pain that worsens with a deep breath, the differential diagnosis includes splenic abscess, perisplenitis, and splenic infarction.

CLINICAL PRESENTATION

Factors to consider when evaluating a patient with LA include history, age, duration of enlarged nodes, associated signs and symptoms, and location. General categories of LA may be remembered by using the acronym CHI-CAGO: *c*ancers, *h*ypersensitivity syndromes, *i*nfections, *c*onnective tissue diseases, *a*typical lymphoproliferative disorders, *g*ranulomatous disorders, and *o*ther. The most important factor in determining the probability of a benign or malignant cause for LA is age. In patients younger than 40 years, the presence of LA is usually benign. Older patients more frequently have malignancies, such as non-Hodgkin's lymphomas (NHL) and metastatic solid tumors. Hodgkin's disease has a bimodal distribution at 20 to 25 years of age and over 65 years of age. Patients older than 40 years have a more than 20 times higher risk of LA's being related to a malignancy or granulomatous disease compared with younger patients. LA of less than 15 days' duration is usually caused by infection. If LA persists for longer than 1 year, then the etiology is usually benign but may include tuberculosis, chronic lymphocytic leukemia, low-grade NHL, and Hodgkin's disease. A partial list of diseases associated with LA and fever includes infectious mononucleosis, cytomegalovirus (CMV), toxoplasmosis, histoplasmosis, syphilis, subacute bacterial endocarditis, typhoid fever, tuberculosis, acquired immunodeficiency syndrome, sarcoidosis, Hodgkin's disease, NHL, angioimmunoblastic LA, Kaposi's sarcoma, systemic lupus erythematosus, rheumatoid arthritis, Kawasaki disease, Whipple's disease, and serum sickness. Viral syndromes may have accompanying arthralgias and myalgias. Streptococcal infection or infectious mononucleosis may be accompanied by a sore throat. Symptoms such as cough, hemoptysis, dysphagia, hematuria, dysuria, stool occult blood, abdominal pain, and menorrhagia may suggest metastatic disease. In Hodgkin's disease and NHL, 30% and 10% of patients, respectively, present with fever, weight loss, night sweats, and pruritus (B symptoms).

The location of the LA gives important clues as to possible etiologies. The cervical chains are the most frequent locations of LA. Cervical LA is typically caused by infection or malignancy. Infections include pharyngitis, infectious mononucleosis, CMV, toxoplasmosis, tuberculosis, otitis media and externa, and adenovirus. Malignancies presenting in the cervical area include head and neck cancers, and thyroid, lung, breast, NHL, and Hodgkin's disease. Sarcoid may also present with cervical LA. Submandibular lymph nodes are typically caused by oral or dental lesions; however, cat-scratch disease or NHL may also present with submandibular LA. Anterior auricular LA can be seen in ocular diseases, whereas posterior auricular and occipital LA can be present in rubella. An infection of the scalp is often the cause of suboccipital LA but may also be seen in infectious mononucleosis, tick bites, toxoplasmosis, pediculosis capitis, and NHL.

Nonspecific LA is rarely located in the supraclavicular area. Tuberculosis is the most common infectious cause, whereas toxoplasmosis or sarcoid can also cause supraclavicular LA. Virchow's node is an enlarged left anterior supraclavicular lymph node that is associated with abdominal or thoracic malignancy. Causes include lung, breast, genital, and gastrointestinal cancer. Axillary LA is often caused by injuries and infections of the upper extremities, typically caused by staphylococcus and streptococcus. Other infectious causes include cat-scratch disease, tularemia, tuberculosis, toxoplasmosis, infectious mononucleosis, and sporotrichosis, whereas neoplastic causes include breast cancer, melanoma, lung cancer, NHL, and Hodgkin's disease. Epitrochlear lymph nodes may be enlarged in lymphoma, chronic lymphocytic leukemia, and infectious mononucleosis. More rare causes of epitrochlear LA include sarcoidosis, HIV, tularemia, secondary syphilis, pyogenic infections, and rubella. Palpable small inguinal lymph nodes are a common finding in healthy adults; however, enlarged inguinal nodes are seen in patients with injuries and infections of the lower extremities. Other infectious causes for inguinal LA include primary syphilis, lymphogranuloma venereum, chancroid, and genital herpes, whereas neoplastic causes include NHL, Hodgkin's disease, squamous cell carcinoma of the penis or vulva, and malignant melanoma.

Hilar or mediastinal LA may be suspected when a chest radiograph reveals a hilar prominence. Unilateral LA is often due to pneumonitis or neoplasia. Infectious causes of unilateral hilar LA include bacterial pneumonia, tuberculosis, granulomatous disease, atypical mycobacterial infections, coccidioidomycosis, histoplasmosis, tularemia, psittacosis, and pertussis. Neoplastic diseases, such as bronchogenic carcinoma, NHL, Hodgkin's disease, and breast and gastrointestinal cancer, can present with unilateral or bilateral LA. Diseases that typically cause bilateral hilar LA include berylliosis, chronic granulomatous infections, sarcoidosis, and malignancies. The differential diagnosis for mediastinal LA is similar to that for hilar LA, but other causes, such as esophageal rupture, hemorrhage, or mediastinitis, need to be considered in the appropriate clinical setting. LA limited to the abdomen is often malignant. The Sister Mary Joseph nodule (periumbilical anterior abdominal lymph node or metastatic nodule) is a classic sign of gastric adenocarcinoma, although it may be seen in other malignancies. Causes of mesenteric and retroperitoneal LA include gastric adenocarcinoma, other metastatic adenocarcinoma, bladder transitional cell carcinoma, NHL, Hodgkin's disease, tuberculosis, and chronic lymphocytic leukemia. Causes of generalized LA include lymphomas and chronic lymphocytic leukemia. Infectious causes include infectious mononucleosis, toxoplasmosis, CMV, and tuberculosis. Connective tissues diseases, such as rheumatoid arthritis and systemic lupus erythematosus, may cause generalized LA.

The most common cause of splenomegaly is portal hypertension, usually caused by cirrhosis. Other causes include lymphoma, infections, congestive heart failure, and splenic vein thrombosis. Massively enlarged spleens are typically seen in myelofibrosis, Gaucher's disease, acquired immunodeficiency syndrome with *Mycobacterium avium* complex, kala-azar, malaria, and thalassemia major. Diseases that present with both LA and splenomegaly include infectious mononucleosis, NHL, Hodgkin's disease, and chronic lymphocytic leukemia. Solid tumors rarely metastasize to the spleen.

DIAGNOSIS

The clinical presentation helps to guide the initial choice of laboratory studies. Initial studies may include a complete blood count with a differential, chemistry panel, chest radiograph, blood cultures, tuberculin skin test, erythrocyte sedimentation rate, titers for histoplasmosis and toxoplasmosis, serologies for Epstein-Barr virus and CMV, HIV testing, antinuclear antibody, rapid plasma reagent, computed tomography, and ultrasound.

MANAGEMENT

If blood and serologic tests are unrevealing, a biopsy of an enlarged lymph node should be performed. Fine-needle aspiration is adequate to diagnose solid tumors; however, if lymphoma is suspected, the patient should undergo an excisional biopsy of the node.

Chapter 54

HEMOGLOBINOPATHIES

Ashwin Balagopal

OVERVIEW

The hemoglobinopathies are a group of congenital disorders affecting the structure, function, or production of hemoglobin. Hemoglobinopathies are the most common genetic disorders in the world. They originate geographically around the "malaria belt" of the Mediterranean, Middle East, India, and Southeast Asia, and there is evidence to suggest that the heterozygous state is protective against malarial infection. Patients with hemoglobinopathies may have complication of illness as well as complication from their therapy. Hemoglobinopathies can be divided into those affecting hemoglobin structure, such as sickle cell disease; those affecting production, such as the thalassemias; and those affecting hemoglobin function, such as methemoglobinemia.

PATHOPHYSIOLOGY

In sickle cell disease, hemoglobin S (HbS) is the product of a single A→T nucleotide switch in the β-globin gene of hemoglobin. This results in a glutamate→valine substitution in the sixth codon of β-globin. The consequence is a greater tendency than normal for HbS to form a polymer when it is deoxygenated. This polymer leads to sickling of the red blood cell (RBC) into a less deformable state, which in turn increases blood viscosity and causes vaso-occlusion in the capillaries. This polymerization can be induced by oxidative stress, such as higher altitudes, dehydration, infections, and acidosis.

The thalassemias arise from decreased or absent production of either the α-globin or the β-globin chains. There are two copies of the α-globin gene on each chromosome 16, so that α-thalassemia can be caused by several genotypes (αα/αα, normal; αα/α–, silent carrier; α–/α– or αα/– –, thalassemia trait; α–/– –, hemoglobin H; – –/– –, hydrops fetalis). There is only one copy of the β-globin gene on each chromosome 11, so patients with β-thalassemia can either be heterozygous or homozygous for the condition. As hemoglobin A (HbA), the predominant adult hemoglobin, is formed from two α-chains and two β-chains ($\alpha_2\beta_2$), the result of mutations in either α or β globin is decreased tetramer formation and precipitation of the insoluble excess globin chains, which leads to the intramedullary death of RBC precursors.

Methemoglobinemia normally occurs when the iron group in heme partially lends an electron to the oxygen it acquires in the lungs. Ferrous (Fe^{2+}) iron is thereby changed into a transient ferric (Fe^{3+}) state. Normally occurring in small percentages, when induced by toxins, such as nitrites, nitrates, sulfa drugs, or nitroprusside, it can form more than 30% of the total hemoglobin pool, leading to deleterious effects.

CLINICAL PRESENTATION

There are myriad presentations of sickle cell disease, many of them age dependent. Chronic anemia, with acute decreases in hemoglobin during infection (e.g., parvovirus B19) is a common feature in children and adults. Growth is often stunted. Patients are subject to infections, especially with encapsulated organisms, as they are functionally asplenic from recurrent infarctions by age 4. Vaso-occlusion, causing painful crises in bones and digits, is often preceded by periods of oxidative stress. Other vaso-occlusive complications include transient ischemic attacks, cerebrovascular accidents, acute chest syndrome, pulmonary embolus, avascular osteonecrosis, and priapism in men. The chronic hemolytic anemia leads to gallstones and cholecystitis. Renal complications include isosthenuria, papillary necrosis, and hematuria.

Clinically, β-thalassemias are divided by severity into thalassemia major, intermedia, and minor. Thalassemia major causes severe anemia that manifests in the first year of life, poor growth, and marked hepatosplenomegaly. Extramedullary hematopoiesis leads to expansion of marrow spaces, especially of the skull, resulting in the typical facies of these patients and other skeletal deformities, and severe osteoporosis. The chronic blood transfusions lead to iron overload because the body does not have the ability to excrete iron. Iron in the heart, liver, and endocrine organs causes congestive heart failure, liver fibrosis, and polyglandular failure, respectively. Patients with thalassemia intermedia have a moderate hemolytic anemia and need few or no transfusions. Thalassemia minor results in mild microcytic anemia and, sometimes, asymptomatic splenomegaly. Carriers of the α-thalassemias are asymptomatic, whereas those with thalassemia trait have splenomegaly and microcytic anemia. Hemoglobin H patients have moderate anemia and splenomegaly, and those with hydrops fetalis are stillborn.

At low concentrations, the only manifestation of methemoglobinemia is cyanosis without hypoxemia (i.e., normal PaO_2). At higher concentrations, symptoms and signs of hypoxemia prevail, such as mental status change, loss of consciousness, and, without treatment, coma and death.

DIAGNOSIS

Anemia is the salient feature in most hemoglobinopathies. In sickle cell disease, anemia is present because of both intravascular and extravascular hemolysis. The peripheral smear shows sickled RBCs and target cells. If present, Howell-Jolly bodies (cytoplasmic inclusion bodies in the RBC, representing nuclei of precursors, which have not been cleared by splenic macrophages) are evidence of functional asplenia. Sodium phosphate preparations induce sickling. In thalassemia, the patient's peripheral blood smears exhibit a hypochromic, microcytic anemia, with normoblasts, target cells, and basophilic stippling. Methemoglobinemia should be suspected if the patient's blood appears brown, but there are no specific abnormalities on the smear in toxic methemoglobin-emia. Patients with congenital methemoglobinemia may have polycythemia from chronic anoxia. An important diagnostic distinction between methemo-globin and normal hemoglobin is that light is absorbed through them on the mass spectrophotometer at different wavelengths.

Hemoglobin electrophoresis in patients with sickle cell disease reveals an abnormal band, representing HbS, and no HbA band, and has a variable amount of hemoglobin F (HbF) ($\alpha_2\gamma_2$). In patients with β-thalassemia trait, a reduced percent of HbA is found, with compensatory increases in HbF and HbA$_2$ ($\alpha_2\delta_2$). β-Thalassemia major gives a very narrow band of HbA, and a large amount of HbF and HbA$_2$. α-Thalassemia can be diagnosed by molecular techniques, but the hemoglobin electrophoresis is normal, as these patients cannot mount a compensatory increase in HbF and HbA$_2$ (which both contain α-chains). Methemoglobin exhibits altered motility on the electrophoresis gel, this being heightened when ferricyanide is added to convert all hemoglobin to methemoglobin before running the gel. In sickle cell disease and thalassemia, the techniques of restriction fragment length polymorphism/polymerase chain reaction can be used to identify defective codons on each allele. These tests can also be used for congenital methemo-globinemia.

MANAGEMENT

Because of its severity and chronicity, the optimal management of a patient with sickle cell disease is through a team of doctors and nurses with whom the patient is familiar. Routine prevention of complications includes ade-quate hydration, prompt treatment of infections, avoidance of acid loads (acetaminophen, not aspirin, for fever), pneumococcal and *Haemophilus influenzae* type B vaccines, and administration of folic acid. Repeated transfu-sions to keep the HbS fraction less than 30% of total are indicated to prevent recurrent strokes in patients who have had transient ischemic attacks and cerebrovascular accidents. Iron chelation may be necessary. Hydroxyurea is used to boost the proportion of HbF, effectively lowering the relative concen-tration of HbS, and can prevent vaso-occlusive episodes in these patients. Cura-tive approaches, such as bone marrow transplant and gene therapy, are currently being investigated. Acute pain crises are treated with intravenous hydration and opiates. Early diagnosis and treatment of infections are cru-cial. Acute chest syndrome, the constellation of dyspnea, chest pain, fever, raised white blood cell count, and a pulmonary infiltrate, is aggressively treated with intravenous hydration, antibiotics, and blood exchange to lower the percent of HbS to below 30%. Genetic counseling should be provided to families when sickle cell disease or sickle cell trait is found.

Routine transfusions have dramatically lengthened the lives of thalas-semia patients. Because of constant transfusions, total body iron stores are approximately seven to eight times normal by adolescence. To prevent this iron overload, parenteral deferoxamine is used. Splenectomy should be considered in patients with signs of hypersplenism. As with sickle cell dis-ease, genetic counseling should be provided to carriers of the thalassemia traits.

In treating toxic methemoglobinemia, methylene blue, 1–2 mg per kg IV, is given rapidly in a 1% saline solution. Methylene blue activates nicotinamide adenine dinucleotide phosphate reductase, which lends an electron back to ferric iron, converting it to its ferrous form. Although this process returns the oxygen-carrying capacity to normal, it may not cure the cosmetic cyanosis that afflicts congenital patients.

Chapter 55

HYPERCOAGULABLE STATES

Stephen E. Possick

OVERVIEW

Deep venous thrombosis (DVT) and pulmonary embolism (PE) are relatively common clinical entities. Thrombosis forces the clinician to make difficult decisions regarding anticoagulation and other interventions that carry a significant risk of morbidity. Multiple acquired and inherited hypercoagulable states predispose patients to thrombosis.

PATHOPHYSIOLOGY

Abnormalities in blood flow, the blood vessel, and the blood itself (Virchow's triad) contribute to the formation of venous clots. A number of conditions, both inherited and acquired, increase the risk for thrombogenesis. Congenital predisposition to thrombophilia is being increasingly recognized. Factor V Leiden contributes to up to 40% of DVTs. The factor V Leiden mutation is a mutation in factor V that renders it resistant to activated protein C, the most potent endogenous anticoagulant. In the Physicians Health Study, this mutation conferred a 2.7-fold increased risk of DVT. This risk is dramatically increased in the presence of other hypercoagulable states. Patients with factor V Leiden who use oral contraceptives have a risk of DVT that is 35-fold that of the general population. Approximately 5% of the white population carries the factor V Leiden mutation. Although the risk of thrombosis in patients heterozygous for the mutation is almost three times that of the general population, most authorities do not currently recommend prophylactic lifelong anticoagulation in these individuals.

Hyperhomocysteinemia is another common condition that increases thrombogenesis in both arteries and veins. It is believed to contribute to 15% of DVTs. Alone, hyperhomocysteinemia confers a two- to threefold increased risk of DVT, depending on its severity. When present in concert with factor V Leiden, the risk of DVT is ten times as great as for the general population. Homocysteine levels can be reduced with the administration of folate and vitamin B_{12} supplementation.

The prothrombin gene mutation, a substitution of A for G at position 20210, increases plasma prothrombin levels and is found in approximately

2% of the white population. When the prothrombin mutation occurs in the setting of factor V Leiden, the risk of thrombosis appears to be additive, with a relative risk of 4 compared with the general population.

Antithrombin III (ATIII) deficiency, protein C deficiency, and protein S deficiency are relatively rare inherited causes of hypercoagulability. Estimates of the prevalence of these deficiencies in the general population range from 0.02% for ATIII to 0.1% to 0.2% for protein C and S deficiency. ATIII deficiency increases the risk of thrombosis significantly, with a risk of clots 15-fold to 20-fold higher than for the general population. Warfarin decreases the levels of proteins C and S, which are vitamin K–dependent factors, and therefore induces a transient prothrombotic state, particularly in individuals with protein C or S deficiency. Pregnancy and oral contraceptives also reduce protein S levels. High levels of factor XI have recently been identified as a risk factor for DVT. The antiphospholipid antibody results in increased venous and arterial clots, cerebrovascular accidents, and recurrent miscarriages. The significant morbidity of this condition necessitates lifelong anticoagulation.

A number of acquired conditions result in an increased thrombotic risk. Neoplasia is a common cause of acquired hypercoagulability. Neoplastic cells are thought to cause arterial and venous thrombosis through a number of mechanisms, including direct activation of the clotting system via tissue factor or other thromboplastins, and vessel wall injury. Mucin-secreting adenocarcinomas, brain tumors, acute promyelocytic leukemia, and myeloproliferative disorders are the most common malignancies associated with clots. The current guidelines recommend age-appropriate cancer screening in patients with evidence of thrombosis, although an extensive search for occult cancer is not warranted. Tobacco use and hypertension were associated with an increased risk of thrombosis in the Nurses Health Study. Pregnancy and oral contraceptives have long been known to increase the risk of venous thrombosis. The second-generation oral contraceptives have been found to confer a risk of DVT approximately three times that of controls. Hormone replacement therapy has been shown to increase the risk of thrombosis in the first few years of therapy. Chronic inflammatory disorders, such as ulcerative colitis, have also been shown to be thrombophilic. Heparin may induce venous and arterial thrombosis in the setting of heparin-induced thrombocytopenia.

CLINICAL PRESENTATION

Hypercoagulable states usually come to clinical attention after an individual has experienced a thrombotic event. In some cases, family members are discovered to have a congenital thrombophilic state through screening when a relative experiences a thrombotic event and is discovered to carry a congenital hypercoagulable condition.

DIAGNOSIS

The following situations should prompt testing for congenital hypercoagulable states: idiopathic DVT, such as DVT in the absence of surgery, trauma, prolonged immobilization, or metastatic neoplasia; thrombosis in those younger than age 50 years; unusual site of thrombosis; massive, life-threatening DVT; or recurrent DVT. Screening tests that should be sent include factor V Leiden, the prothrombin gene mutation, homocysteine, and antiphospholipid antibody. It is reasonable to look for proteins C and S and antithrombin deficiencies in patients with thrombosis in atypical areas or in those who are young at the age of first thrombosis.

MANAGEMENT

Hyperhomocysteinemia may be treated with folate and vitamin B_{12}, but it is not yet clear if this decreases the thrombotic risk associated with increased homocysteine levels. Anticoagulation for DVT and PE are discussed in Chapter 36. Inherited and acquired hypercoagulable states may affect both the duration and intensity of anticoagulation. Patients with factor V Leiden or the prothrombin gene mutation may require longer or lifelong anticoagulation if recurrent DVT or PE occurs. Patients with both mutations should be anticoagulated for at least 6 months after a venous clot. Patients with malignancy who experience a DVT or PE should receive long-term anticoagulation if not contraindicated. Patients with the antiphospholipid antibody who experience DVT, or arterial thrombosis should receive long-term anticoagulation.

Chapter 56

HODGKIN'S DISEASE

Richard Mark White

OVERVIEW

There is a bimodal age distribution in Hodgkin's disease (HD), with the first peak between the ages of 20 and 30 years and the second peak after the age of 50 years. There is a higher incidence seen in men than in women, and the incidence is higher among the white population. It classically occurs in increased frequency in small families with a high standard of living and first-born individuals. The incidence in the United States is approximately 7,500 cases annually, with 1,500 deaths per year.

PATHOPHYSIOLOGY

Although Reed-Sternberg cells constitute only 1% to 2% of the cells in a pathologic sample, they are thought to represent the malignant clone. They appear to be cells derived from the B-cell lineage. The specific defect in these cells has not been clearly identified, but mutations in the variable region of the immunoglobulin heavy chain have been observed. It has been postulated that a transforming event involving the Epstein-Barr virus renders these cells resistant to apoptosis. In cases in which Epstein-Barr virus is not present, some cells demonstrate mutations in the p53 tumor suppressor gene.

The four subtypes of HD include lymphocyte predominance, nodular sclerosis, mixed cellularity, and lymphocyte depletion. The most common subtype, especially in patients younger than 40 years of age, is the nodular sclerosis type, in which broad bands of collagen appear in a cellular focus, containing plasma cells, eosinophils, neutrophils, and lymphocytes.

CLINICAL PRESENTATION

The lymph nodes in HD tend to be painless, and the malignancy typically spreads from one lymph node station to the next. Mediastinal lymphadenopathy may be associated with pulmonary, pericardial, or chest wall involvement. Splenic lymphadenopathy indicates likely hepatic involvement. Bone marrow involvement occurs in 5% to 20% of patients. Systemic symptoms, termed *B symptoms*, include low-grade fevers, occasionally in the classic cyclic or Pel-Ebstein pattern; drenching night sweats; and more than 10% weight loss. Other symptoms may include pain in involved lymph nodes after alcohol intake and complaints of pruritus.

DIAGNOSIS

The physical examination should focus on lymph node evaluation, with diseased nodes often being nontender and rubbery. The chest wall, vertebral column, liver, and spleen should be palpated. Laboratory studies include a complete blood count; erythrocyte sedimentation rate, which correlates with advanced disease; chest radiograph to look for mediastinal lymph nodes; and, following that, a computed tomography scan of the chest, abdomen, and pelvis, given that computed tomography provides the best sensitivity for detecting nodes in these areas. Obtaining a lymph node biopsy is essential; open biopsy is essential, as it preserves the architecture of the tissue. A bone marrow biopsy is performed in most patients. Gallium scans are useful for following response to treatment, as diseased areas avidly take up gallium. The staging of HD is as follows: I, one nodal site; II, two or more nodal sites on the same side of the diaphragm; III, lymph nodes on both sides of the diaphragm; IV, disease involving the bone marrow, liver, lung, or other extralymphatic organs; A or B, absence or presence, respectively, of B symptoms; E, involvement of a single extranodal site contiguous to a known nodal site.

MANAGEMENT

For stages I and IIA, radiation therapy traditionally has been the treatment of choice and has produced an 80% relapse-free survival rate. The increased incidence of secondary tumors from radiation has led to the development of combination regimens using several courses of standard chemotherapy, such as doxorubicin (Adriamycin) bleomycin, vinblastine, and dacarbazine (ABVD); or mechlorethamine, vincristine, procarbazine, and prednisone (MOPP), plus limited-field radiation with similar cure rates. In stage III or IV disease, combination chemotherapy is used, with cure rates dependent on age and tumor burden. For stage IIIA disease, ABVD is well tolerated and cures 65% to 70% of patients. For stage IIIB disease, combination chemotherapy with ABVD or MOPP, with or without radiation depending on tumor bulkiness, has an expected cure rate of 70% to 75%. Patients who relapse after radiation do well when treated with combination chemotherapy, such as MOPP or ABVD. Failure to achieve initial remission or relapse within 12 months of treatment is a poor prognostic sign, and the use of high-dose chemotherapy with autologous hematopoietic stem cell rescue may offer long-term survival for these patients.

Chapter 57

NON-HODGKIN'S LYMPHOMA

Richard Mark White

OVERVIEW

The name *non-Hodgkin's lymphoma* (NHL) refers to a diverse group of neoplasms of lymphoid tissues. Eighty-five percent of these lymphomas originate from B lymphocytes, whereas the rest originate from T lymphocytes. The NHLs are increasing in frequency in the United States, doubling in the past 20 years. They typically have a peak incidence in the fifth decade of life. The reasons for the increasing frequency are likely multifactorial. The human immunodeficiency virus (HIV) epidemic is certainly responsible for some of this increase, but other chronic immunosuppressive states, such as post organ transplantation and prior Hodgkin's disease treatment, likely are important.

PATHOPHYSIOLOGY

There are no known unifying etiologic mechanisms for the NHLs, which likely explains their diverse clinical and pathologic presentations. Some autoimmune conditions, most notably Sjögren's syndrome, and infections, such as *Helicobacter pylori*, Epstein-Barr virus (EBV), and Kaposi's sarcoma–associated virus, are known to predispose individuals to the NHLs. Genetic mutations that are commonly and consistently seen in various subtypes include karyotypic abnormalities at t(8;14), t(14;18), and t(11;14), but the relationship of these translocations to malignant transformation is not completely understood. An association between overexpression of the antiapoptotic gene mutations of the bcl-2 gene, present on chromosome 18, and follicular lymphomas is well established. The 11;14 translocation is seen in mantle cell lymphoma and results in overexpression of cyclin D1, one of the regulators of the cell cycle. The 8;14 translocation results in the overexpression of the cmyc protooncogene.

CLINICAL PRESENTATION

There are two main concepts regarding the classification of NHLs. *Grade* refers to the histopathologic, molecular, immunologic, and phenotypic specificities of the cells involved. There are currently two main systems: the older Working Formulation (WF) system, and the newer World Health Organization (WHO) classification. The WHO system provides an updated version of all the information contained in the WF. The WF grouped all of the major NHLs into low, intermediate, and high-grade lymphomas, with lower grades being more indolent, but incurable in most cases, and higher grades more aggressive, although curable. The newer WHO classification functionally retains this system. The *stage* refers to the extent of disease throughout the body. The following listing includes the WHO subtype (with the WF subtype in parentheses) and important clinical manifestations of the most common types of NHLs but is not inclusive of all types. It also designates whether it is commonly thought to be low, intermediate, or high grade.

1. Follicular lymphomas (WF: follicular, small cleaved, mixed or large cell): Composed of variable numbers of small cleaved cells and large non-cleaved cells. The WHO grade (I, II or III) refers to the proportion of large noncleaved cells. This type typically affects older adults, who present with widespread nodal, splenic, and bone marrow disease. These are the typical "indolent" or "low-grade" lymphomas, and patients often have a median survival of 7 to 10 years. Higher grades, particularly grade III, have a tendency to transform into aggressive diffuse large B-cell lymphomas (Richter's transformation).

2. Diffuse large B-cell lymphomas (WF: diffuse large cell, large cell immunoblastic, occasionally diffuse mixed small and large cell): This type is composed of large cells expressing B-cell markers. Approximately 30% of these tumors show overexpression of bcl-2 and the 14;18 translocation.

   Clinically, these account for 30% of all adult NHLs and have a broad age distribution, with a peak in the sixth decade. They often present as single or multiple, rapidly enlarging masses in either lymph nodes or extranodal sites. The most common extranodal masses are in the stomach, central nervous system (CNS), bone, kidney, and testis. These NHLs are the typical "aggressive" NHLs, which can be cured in some cases but can be rapidly fatal if untreated. When these tumors arise from a previously "indolent" lymphoma (i.e., follicular lymphoma or chronic lymphocytic leukemia), it is referred to as *Richter's syndrome*, and it typically has a worse overall prognosis.

3. Mantle cell lymphomas (WF: usually diffuse small cleaved-cell lymphoma): Composed of small to medium-sized cells with "cleaved" nuclei. These cells typically show overexpression of cyclin D1, which is a useful diagnostic marker.

   Clinically, these NHLs usually present in older men with very widespread disease, including both nodal and extranodal sites (Waldeyer's ring, stomach, bone marrow, and spleen). Although morphologically they seem low grade, they are associated with a median survival of only 3 to 5 years.

4. Mucosa-associated lymphoid tissue (MALT) lymphomas (WF: not specified): These NHLs are composed of small lymphocytes, marginal zone B cells, and plasma cells making up a tumor mass in an extranodal site.

   Clinically, these tumors usually arise in patients who have chronic stimulation of MALT tissue, such as in the stomach (due to *H. pylori* infection), salivary glands, the orbits, lungs (due to Sjögren's syndrome or other autoimmune diseases), or the thyroid (due to Hashimoto's thyroiditis). These tumors are usually "indolent," especially early on, although they may transform into "aggressive" diffuse large B-cell lymphomas.

5. Burkitt's lymphoma (WF: small noncleaved cell of the Burkitt's type): Composed of medium-sized cells with basophilic cytoplasm and round nuclei (thus noncleaved). Biopsies have a characteristic "starry-sky" appearance due to macrophages that infiltrate the tumor and then apoptotic tumor cells. Clinically, these tumors fall into two major categories: endemic (African) and nonendemic. The endemic African type is associated with EBV infection and often presents in the jaw and other facial bones. The nonendemic, non-African type seen in the United States has less association with EBV and most commonly presents in the abdomen, although the kidneys or ovaries may be involved.

   These tumors are typically highly aggressive with a rapid doubling time. They are highly curable, especially in children, but have a significant risk of tumor lysis syndrome.

   Overall, the prognosis of lymphoma is related to both tumor type and stage. For indolent, low-grade lymphomas, median survival is approximately 7 to 10 years, regardless of therapy. For aggressive, high-grade lymphomas, survival may be as little as weeks to months without treatment; however, patients with high-grade disease are able to achieve complete cures.

DIAGNOSIS

The history and physical examination are geared toward eliciting complaints of B symptoms, such as night sweats, fever, and weight loss, and pointing toward likely sites of disease involvement. Complaints of pain, fullness, or discomfort, especially in the abdomen or chest, indicate likely involvement in these sites. A thorough examination of the lymph nodes must include sites such as the epitrochlear and preauricular nodes. Patients with preauricular involvement also must be screened for involvement of Waldeyer's ring. Laboratory evaluation includes complete blood count (NHL is associated with Coombs'-positive hemolytic anemias and immune thrombocytopenia), as well as electrolytes and tests of renal and liver function. Lactate dehydrogenase has important prognostic significance as an indicator of disease burden. Standard imaging typically includes computed tomography of the chest, abdomen, and pelvis to ascertain occult involvement of these areas and complications caused by bulky lymphadenopathy, such as obstructive uropathy. Magnetic resonance imaging scanning is primarily used for evaluation of the CNS, orbits, and sinuses. Gastrointestinal endoscopy or contrast studies are indicated for those patients suspected of having gastric or small intestine involvement, either of which is commonly associated with Waldeyer's ring disease. Bone marrow aspiration and biopsy are part of the staging and should be performed in most patients. It is important to obtain both an aspiration and flow cytometry of the aspirate, and an adequate biopsy specimen with representative architecture.

MANAGEMENT

The mainstay of treatment of the NHL is chemotherapy, either single-agent or combination regimens. Radiation therapy may be used in selected patients with bulky disease, either alone or in combination with chemotherapy. Because of the indolent nature of many of the NHLs, a "watchful waiting" approach is advocated for many patients and is considered an acceptable form of treatment for some patients.

Specific treatments for the more common types of NHL are presented in the following:

1. Follicular lymphomas (WF: follicular, small cleaved, mixed or large cell): For patients with grade I or II, "watchful waiting" is often the accepted initial treatment regimen, especially if the patient has only limited-stage involvement, such as one or two sites. For these patients, palliative site-directed radiation or single-agent chemotherapy might be the best option. Radiation therapy may be curative in patients with stage I and II disease. For patients with grade I or II but more extensive stage and tumor burden, the correct initial therapy is controversial, primarily because no specific regimen has been demonstrated to improve survival. Most patients, however, with extensive disease will require some type of therapy, either single-agent chemotherapy or combined chemotherapy, for disease palliation. For patients with grade III follicular lymphoma at presentation, the treatment is usually the same as for the diffuse large B-cell lymphomas.

2. Diffuse large B-cell lymphomas (WF: diffuse large cell, large cell immunoblastic, occasionally diffuse mixed small and large cell): Localized and dif-

fuse disease is typically treated with an anthracycline-containing regimen, such as CHOP (cyclophosphamide, doxorubicin, vincristine, and prednisone). A multicenter trial compared the efficacy and tolerability of CHOP with more toxic chemotherapy regimens and found that CHOP was as effective and better tolerated than the "second-generation" or "third-generation" regimens. CHOP will cure only approximately 30% to 40% of patients with advanced disease. Patients who relapse should be considered for autologous stem cell transplantation.

3. Mantle-cell lymphomas (WF: usually diffuse small cleaved cell lymphoma): Mantle-cell lymphoma tends to have a more aggressive course, with a median survival significantly less than the follicular, low-grade lymphomas (3 years vs. 7–10 years). Thus, these lymphomas may be treated as the more aggressive lymphomas, typically using CHOP.

4. MALT lymphomas (WF: not specified): Because these tumors are indolent and may remain localized for long periods of time, the approach to therapy is mainly that of local disease control, using site-directed radiation or surgery, especially for tumors of the thyroid, lung, or salivary gland. The treatment of gastric MALT has undergone significant changes since the recognition of the strong association with *H. pylori* infection. These patients should be treated with antibiotic therapy alone, and tumor regression and bacterial eradication have been documented.

5. Burkitt's lymphoma (WF: small noncleaved cell of the Burkitt's type): These tumors are usually treated with high-dose combination chemotherapy. Because there is a propensity for CNS involvement, cranial irradiation and intrathecal chemotherapy are included in all regimens. Complications of therapy include severe tumor lysis syndrome, and some patients may require temporary hemodialysis to manage hyperkalemia, hyperphosphatemia, acidosis, and acute renal failure.

6. HIV-associated lymphomas: The finding of lymphoma in a patient with HIV disease carries a poor prognosis, with a median survival of less than 1 year. These patients have a higher than expected rate of CNS involvement. Treatment options are limited in these severely immunocompromised patients, but for patients with CD4 counts higher than 200 and lymphoma as their presenting acquired immune deficiency syndrome condition, prognosis may be significantly improved by use of CHOP or similar regimens.

Chapter 58

THROMBOCYTOPENIA, THROMBOTIC THROMBOCYTOPENIC PURPURA, AND DISSEMINATED INTRAVASCULAR COAGULATION

Jared G. Selter

OVERVIEW

Few clinical scenarios are as challenging as those involving thrombocytopenia (TCP). Furthermore, platelet disorders are common. For example, more than 50 medications can cause TCP; disseminated intravascular coagulation (DIC) occurs in up to 50% of patients with amniotic fluid emboli; between 5% and 10% of patients treated with heparin develop heparin-induced thrombocytopenia (HIT), and up to 50% of these patients will develop clots. This review focuses on the pathophysiology of TCP, with an emphasis on drug-induced and immune-mediated TCP, and on consumptive coagulopathies, and discusses the diagnosis and treatment of these disorders.

PATHOPHYSIOLOGY

Before establishing the diagnosis of TCP, one must rule out pseudo-TCP. Pseudo-TCP is an *in vitro* agglutination artifact that occurs when whole blood is anticoagulated with ethylenediaminetetraacetic acid in the tube used to perform complete blood count (CBC) analysis. The diagnosis is made by reviewing the peripheral blood smear and demonstrating platelet clumps. The CBC should then be repeated using a different anticoagulant, such as heparin, which should result in a normalization or improvement of the platelet count.

Derangements in platelet production can be congenital, which are not discussed in this review, or acquired. Both viral and bacterial infections can affect platelet production. Viral infections, particularly rubella, cytomegalovirus, Epstein-Barr virus, and human immunodeficiency virus, cause decreased platelet production via megakaryocyte (MKC) infection or inhibition. Three nutritional deficiencies, cyanocobalamin (vitamin B_{12}), folate, and, very rarely, iron, can all cause TCP. Usually, though, all cell lines are involved, as platelet involvement occurs in late-stage disease. Any process that destroys or replaces the bone marrow can cause TCP by limiting the number of functional MKCs available for platelet production. Three classes of drugs, chemotherapeutic agents, thiazides, and estrogens, cause decreased platelet production via a mechanism separate from drug-induced TCP (see related paragraph), although the exact mechanism is unclear. Last, ingested toxins, such as cocaine and ethanol, in isolation of nutritional deficiencies, can limit platelet production.

The primary disease state that alters platelet distribution is hypersplenism of any cause. Hypersplenism causes a pancytopenia in most cases. Platelets are sequestered in the spleen, rather than destroyed, and can be mobilized during times of stress. Hypothermia (<25°C), via exposure or therapeutic procedures (cold cardioplegia), causes a thrombocytopenic state that is reversible on rewarming.

Platelet destruction can be immune mediated, consumptive, or microangiopathic. MKC can increase production threefold before TCP is seen. True autoimmune TCP is fairly common in adult women (women to men ratio, 3:1) in their 20s to 40s and is rarely life threatening. It can be seen in association with disease states such as lupus, in which 20% of patients (particularly those with the anticardiolipin antibody) will develop idiopathic thrombocytopenic purpura (ITP), lymphoproliferative disorders, and other solid tumors. In these conditions, an autoantibody (Ab) to GpIIb/IIIa and GpIb/IX (immunoglobulin G and rarely immunoglobulin M or complement) adheres to the platelet membrane, leaving the Fc portion available to bind to receptors within the reticuloendothelial system (RES). This binding induces phagocytosis and destruction of the affected platelets. A similar process is involved in viral infections.

Drug-induced TCP is mediated by one of two pathways. The first involves a drug-platelet hapten that is then phagocytosed by the RES. Platelets can also be destroyed in an "innocent bystander" fashion when drug-Ab complexes activate complement and cause RES or complement-mediated destruction. HIT warrants special consideration. Heparin can cause mild platelet activation, resulting in platelet factor (PF) 4 release. Immunoglobulin G Ab's against the heparin-PF4 complex are created and bind to platelet FcγIIa receptors, resulting in platelet clumping and activation, as well as endothelial activation and thrombin generation. Thus, although HIT is mediated by the immune system, the TCP is a consumptive process.

Two other forms of platelet destruction involve consumption: the microangiopathic hemolytic anemias (MHAs) and DIC. There are multiple causes for MHA, but the common result is endothelial damage, red blood cell fragmentation and destruction, complement activation, and platelet consumption. In DIC, a triggering event results in cytokine (TNF α and interleukin-6) release and extrinsic clotting pathway activation. Thrombin is generated, the fibrinolytic pathway is inhibited, and fibrin and platelet clots form, resulting in a consumptive TCP. Bleeding is promoted by TCP, depletion of clotting factors, and fibrin cleavage and fibrin split products' inhibition of platelet activity.

CLINICAL PRESENTATION

The clinical presentation and physical examination can often point the clinician to the possible etiologies of the TCP. In decreased production states, physical signs of the underlying disease process can aid the clinician in diagnosis. In splenic sequestration, a palpable spleen is mandatory for the diagnosis. Signs and symptoms of ITP are usually limited to the bleeding manifestations caused by the TCP. HIT patients are at risk for systemic thrombosis (3:1 venous to arterial), acral tissue necrosis, and limb gangrene. Ten percent to 20% of patients with HIT can develop skin lesions ranging from painful erythematous plaques to skin necrosis. Additionally, patients can have acute systemic reactions to heparin, presenting as rigors, fever, tachycardia, hypertension, tachypnea, chest pain, diaphoresis, nausea, vomiting, and diarrhea. The MHAs have variable clinical presentations, depending on the cause, and can include jaundice, HELLP syndrome (*h*emolysis, *e*levated *l*iver enzymes, *l*ow *p*latelets), fever and confusion [thrombotic thrombocytopenic purpura (TTP)], and renal failure (hemolytic uremic syndrome and, less frequently, TTP). Patients with DIC usu-

ally have multiple signs and symptoms related to the underlying disorder causing the DIC, and they may include fevers, hypotension, acidosis, proteinuria,
hypoxia, petechiae and purpura, hemorrhagic bullae, acral cyanosis, and bleeding from multiple sites.

DIAGNOSIS

Determining the etiology of TCP is based predominantly on the clinical scenario in which the patient presents. The first step involves a thorough medical history that includes a review of systems, an extensive drug history
(prescription and over the counter), and personal and family histories of
bleeding disorders. Physical examination should focus on signs of bleeding
(e.g., petechiae) clots, splenomegaly, signs of nutritional deficiencies, and
rashes. A full CBC with differential must be obtained. The peripheral smear
must be reviewed to confirm the TCP and rule out pseudo-TCP, evaluate
platelet morphology, and look at other cell lines. Evidence for microangiopathic disorders should be sought. If other cell lines are affected, then a
bone marrow biopsy should be considered. If the patient has TCP with
abnormal coagulation studies (activated partial thromboplastin time, prothrombin time) in the right clinical setting, DIC becomes increasingly likely.
In this scenario, further studies, including D-dimers (a byproduct of fibrinogen degradation; 93% sensitive if the DP-3B6/22 Ab is used), and fibrin split
products should be obtained. Fibrinogen has long been advocated in the
workup of DIC, but it is an acute phase reactant and sometimes difficult to
interpret. If the patient is receiving heparin, HIT becomes likely. Classically,
patients who have HIT have a platelet count of less than 150×10^9 or at least
a 50% decline in their platelet count after 5 days of heparin therapy. Patients
may have a nonimmune-mediated decline in platelets that is much less
severe in its decline and pathology. Patients who have been previously sensitized to heparin can have an earlier, precipitous decline in platelets. Multiple
HIT-related assays are available at reference laboratories and have variable
sensitivities and specificities. These assays are not readily available, however,
and interventions must be initiated before results are ready, thus limiting the
assays' applicability. If all above evaluations prove negative, then a drug-
induced TCP needs to be reconsidered and a thorough medication review
repeated.

MANAGEMENT

In cases of defects of platelet production, unless the underlying medical problem can be reversed (e.g., treating malignancies, infections) then supportive
measures with platelet transfusions are the mainstay of therapy. No absolute
recommendations have been made as to when transfusions must be initiated,
but evidence suggests that in patients who are not bleeding, the chances of
bleeding with a platelet count higher than 10,000 are low, and transfusions
need not be initiated. In altered distribution, therapy is usually not required,
as TCP is often mild, platelet function normal, and platelet release in stress
adequate. If necessary, splenectomy or splenic artery embolization may be
performed, but such therapy is rarely indicated. If drug-induced TCP is suspected, then all potential offending agents should be eliminated. ITP, HIT,
DIC, and TTP require specific therapies. In ITP, therapy is directed at lowering Ab production or interfering with RES function. Steroids (e.g., prednisone, 1 mg/kg or greater) are the mainstay of therapy and decrease Ab
production. Approximately 80% of patients respond to therapy within 1 to 2
weeks. Steroids should then be slowly tapered over 6 to 8 weeks. High-dose

immunoglobulins are also effective in ITP and can result in a rapid response, sometimes within 24 to 48 hours. Alternative therapies, aimed at limiting RES function, include anti-rho globulin, vincristine, danazol, and several immune suppressants, but should only be used under the direction of an experienced hematologist. If medical therapies fail or have unacceptable side effects, then the patient should undergo splenectomy. Therapy of HIT includes immediate termination of all exposure to heparin; however, as 50% of patients with HIT Ab will develop clots within 30 days, short-term anticoagulation with direct thrombin inhibitors, such as lepirudin or argatroban, should be considered. Patients requiring long-term anticoagulation should receive warfarin (Coumadin), but with overlapping parenteral anticoagulation to limit the possibility of skin necrosis. In DIC, the critical step in management is identifying and reversing the underlying cause. In patients with clots, heparin therapy should be used. Bleeding patients should receive replacement therapy with plasma and cryoprecipitate. In HELLP and preeclampsia, delivery of the baby almost universally corrects the problem. Treating the hypertension can relieve the TCP in malignant hypertension. TTP requires swift initiation of plasmapheresis and plasma transfusions. We now know that acquired TTP is caused by an inhibitor to a metaloprotease that cleaves von Willebrand factor multimers. Plasma exchange removes this inhibitor and replaces the missing protease. Platelet transfusions are contraindicated in TTP, as they can worsen the microthrombi and induce more tissue ischemia.

Chapter 59

SUPERIOR VENA CAVA SYNDROME

Lynn E. Sullivan

OVERVIEW

Superior vena cava (SVC) syndrome is a medical emergency in which the SVC is obstructed. Although the presentation of SVC syndrome is sometimes confused with allergic or infectious etiologies, it is important to consider this diagnosis in patients who have a known malignancy and to look for malignancy in patients with symptoms consistent with SVC syndrome.

PATHOPHYSIOLOGY

The SVC is the major blood vessel that drains venous blood from the head, neck, thorax, and upper extremities. It is an easily compressible vessel and therefore is susceptible to being occluded by tumor or lymph nodes adjacent to it. In addition, SVC syndrome can occur from the presence of a mass or a clot within the SVC itself. Obstruction of the venous return of the SVC causes a venous collateral circulation to develop, the azygos system being the most important. Patients typically present with engorged neck and chest veins secondary to increased circulation in the subcutaneous veins in the neck and thorax. Patients also complain of swelling around the face, particularly around the eyes; swelling of the neck and upper extremities; dyspnea; cough; hoarseness; dysphagia; and headache. The physical examination is notable for plethora, dilated neck veins, collaterals on their chest, and signs and symptoms that worsen when the patient bends forward or lies down.

In 90% to 95% of cases, malignancy is the cause of SVC syndrome and the syndrome is a presenting feature of lung cancer, lymphoma, and other malignancies. The tumors are primary mediastinal tumors or metastatic disease to the area. Eighty-five percent of these malignancies are lung cancers, one-half being small-cell carcinoma. The remaining 15% are lymphomas and germ cell and breast cancers. Although less common, benign causes include tuberculosis, syphilis, a goiter, aortic aneurysms, histoplasmosis, fibrotic mediastinitis, and thrombus secondary to a central venous catheter. Symptoms of recent onset are more likely to be malignant in etiology, whereas long-standing symptoms are more likely to be nonmalignant.

DIAGNOSIS

Chest radiography typically shows a mass on the right side of the chest. Fifty percent of patients have hilar adenopathy, and 25% have a pleural effusion. A diagnostic evaluation of the mass itself significantly impacts treatment, and a tissue diagnosis can be made via sputum cytology, lymph node biopsy, bone marrow aspiration, thoracentesis, bronchoscopy, mediastinoscopy, or thoracotomy.

MANAGEMENT

SVC syndrome is considered a medical emergency when the patient is experiencing respiratory distress or has evidence of laryngeal or cerebral edema. In these cases, patients require emergent treatment with diuretics and radiation treatment. The use of steroids in these cases is still considered controversial. In nonemergent situations, the diagnosis first should be confirmed, and then local radiation therapy is the usual approach; chemotherapy should be considered when chemosensitive tumors, such as small-cell lung cancer or lymphoma, are present. Patients with an obstructing thrombus should receive anticoagulation. Percutaneous stenting occasionally can be used to palliate SVC syndrome. A balloon catheter is used to dilate the vein, followed by placement of a stent. Recent studies revealed good response rates and low recurrence rates.

Chapter 60

SPINAL CORD COMPRESSION

Kathleen Stergiopoulos

OVERVIEW

Spinal cord compression (SCC) is a major cause of morbidity in patients with cancer and often renders a previously functioning patient bedridden or requiring a chronic care hospital for the rest of his or her life. Malignant SCC is a medical and surgical emergency that requires urgent diagnosis and treatment, because a delay can result in irreversible paralysis or loss of sphincter function, or both. In acute SCC, irreversible neurologic damage can occur within hours. It is crucial to diagnose SCC before the patient loses the ability to walk, because patients with SCC who are able to ambulate at presentation have a greater than 90% likelihood of walking after treatment. Patients who already have lost neurologic function are much less likely to walk after treatment. Thus, functional outcome depends on the functional status at the time of treatment. Prevention of complications is the goal of aggressive treatment, given that reversal of the primary process is usually not an option.

PATHOPHYSIOLOGY

SCC from metastasis occurs in 1% to 2% of all cancer cases, most commonly in lung, breast, and prostate cancers and lymphoma, although primary tumors of the central nervous system also should be considered. Less common cancers to metastasize to the vertebral bodies are renal cell carcinoma and sarcoma. Single or multiple lesions extend from the vertebral bodies posteriorly, invading the epidural space and eventually compressing the spinal cord. The hallmark of spinal cord dysfunction is usually demonstrated by motor, sensory, or autonomic dysfunction below an anatomic spinal level, although falsely localizing sensory signs should be evaluated. The sites of lesions are thoracic in 70% of patients, lumbar in 20% of patients, and cervical in 10% of patients.

CLINICAL PRESENTATION

SCC typically presents with back pain at the level of the compression, although some lesions may be painless. Back pain in patients with a history of a solid tumor should be taken very seriously, especially if new characteristics about the pain develop. The progression from back pain to SCC may follow an unpredictable time course. Other presenting symptoms are progressive difficulty walking secondary to weakness of both lower extremities, sensory loss and autonomic dysfunction manifested in urinary retention with overflow incontinence, and decreased anal sphincter tone with loss of stool continence. Cauda equina syndrome occurs from compression of the lumbar and sacral roots, producing sensory loss in a saddle distribution, termed *saddle anesthesia*; bilateral lower extremity weakness; decreased deep tendon reflexes; and bladder and bowel incontinence.

DIAGNOSIS

A thorough neurologic examination may reveal myelopathic signs, including a band of dysesthesia at the level of a lesion, with bilateral sensory and motor loss as well as diminished tone and reflexes below the level of the lesion. Rectal tone also should be evaluated.

Emergent magnetic resonance imaging (MRI) is indicated when SCC is suspected. MRI is the imaging modality of choice for evaluation of the spinal canal because of its ease of performance, superior contrast resolution, multiplanar capabilities, lack of ionizing radiation, and ability to detect multiple lesions. The entire spine should be imaged, because in 40% to 50% of patients, there are multiple sites of impingement. Myelography or computed tomography should only be used if MRI is not available. Myelography or computed tomography is inferior to MRI because of the additional risks of contrast material and the invasiveness of the procedure, with spinal needle placement and the possibility of exacerbating a SCC by removing cerebrospinal fluid below the level of a spinal cord compromise.

MANAGEMENT

Dexamethasone is indicated for patients with back pain or neurologic symptoms, or both (10 mg IV bolus, followed by 4–6 mg IV q6h) without delay. Emergent neurosurgical consultation is required, as well as involving the radiation oncology service. Treatment options include emergent neurosurgical decompression with laminectomy or high-dose steroids combined with emergent radiotherapy. There are no valid results confirming that surgery is superior to radiotherapy. Surgery is indicated if the patient already has received radiation therapy to the area, if the SCC is acute and progressing rapidly, or if there is progression despite treatment with steroids and radiation; however, combined high-dose steroids and radiotherapy are usually indicated for SCC secondary to malignancy. Important clinical parameters affecting treatment decisions and outcomes are ambulatory status at the time of diagnosis and the extent to which the tumor is radiosensitive. Other factors, such as the patient's general condition, multiple spinal compression sites, and metastases to major organs, such as brain and liver, must be considered. Acute and long-term supportive care includes airway management, diagnosing and treating pulmonary and urinary infections early, and prevention of contractures, pressure ulcers, and skin breakdown.

Chapter 61

PANCYTOPENIA AND APLASTIC ANEMIA

Melinda M. Mesmer

OVERVIEW

Pancytopenia is the decrease of all three cellular elements of the peripheral blood, the leukocytes, erythrocytes, and platelets. It describes a triad of findings rather than a disease state itself. Causes of pancytopenia include infiltration of the bone marrow space by fibrosis or a neoplastic process; peripheral loss of cells at the spleen, termed *splenic sequestration*; ineffective hematopoiesis; or a hypocellular or aplastic marrow. Aplastic anemia is diagnosed in the presence of pancytopenia with an "empty" or aplastic bone marrow. The primary defect is a deficiency in stem cells that results in aplasia and pancytopenia. Congenital stem cell defects can cause an aplastic marrow, but acquired aplasia is much more common. Fanconi's anemia is a congenital cause of aplastic anemia that is accompanied by skeletal deformities, skin changes, and short stature.

PATHOPHYSIOLOGY

Aplastic anemia is a pancytopenia caused by a hypocellular or acellular marrow. In severe cases, neutrophil counts may be depressed to less than 500 per mm^3, with platelet counts of less than 20,000 per mm^3, and reticulocytes of less than 40,000 per mm^3. In the marrow, there are hematopoietic precursors. Stem cells, which usually account for 1% of the marrow, cannot be recognized. Immunochemistry has shown that progenitor cells characteristically display CD34 and can be detected with flow cytometry. In cases of aplastic anemia, these CD34 cells are virtually absent in the marrow. The most common cause of aplastic anemia is iatrogenic, chemotherapy and radiation being the most typical provocative agents. In community-acquired cases of aplastic anemia, drug toxicity, alcohol use, and immune-mediated mechanisms are much more likely. Chemical exposures to compounds, such as benzene or hexachloride; ionizing radiation; and viral infections may all cause hypocellularity of marrow. An immune disorder can precipitate destruction of the marrow, as is the case of aplastic anemia associated with pregnancy. Radiation causes direct stem cell damage in a dose-dependent fashion. Cytotoxic agents used in chemotherapy are common identifiable causes of marrow toxicity and consequent bone marrow failure. Of the disorders causing infiltration of the bone marrow, neoplastic processes are most common. Other causes include myelofibrosis, agnogenic myeloid metaplasia, collagen vascular disease, alcohol, myelodysplasia, and changes associated with osteoporosis. In cases of bone marrow production, splenic sequestration becomes a more likely etiology. A metabolic abnormality, such as Gaucher's disease or Niemann-Pick disease, may infiltrate the spleen. Occasionally, an infectious agent can cause hypersplenism. Traditionally, miliary tuberculosis or other mycobacterium, syphilis, and brucellosis have been implicated as infiltrating the bone marrow or as infecting the spleen and causing a reactive pancytope-nia. The presence of splenomegaly is typically an indication that aplastic ane-mia is not present. Causes of ineffective hematopoiesis include folate and vitamin B_{12} deficiency. Dysfunctional marrow may also result from chronic disease or overwhelming infection. Systemic lupus erythematosus can some-times cause pancytopenia and must be excluded in a patient with pancytope-nia. Bicytopenia is the relative decrease of two of three of the formed elements in the blood. Although less common than pancytopenia, bicytope-nia may represent a progression toward pancytopenia or an entity in itself.

CLINICAL PRESENTATION

Aplastic anemia usually manifests with an insidious onset of anemia, thrombo-cytopenia, and leukopenia. The anemia causes excessive fatigue or decreased exercise tolerance. Thrombocytopenia associated with aplastic anemia may manifest as petechiae, easy bruisability, or bleeding. Leukopenia, particularly neutropenia, can lead to recurrent infections. A patient may present with splenomegaly, lymphadenopathy, or other signs and symptoms suggestive of a particular etiology, such as signs of vitamin deficiency in vitamin B_{12} and folate deficiencies.

DIAGNOSIS

A detailed history and physical examination can reveal many clinical signs and symptoms suggestive of the etiology of the pancytopenia. If the patient has splenomegaly, then leukemia, lymphoma, myelofibrosis, or congestive splenomegaly is the more likely diagnosis. The presence of lymphadenopathy is suggestive of systemic lupus erythematosus, leukemia, or lymphoma. If there is no lymphadenopathy or nutritional deficiency, such as vitamin B_{12} or folate insufficiency, then aplastic anemia should be considered. Nucleated red cells in the periphery, teardrops, and immature leukocytes are clues that an infiltrative disease is present. In most cases, a bone marrow aspirate with biopsy is required. Aplastic anemia characteristically displays pronounced hypocellular marrow with fatty infiltration and increased marrow stroma. The remaining progenitor cells are morphologically normal, and there should be no evidence of megaloblastic hematopoiesis. Dysplasia is not part of aplastic anemia and warrants investigation for myelodysplastic syndrome or aleuke-mic leukemia. Careful examination of the marrow is necessary to rule out malignant infiltrates and fibrosis, which would exclude the diagnosis of aplas-tic anemia.

MANAGEMENT

The initial intervention for any pancytopenia should be the identification and removal of the agents damaging the marrow. Supportive measures are the mainstay of treatment, but blood and platelet transfusions are often required. All transfusions should be administered very conservatively in patients who are candidates for bone marrow transplantation so as to prevent alloimmunization. The severity of aplastic anemia should be assessed to deter-mine prognosis and appropriateness of bone marrow transplantation.

Patients with severe or very severe aplastic anemia should be considered for bone marrow transplantation. Severe aplastic anemia is defined by a mar-row that is less than 30% cellular and at least two of the following peripheral blood criteria: an absolute neutrophil count of less than 500 per mm^3, a plate-let count of less than 20,000 per mm^3, and a reticulocyte count of less than 40,000 per mm^3. Very severe aplastic anemia is characterized by an absolute neutrophil count of less than 200 per mm^3. The overall prognosis of severe and very severe aplastic anemia is 70% mortality in untreated patients at 1 year. The elderly tend to have a worse prognosis. If the patient is younger than 45 years old and has a good functional status, then a related human leukocyte antigen–matched allogenic bone marrow transplant should be considered. Patients who lack an appropriate donor or who are too old for transplantation should be considered for immunosuppressive therapies. Licensed for use in the United States, antithymocyte globulin (ATG) produces hematologic responses in 40% to 50% of those patients who receive this treatment. The use of ATG leads to significantly improved blood counts, such that the patient is no longer susceptible to infection and does not require continued blood product transfusions. The addition of cyclosporine to the ATG is typically needed in cases of severe aplastic anemia, and this combination of therapies leads to improved rates of response and survival.

Chapter 62

MYELODYSPLASIA, LEUKEMIA, AND BLAST CRISIS

Melinda M. Mesmer

OVERVIEW

Leukemias arise from the expansion of a neoplastic clone of hematopoietic cells. Often this results in a large dysfunctional population of blood cells with the suppression of the production of normal blood cells. As a result, patients have recurrent infections, bleeding, anemia, or hyperviscosity, or a combination of these. Not all leukemias result in high numbers of circulating blood cells, and some patients present with cytopenia. Leukemias are categorized as acute or chronic on the basis of their clinical behavior and the amount of immature cells in the blood and bone marrow.

Acute leukemias may evolve *de novo*, from antecedent myelodysplasia, or from chronic myelogenous leukemia. Of the *de novo* acute leukemias, acute myelogenous leukemia (AML) is most common in patients older than 55 years, and acute lymphocytic leukemia (ALL) is most common in patients younger than 15 years. In acute leukemia, per definition, the bone marrow contains at least 20% blasts.

Chronic leukemias are malignancies resulting in the overproduction of myeloid cells (CML) or lymphocytes (CLL). The dominant clone of malignant cells in both cases maintains the ability to differentiate; hence, they produce large numbers of mature cells, in contrast with the overabundance of immature cells in acute leukemias. In the early stages of CML, cells are immunocompetent; therefore, the clinical course of the disease is often mild at this

detect the bcr/abl translocation. The prognosis of CML can be affected by the presence or absence of either the Philadelphia chromosome or the bcr/abl translocation.

The diagnosis of CLL may be incidental and based on an asymptomatic lymphocytosis on peripheral blood. In less than 10% of cases, an autoimmune hemolytic anemia or thrombocytopenia is present at diagnosis. For diagnostic purposes, the test of choice is flow cytometry, which reveals the typical immunophenotype of these cells.

MANAGEMENT

Acute leukemia is a medical emergency. The functional status of each patient should be weighed against the morbidity associated with the treatment. Treatment is targeted at decreasing the amount of leukemic cells, and enabling the normal hematopoietic clones to repopulate the bone marrow. Elimination of the malignant clone is the ultimate goal. In AML, current therapies use two chemotherapeutic agents (an anthracycline or anthraquinone and cytarabine). If remission is not achieved after the first cycle, a second, similar regimen is used. Tretinoin (all-*trans*-retinoic acid) is added at induction in acute promyelocytic leukemia.

With ALL, typically adults are induced with vincristine, prednisone, daunorubicin, and asparaginase. Hydroxyurea may be used as a temporizing measure to reduce the white blood cell count. Therapy with alpha-interferon, with or without low-dose cytarabine, may also result in remission and delay progression of disease, but it is poorly tolerated and less effective than imatinib. The only curative treatment is allogeneic bone marrow transplant, and this approach should be offered to the younger patient with a human leukocyte antigen–matched sibling.

Treatment of CLL is palliative and is reserved for patients with anemia, thrombocytopenia, recurrent infections, systemic symptoms, or bulky lymphadenopathy. Active chemotherapy agents include chlorambucil, fludarabine, and other agents used for the treatment of lymphomas, usually in combination with steroids. Rituximab and other monoclonal antibodies are emerging as effective and well-tolerated agents in this disease.

Chapter 63

MYELOPROLIFERATIVE DISORDERS

Richard Mark White

OVERVIEW

The term *myeloproliferative disorder* refers to a group of related disorders that are characterized by an abnormal proliferation of a pluripotent stem cell that leads to overproduction of various hematologic cell types. There are four main variants of myeloproliferative disorder: polycythemia vera (PV; red cell overproduction), essential thrombocythemia (ET; platelet overproduction), agnogenic myeloid metaplasia (AMM) with myelofibrosis (marrow fibrosis with extramedullary hematopoiesis), and chronic myelogenous leukemia (CML; neutrophil overproduction). Although usually clinically distinct, there is significant clinical overlap between these disorders. Epidemiologic studies have shown an incidence trend of PV of 2.3 per 100,000. There is a slight male predominance, and it most commonly occurs in ages 50 to 70 years. ET is generally most common in middle age and more frequently seen in women. The estimated annual incidence of AMM is 0.5 per 100,000. The incidence of CML is approximately 1 in 100,000, and it increases with age. Most cases of CML are diagnosed during middle age, with a median age at diagnosis of 53 years; there is a slight male predominance (1.5:1.0), and the incidence may also be affected by exposure to radiation.

PATHOPHYSIOLOGY

The clonal basis of most myeloproliferative disorders has been established by several methods. Thus, it is likely that all of these disorders are a result of mutations in single stem cell precursors, although the particular stem cell type in each disorder may vary. Various cytogenetic abnormalities, most commonly trisomy 8 and 9, have been identified in 12% to 40% of patients with PV, depending on the stage. Several groups have demonstrated that the erythroid precursor colony-forming units from patients with PV do not require the presence of erythropoietin (EPO) for growth, in contrast to those from healthy individuals. This finding suggests abnormalities in EPO sensitivity or receptor function in PV, and in fact, the erythroid colony-forming units from PV patients only express the low affinity form of the EPO receptor. Little is known about the genetic or pathogenic mechanisms in ET. There is an increase in the megakaryocyte pool, and there is dysregulation of platelet production. No specific cytogenetic or oncogenic mutations have been described. AMM has been etiologically linked with exposure to both petroleum derivatives, such as toluene or benzene, and to ionizing radiation. These exposures likely initiate a mutagenic course in susceptible hematopoietic stem cells, which then gives rise to the characteristic clonal nature of the disease. The fibrosis seen in the marrow of patients with AMM is thought to be reactive phenomena, and the fibroblasts in the marrow mediating the fibrosis are not clonal. The occurrence of CML is clearly linked to the presence of the Philadelphia chromosome, which represents a translocation between the protooncogene ABL (on chromosome 9) to the BCR locus (on chromosome 22). This translocation results in the production of the abnormal fusion protein bcr-abl, which is a tyrosine kinase. Cells expressing this bcr-abl protein are less responsive to normal growth-inhibitory signals (i.e., adhesion or stromal cell interactions) and undergo slightly more divisions when compared to normal cells. Therefore, the overall effect of the Philadelphia chromosome is to enhance proliferation of a clone of myeloid cells that has growth advantages over normal hematopoietic cells.

CLINICAL PRESENTATION

The classic patient with PV has a ruddy complexion, conjunctival suffusion, and pruritus after a hot bath. As the disease progresses, the major complications arise from increasing whole-blood viscosity, leading to occlusive arterial or venous lesions in the cerebral, cardiac, portal venous, or peripheral venous systems. The expanded red cell mass can also lead to central nervous system symptoms, such as headache, vision changes, dizziness, and a marked increase in the risk of cerebrovascular accidents. Other characteristic findings in PV include systemic hypertension and peptic ulcer disease, although the etiology of both of these is unclear. The majority of patients with ET are symptomatic at diagnosis, although a significant number are found incidentally by automated routine complete blood counts. The clinical picture of ET is characterized by episodes of both thrombosis and hemorrhage. An increased risk of hemorrhage occurs especially when the platelet count is more than 1,000,000. Erythromelalgia is a characteristic symptom of both ET and PV, in which micro-occlusions of the vasculature of the extremities cause warm, red, congested extremities with burning pain. Major sites of thrombosis are the central nervous system arteries (producing stroke), coronary arteries, peripheral deep veins, splanchnic system, and portal veins. The most common site of hemorrhage is the gastrointestinal tract, but patients may also bleed from the skin and mucosal sites. In AMM, patients are asymptomatic at presentation in 25% of cases. The most common symptoms reported include those related to a hypermetabolic state, such as fever, fatigue, weight loss, night sweats, and attacks of gout. As the disease progresses, patients may complain of symptomatic splenomegaly (described as a mass in the abdomen or early satiety), bleeding complications, or symptoms related to anemia. Most patients have significant splenomegaly, and 50% may have hepatomegaly as well. The organomegaly is secondary to extramedullary hematopoiesis. The symptomatology in CML is directly related to the stage of the disease. As the disease progresses through the chronic, accelerated, and finally blastic stages, symptoms become progressively more severe. Early on, most patients are asymptomatic, and their disease is detected on routine blood counts. Later, patients may present with symptoms and signs of a hypermetabolic state, as seen in AMM. Splenomegaly generally correlates with the degree of white blood cell elevation, and thus may not be a prominent finding early in the disease. In contrast to AMM, hepatomegaly is less common. Finally, patients may also present with bleeding, thrombosis, or anemia, depending on the degree of leukocytosis and suppression of normal hematopoiesis.

DIAGNOSIS

The characteristic finding in PV is an increase in all cell lines, but most prominently in the erythroid lines. An increase in the red blood cell mass is required for diagnosis. The red cells are usually morphologically normal, but occasional normoblasts may be seen in the peripheral smear. Most patients also have a moderate leukocytosis and thrombocytosis at the time of diagnosis. The leukocyte alkaline phosphatase is elevated in PV, in contrast to that seen in CML. Other laboratory findings include pseudohyperkalemia due to high platelet counts and hyperuricemia secondary to increased cell turnover. The bone marrow of these patients shows diffuse hypercellularity affecting all cell lines. Patients with ET have thrombocytosis. A mild leukocytosis is common, but the hematocrit is usually normal. Pseudohyperkalemia may be observed from the elevated platelet count. Bleeding time, prothrombin time, and partial thromboplastin time are usually normal, although many patients demonstrate hemorrhagic complications. The platelets are often bizarre, large, and abnormal in structure. The bone marrow reveals megakaryocyte hyperplasia but without fibrosis, and with adequate iron stores. The characteristic peripheral blood finding of AMM is leukoerythroblastosis, reflecting an increase in release of early precursors from both the marrow and sites of extramedullary hematopoiesis. Bone marrow aspiration is usually a "dry tap" due to increased fibrosis, and when it is obtained, shows increased reticulin in the setting of trilineage hyperplasia. Depending on the stage of disease, various degrees of anemia, thrombocytopenia, and leukopenia may develop owing to ineffective hematopoiesis. This finding is also reflected in the increased uric acid and lactate dehydrogenase levels. Some patients also have clinical or subclinical episodes of hemolytic anemia, which may contribute to the overall decrease in hematocrit seen at various stages of disease. The peripheral blood findings during the chronic phase of CML consist of a left-shifted neutrophilia containing all stages of neutrophil differentiation, as well as basophilia and eosinophilia. Pseudo Pelger-Huët cells may be seen. Blasts are less than 20% in the chronic phase. A mild thrombocytosis is usually present, and anemia of chronic disease is not uncommon. The leukocyte alkaline phosphatase level is low, despite the high numbers of circulating leukocytes. As the disease progresses to the accelerated, or blast, phase, the percent of blasts in the bone marrow increases. In approximately two-thirds of patients with CML who develop acute leukemia, it is of the myeloid lineage, whereas in one-third, the blast crisis is of the lymphoid lineage. The most characteristic finding of CML is the presence of the Philadelphia chromosome. Although classically demonstrated by cytogenetic translocation of the ABL locus on chromosome 9 to the BCR locus on chromosome 22, some patients may have subtle translocations not readily appreciated by cytogenetics; however, the presence of an abnormal bcr-abl fusion protein is demonstrable by polymerase chain reaction or by fluorescence *in situ* hybridization in most of these patients.

MANAGEMENT

The most widely used therapy for PV is phlebotomy, with or without antiplatelet therapy. The goal is obtaining a normal hematocrit of 42 to 46. For long-term management, phlebotomy has been shown to be superior to alkylating agents or radioactive phosphorus. The benefits are somewhat offset by the increased risk of thrombosis in the phlebotomy group, however. This occurrence is of greatest concern in those patients with a history of coronary disease or previous evidence of thrombotic disease. The use of antiplatelet agents to decrease this risk has shown mixed results. Alkylating agents currently have only a limited role in PV, as they are associated with a significantly increased risk of transformation to acute leukemia. Similarly, radioactive phosphorus also increases the risk of acute leukemia; however, it may be appropriate for elderly patients who are not compliant with chronic oral therapy. Hydroxyurea is one of the most useful agents in PV, as it decreases the counts in all three cell lines, in contrast to phlebotomy, and decreases the risk of thrombotic complications. Major side effects include anemia, thrombocytopenia, and leukopenia if the dose is not adjusted appropriately; diarrhea, and leg ulcers. It may be associated with a slightly increased risk of leukemia. In ET, aspirin reduces or eliminates the symptoms of erythromelalgia and central nervous system microvascular occlusions. Long-term therapy with hydroxyurea is clearly effective in terms of reduction in thrombotic event rates. Anagrelide is a relatively new drug of unknown mechanism of action that lowers platelet counts in 90% of patients. It appears to have cardiovascular side effects, including peripheral edema, palpitations, arrhythmias, and congestive heart failure. The exact role of this agent, and how it fits into the treatment scheme, is an area of ongoing study. Finally, for patients presenting with acute, life-threatening thromboses, platelet pheresis is the most rapid, efficient mechanism to acutely lower the platelet count. This approach can be combined with hydroxyurea to produce a sustained reduction in platelet counts after the acute event has resolved. Therapy for CML has undergone a major advance over the last 4 years, with the development of imatinib mesylate (Gleevec), which is a selective inhibitor of the abnormal tyrosine kinase produced by the bcr/abl fusion gene. This oral therapy induces remissions in the majority of patients and delays the transformation to blast crisis. Allogeneic matched-sibling stem cell transplant (SCT) is indicated in recently diagnosed younger patients, ages 30 to 40 years old, who are in the chronic phase of CML. "Cure" rates of 50% to 55% at 10 years can be seen. The transplant-associated mortality rate for older patients is 30% to 50%. Ten percent to 20% of patients who receive allogeneic SCT have a disease relapse, usually occurring within 3 years of transplant. Subsequent treatment choices include a second SCT, alpha-interferon (INF), or infusion of donor lymphocytes. Alpha-INF produces complete hematologic remission and complete cytogenetic remission within a median time of 6 to 7 months and 12 to 17 months, respectively. Survival rates with alpha-INF have exceeded 9 years in patients with low-risk disease. In addition, 80% of patients with complete cytogenetic response survive for more than 10 years. Donor lymphocyte infusion induces complete remission via a graft-versus-tumor effect in 60% to 80% of patients who relapse with CML and is most effective when given within 2 years of SCT.

Chapter 64

MULTIPLE MYELOMA

Richard Mark White

OVERVIEW

Multiple myeloma (MM) is the prototype of a group of disorders characterized by overproduction of immunoglobulin chains. The clinical spectrum of these diseases, (which include overt myeloma, monoclonal gammopathy of undetermined significance, Waldenström's macroglobulinemia, and plasmacytomas), is dependent on the particular type and amount of immunoglobulin produced, the burden of disease, and the biology of the individual proliferating cell types.

MM accounts for 1% of all malignancies in the United States. It is relatively rare in people younger than 40 years of age, and the peak incidence appears to occur in the mid-sixties. It is two times as common in men and in blacks.

Numerous environmental risk factors have been implicated, but never proven, as risk factors for MM. They include exposure to benzene, ionizing radiation, and pesticides. Recently, it has been suggested that MM may be due to an infection with the human herpesvirus 8, as this virus may be demonstrated in the dendritic cells of some patients with MM. To date, however, no clear evidence of viral oncogenesis has been demonstrated, and it remains an area of speculation. Genetic factors leading to MM were originally suggested by the finding of increased incidence of MM in blacks versus whites; however, classic cytogenetic studies have demonstrated abnormalities in only 20% of cases, usually involving loss of portions of chromosome 13.

PATHOPHYSIOLOGY

The critical difference between overt MM and monoclonal gammopathies of undetermined significance likely lies in the transformation of a single clone of plasma cells into a malignant phenotype in the former. Thus, the distinguishing characteristic of MM is overproduction of an immunoglobulin (Ig) molecule containing two identical heavy chains (most commonly of the IgG, IgA, or IgM types) with two identical light chains (kappa or lambda). The critical steps in malignant transformation appear to be linked to overproduction of interleukin (IL)-6, which prevents normal apoptotic mechanisms in the plasma cells. The IL-6 originates from the supporting stromal cells in the bone marrow, likely demonstrating the importance of the bone marrow microenvironment in the development of MM. Other mutations in such genes as bcl-2, p53, and ras also likely contribute to prevention of apoptosis in the malignant clone and allow the disease to progress.

Survival is directly related to stage of disease. Thus, for patients in stage IA (low M-protein concentration, absence of hypercalcemia or renal failure), the median survival is 5 years. In contrast, in older series, patients with markedly elevated M proteins and numerous skeletal lesions, even in the absence of renal insufficiency (stage III), had a median survival of only 15 months. The median survival of patients with MM has improved significantly over the last few decades, however, with the availability of multiple new therapeutic agents.

CLINICAL PRESENTATION

Many patients with MM are asymptomatic at diagnosis, and the disease is found in the workup of unexplained anemia or renal failure; however, patients can present with a variety of symptoms, including pathologic bone fractures, pain, fatigue, acute renal failure, and recurrent infections. Normocytic, normochromic anemia is seen in the majority of patients. It is usually due to a combination of marrow replacement, renal failure, and anemia of chronic disease. Bleeding may be seen late in the disease and likely is related to attachment of immunoglobulin to platelet membranes. Diffuse, lytic bone lesions are a hallmark of the disease. These changes are primarily due to the action of IL-6, which results in osteoclast activation. Generalized osteopenia is the most common bony manifestation of MM and is found in most patients. Vertebral body involvement may result in compression fractures that can cause cord compression. Impending fractures are often heralded by persistent pain, particularly with movement, and may require emergent radiation or surgical pinning.

At least 25% of patients present with a serum creatinine over 2.0 mg per dL. Renal failure is most commonly due to "myeloma kidney," which is caused by precipitation of myeloma proteins (Bence-Jones proteins) within the tubules. The condition is worsened by dehydration, contrast agents, and urinary acidification (e.g., from vitamin C). Other causes of renal failure include hypercalcemia, dehydration, urate nephropathy, obstructive uropathy (e.g., from plasmacytoma or spinal cord compression), or rarely from amyloidosis of the AL subtype.

Increased susceptibility to encapsulated organisms (*Streptococcus pneumoniae, Haemophilus influenzae, Staphylococcus epidermidis*) is seen early in the disease because of decreased production of normal immunoglobulins in favor of the monoclonal immunoglobulin. Hypercalcemia is directly related to osteoclast activation and bony destruction. "Spurious" hypercalcemia may be observed in some cases owing to binding of calcium to the immunoglobulins, and thus ionized calcium should be checked before ascribing symptoms to elevated calcium.

Plasmacytomas may present with local symptoms, such as spinal cord compression. Rarely, monoclonal immunoglobulin production may be associated with the POEMS syndrome (*p*olyneuropathy of the sensory type, *o*rganomegaly of liver, *e*ndocrinopathy giving diabetes of hypogonadism, *M* spike, and *s*kin changes).

DIAGNOSIS

Pallor is the most common finding on examination. Plasmacytomas commonly present as isolated rib masses or as vertebral masses. Examination for signs of spinal cord compression is essential. Liver enlargement may occur, although splenomegaly is unusual. MM may be diagnosed by the presence of an M spike on serum or urine electrophoresis (typically showing more than 3.5 g per dL of IgG or 2 g per dL of IgA, or more than 1 g of kappa or lambda chains in a 24-hour urine collection), bone marrow with greater than 10% plasma cells, and the presence of hypercalcemia, lytic bone lesions, or otherwise unexplained renal failure. Prognostic indicators include an elevated plasma cell labeling index (PCLI; measures DNA synthesis in plasma cells), elevated IL-6 levels, and increased beta-2-microglobulin levels or C-reactive protein levels (both of which correlate with disease burden). The PCLI is particularly useful and helps to distinguish MM from monoclonal gammopathy of undetermined significance, in which the PCLI is typically low. Urine should be collected for 24 hours and the concentrated specimen examined with electrophoresis. Approximately 75% of patients have elevated urinary light chain excretion (Bence-Jones proteinuria). Between the serum and urine examinations, 98% of patients with MM are found to have an M protein. Because of the absence of osteoblastic activity, radionuclide bone scans are notoriously insensitive for workup of skeletal disease in MM; plain skeletal surveys (which must include the skull and weight-bearing bones) are preferred.

MANAGEMENT

Not all patients with MM are initially treated. A three-tier staging system has been developed, taking into account the level of M protein, number of bony lesions, serum calcium, and degree of renal impairment. Patients with early stages, I or II, may be observed closely for signs of progression or development of worsening signs or symptoms. Many patients require treatment at presentation, however, even without extensive disease burden, owing to pain or renal impairment.

The mainstay of treatment remains the combination of oral melphalan and prednisone (MP). Most patients initially respond to MP with a decrease and then plateau of the M-protein concentration, improvement in hypercalcemia and pain, and reduction in serum creatinine. The major complication of this therapy is myelosuppression and infection. Another commonly used regimen is VAD [vincristine, doxorubicin (Adriamycin), dexamethasone], which is preferred in patients being considered for bone marrow transplant. Relapse after MP is inevitable. Salvage regimens typically consist of VAD, as above, although once the disease has relapsed, it becomes increasingly difficult to treat. Thalidomide, through unknown mechanisms possibly involving cytokine modulation and inhibition of angiogenesis, has been shown to be a well-tolerated and very effective agent in this disease, both as initial therapy, and as a salvage approach. It is commonly combined with steroids, usually dexamethasone.

In selected patients, with good performance status and age under 70 years, high-dose chemotherapy with autologous stem cell rescue has been shown to prolong survival, although it is not curative. There has been recent interest in using high-dose chemotherapy with stem cell rescue early in disease, before any other therapy. This approach is showing promise: 81% of patients in the high-dose arm had responses, compared to only 57% in the standard chemotherapy arm. A large, ongoing trial is examining long-term benefit and survival of this approach. Allogeneic stem cell transplant is potentially curative in MM; however, it is available only to the younger patient with a matched donor.

Focal plasmacytomas respond well to radiation therapy, and it may be curative in rare patients. Radiation is also useful, for pain related to lytic skeletal lesions. Surgical intervention may be required for unstable skeletal lesions.

The bisphosphonates (i.e., pamidronate and zoledronic acid) have been shown to significantly protect against skeletal complications, confer a survival benefit, and treat hypercalcemia. All patients with MM and skeletal disease should be placed on these agents.

Renal insufficiency often improves with institution of therapy against the underlying MM; however, it is important to instruct patients to avoid dehydration, avoid the use of vitamin C or other urinary acidification, and minimize exposure to radiographic contrast. Up to 10% of MM patients may develop evidence of AL amyloidosis and the associated renal disease.

Anemia responds to erythropoietin, especially early in the course of the disease. Prophylactic antibiotics are advocated by some practitioners to avoid the predictable encapsulated organism infections.

Chapter 65

BREAST CANCER

Meredith Talbot

OVERVIEW

Breast cancer is the most common cancer in women and is the second leading cause of cancer death in women. Breast cancer is diagnosed in more than 170,000 women annually, and the American Cancer Society estimates that in 2004, almost one-third of all cancers diagnosed in women will be breast cancers. A woman's average lifetime risk for developing breast cancer is one in eight.

Risk factors for developing breast cancer include age older than 50 [relative risk (RR), 6.5], family history of breast cancer in a first-degree relative (RR, 1.4 to 13.6), atypical hyperplasia on a breast biopsy (RR, 4.0 to 4.4), delayed child bearing (older than age 30) (RR, 1.3 to 2.2), early menarche (younger than 12 years) (RR, 1.2 to 1.5), late menopause (older than age 55) (RR, 1.5 to 2.0), and hormone replacement therapy (RR, 1.0 to 1.5). Age is the most significant risk factor. Assessing a patient's risk for developing breast cancer is important, as it influences decisions regarding screening, hormone replacement therapy, and use of tamoxifen or prophylactic mastectomy to prevent breast cancer. Despite knowledge of risk factors, only 12% of breast cancer patients have an identifiable risk factor.

The prognosis of breast cancer is based on nodal involvement and tumor size. With no nodal involvement, there is a 78% 5-year survival rate and a 65% 10-year survival rate; with nodal involvement, there is a 46% 5-year survival rate and a 25% 10-year survival rate.

PATHOPHYSIOLOGY

The pathophysiology of breast cancer is unknown, but strong evidence links estrogen and its metabolites to the development and growth of breast cancer. Direct effects of estrogen may include the induction of enzymes and proteins involved in nucleic acid synthesis and activation of oncogenes. Indirect effects may include the stimulation of prolactin and production of growth factors, such as epidermal growth factor.

Almost all breast cancers are adenocarcinomas derived from the glandular epithelium of either the mammary lobules (10–15%) or the mammary ducts (72%). Carcinomas are described as either *in situ* (not breaching basement membrane) or invasive. Lobular carcinoma *in situ* confers a 20% to 30% risk of developing invasive cancer over 20 years (one-half of which will be in the contralateral breast), whereas ductal cancer *in situ* confers a 30% risk.

CLINICAL PRESENTATION

Many women are asymptomatic and are diagnosed on screening, and others present with breast masses. Characteristics of masses that favor malignancy are painless, hard lumps with irregular borders. Other concerning physical findings are skin swelling, dimpling (*peau d'orange*), nipple inversion, and bloody, unilateral nipple discharge.

DIAGNOSIS

Diagnosis of breast cancer begins with screening. The American Cancer Society has the following specific guidelines based on age and risk factors:

- Any age with strong family history:
  - Provider preference
- 20 to 39 years:
  - Clinical breast examination every 3 years
  - Self breast examination monthly
- 40 years and older:
  - Clinical breast examination annually
  - Self breast examination monthly
  - Mammogram annually

It has been estimated that screening mammography can reduce breast cancer deaths by 50%.

Breast examination includes inspection in the supine and upright positions to look for retractions, nipple inversion, nipple discharge, or skin changes. Palpation for lymph nodes should occur in the upright position and breast examination in the supine position.

If an abnormality is noted, a mammogram is usually obtained. Ultrasound can be used in young women to rule out the presence of a cyst. If a mass is seen on imaging, a fine-needle aspirate (sensitivity, 82%; specificity, 97%) is usually performed. Core needle and open biopsies may also be obtained. The choice of which to use depends on many factors, such as mass size, location, number of lesions, and how suspicious the mass appears.

MANAGEMENT

Invasive ductal carcinoma is usually treated with lumpectomy or partial mastectomy. Tumors that are large, have microcalcifications throughout the breast, or have a histologic pattern of "extensive intraductal component" are usually treated with mastectomy. Either treatment is accompanied by lymph node evaluation, followed by whole-breast radiation. Because of the morbidity associated with complete lymph node dissection, intraoperative lymph node mapping and sentinel lymph node identification are often used. Adjuvant therapy with chemotherapy, immunotherapy, tamoxifen, or ovarian ablation is usually used in patients with nodal involvement. Usually, premenopausal women receive chemotherapy or ovarian ablation, whereas postmenopausal women are offered tamoxifen. Women with inherited mutations, such as BRCA1 and BRCA2 tumor suppressor genes, have a 50% to 80% lifetime risk of breast cancer. These individuals may benefit from prophylactic mastectomy or tamoxifen.

Chapter 66

LUNG CANCER

Henry Klar Yaggi

OVERVIEW

In the United States, lung cancer is the leading cause of cancer mortality in men and women. Although there has been a decrease in lung cancer incidence and death rates among men in the United States since the early 1990s, the incidence and mortality from this disease have steadily increased in women for the past several decades. A dose-response relationship exists between cigarette smoking and the development of lung cancer. The four major cell types of lung cancer and their approximate relative incidence are adenocarcinoma (31–34%), squamous cell carcinoma (30%), small-cell carcinoma (20–25%), and large-cell carcinoma (10–16%). Bronchoalveolar cell carcinomas (alveolar cell carcinomas) are considered adenocarcinomas and comprise approximately 3% to 4% of lung carcinomas.

PRESENTATION

The average patient with carcinoma of the lung is a heavy cigarette smoker in the sixth or seventh decade of life. Approximately 5% of patients are asymptomatic, and the tumor is discovered on routine radiographic examinations of the chest. Other patients have one or more symptoms related to the presence of the tumor within the thoracic cavity, including cough, hemoptysis, localized wheeze, dyspnea, vague chest pain, hoarseness (recurrent laryngeal nerve involvement), superior vena cava syndrome (compression or invasion of superior vena cava), and Horner's syndrome (superior sulcus tumors involving the brachial plexus). Symptoms caused by metastatic spread include hemiplegia, epilepsy, changes in mental status, and speech deficits caused by intracranial metastases. Less frequently, bone pain and pathologic fractures, abdominal mass, jaundice, and ascites can occur. Symptoms from paraneoplastic syndromes may also occur, usually as a result of secretion of endocrine or endocrinelike substances from the tumor. Common syndromes include Cushing's syndrome (ectopic adrenocorticotropic hormone production), the syndrome of inappropriate antidiuretic hormone secretion, carcinoid syndrome (flushing, diarrhea, tachycardia, wheezing, pruritus), hypercalcemia (excessive secretion of parathyroid hormone–related protein), carcinomatous neuromyopathies, and digital clubbing associated with hypertrophic pulmonary osteoarthropathy (periostitis with elevation of the periosteum and new bone formation).

DIAGNOSIS

Because early-stage lung cancer has significantly better cure rates (as high as 70% and even higher for early stage IA), emphasis has been placed on screening techniques for the early diagnosis. Although there are no official recommendations that advocate screening high-risk patients for lung carcinoma with chest radiography or sputum cytology, promising preliminary data on screening with low-dose chest computed tomography (CT) have been reported, and further trials assessing this approach are under way.

Most lung cancers are detected by the standard chest radiograph or CT scan. It is usually difficult to differentiate benign from malignant lesions radiographically, yet certain radiographic signs, such as spiculation, eccentric calcification, and the presence of lymphadenopathy, may suggest malignancy. Tissue biopsy is commonly obtained either by fiberoptic bronchoscopy with transbronchial biopsy or percutaneous transthoracic needle biopsy. CT or fluoroscopy is used to guide most biopsies. After tissue diagnosis of lung carcinoma is made, the disease is staged to assess extent, select correct therapy, and determine prognosis. The most widely accepted staging system for non–small cell carcinoma is the tumor, node, metastasis or TNM classification system. The staging system commonly used for small-cell carcinoma is simply whether the disease is limited or extensive based on whether it is confined to the ipsilateral hemithorax. The crucial element in staging is whether mediastinal involvement has occurred, which determines in most cases whether surgery is performed. CT remains the procedure of choice for evaluating the mediastinum. Positron emission tomography has been introduced as a useful noninvasive method for diagnosing and staging lung cancer, particularly combined with CT for intrathoracic lymph node staging and as a whole-body test for extrathoracic staging of lung cancer.

MANAGEMENT

Most authorities agree that surgical resection is the proper treatment of lung cancer when there is a reasonable chance of removing all the lung cancer with an acceptable risk of morbidity and mortality; therefore, stages I and II non–small cell lung cancers are usually resected. Patients with clinical IIIA lesions are considered candidates for preoperative chemotherapy with radiation therapy followed by surgical resection, but further randomized controlled trials are awaited to determine the best therapy for IIIA disease. The management of small-cell lung cancer is largely based on systemic treatment with combination chemotherapy rather than on surgical resection, which typically is used for non–small cell lung cancer. Although complete surgical resection remains the cornerstone of therapy for non–small cell lung cancer, curative resection is feasible in fewer than one-third of patients, owing to presence of advanced disease at diagnosis and comorbid illness. For patients not able to undergo surgery, the goal of therapy is to control the tumor both locally and at distant sites. Combined-modality approaches using radiation therapy and chemotherapy are currently recommended for such patients.

Chapter 67

COLORECTAL CANCER

Richard Mark White

OVERVIEW

Cancer of the large bowel and rectum represents a major public health problem that affects adults at every age group, with a median age at diagnosis of 65 years. In Western countries, such as the United States, the number of newly diagnosed cases each year exceeds 131,000. A greater understanding of the process by which this disease develops has led to significant advances in screening, diagnosis, and treatment.

Colon cancer is the second leading cause of cancer death in the United States, behind lung cancer. Overall mortality has not decreased in the past 50 years, although subgroup analysis shows that it has decreased by 20% in white women but increased by 22% in black men for reasons that are unknown. By far, the majority of these tumors are adenocarcinomas (99%), although other histologies, such as lymphoma, carcinoid tumors, and Kaposi's sarcoma, occur. Most cases occur in individuals older than 50 years, and high socioeconomic status is associated with increased risk. Certain familial genetic predispositions (hereditary polyposis coli, Gardner's syndrome, hereditary nonpolyposis coli) markedly increase the risk of colon cancer. These syndromes have provided extensive evidence that specific genetic alterations (e.g., DCC, APC, hMSH2 genes) are important in the pathogenesis of this malignancy.

Diet has long been suggested to be the critical factor in colon cancer, because the incidence is so strikingly different around the world (high in the United States, extremely low in Japan and Africa), and immigrants adopt the risk of their new countries. A low-fiber diet was initially thought to increase risk, but a recent trial of high-fiber diets failed to support this theory. Animal fats are thought to explain some of the dietary risk, as both the Nurses Health Study and the Health Professional Follow-Up Study showed that diets high in animal (generally saturated) fats was associated with increased risk. Other risk factors include inflammatory bowel disease, prior *Streptococcus bovis* septicemia, and tobacco use.

PATHOPHYSIOLOGY

Much has been learned about the development of colon cancer in the past decade. It now appears likely that neoplasms of the colon or rectum arise in what has been called the *dysplastic polyp-to-cancer sequence.*

Colorectal polyps can be classified as juvenile (hamartomas), inflammatory, hyperplastic, or adenomatous. It appears that only adenomatous polyps progress on to cancer. Within the adenomatous polyps themselves, several patterns have emerged. Villous are more likely than tubular adenomas to contain invasive carcinoma, and larger polyps are more likely to have villous (and potentially neoplastic) components. Several lines of evidence have suggested that these adenomatous polyps are the precursors to cancer. First, patients who are found to have them on colonoscopy are at increased risk for later

183

development of invasive colon cancer. Second, inherited syndromes of polyposis are associated with a strikingly increased risk for colorectal cancer. Third, a discrete series of genetic changes occurs during the progression from adenoma to cancer sequence, including point mutations in the K-ras protooncogene; allelic DNA loss, especially at the DCC tumor suppressor gene; and mutations of the p53 tumor suppressor gene. The vast majority of adenomatous polyps does not undergo malignant progression, suggesting that a multitude of genetic alterations must occur, likely in a certain sequence, to result in malignant transformation. Nonetheless, an understanding of this process has allowed for widespread changes in screening for colon cancer, as it is well recognized that early identification and removal of adenomatous polyps significantly reduces the risk of later colorectal carcinoma. This understanding forms the basis of our screening programs.

CLINICAL PRESENTATION

Symptoms primarily depend on the site of the lesion. Proximal tumors in the cecum and ascending colon typically have few obstructive symptoms, as stool is liquid in that portion, and present more often with heme-positive stools and anemia. Transverse colon tumors typically cause pain, cramps, obstruction, and rarely perforation. Tumors in the sigmoid and rectum produce tenesmus, small stool caliber, and hematochezia. There is some degree of overlap among these presentations, and any patient with these symptoms should be evaluated by digital rectal examination and endoscopy.

Once metastatic, colon cancer tends to spread to the liver first, and only then will it spread to lung, supraclavicular nodes, or bone; however, distal rectal tumors, with a blood supply that may bypass the portal system, can have widespread metastases without liver involvement. Colon cancer is now staged using the tumor, node, metastasis or TNM method.

The rationale for colorectal cancer screening is that early detection of adenomatous and preneoplastic polyps reduces the incidence of invasive cancer. Multiple screening strategies currently are in use, none of which is ideal. The current recommendations from the American Cancer Society for asymptomatic people with no risk factors are digital rectal examination from ages 40 to 50 years and fecal occult blood testing and/or flexible sigmoidoscopy every 5 years, or double-contrast barium enema every 5 years or colonoscopy every 10 years begining at age 50 years.

MANAGEMENT

Surgery remains the mainstay of treatment. The goal is to remove the tumor with wide margins. Surgical options include hemicolectomy (ascending and transverse colon tumors), anterior resection with anastomosis (sigmoid and upper rectum), and abdominoperineal resection or colostomy (tumors within 5–7 cm of the anal verge). Although the goal of resection usually is to cure, surgery may be indicated in some patients with metastatic disease to treat bowel obstruction or perforation, or to control bleeding from a tumor. On occasion, patients with metastatic disease may benefit from resection of the metastatic foci. This should only be considered in patients with a good performance status and a small number of small, resectable lesions. Preoperative radiation or chemotherapy, or both, may be used to debulk large rectal tumor masses.

Postoperative radiation is used in stage II and III rectal cancer to reduce the rate of local recurrence, although it does not have a clear impact on long-term survival. Adjuvant chemotherapy (chemotherapy administered after complete surgical resection) improves survival in patients with resected stage III colorectal cancer (who have involved local lymph nodes) and in some high-risk stage II patients. The standard adjuvant treatment regimen consists of 5-fluorouracil plus leucovorin.

The majority of recurrences occurs in the initial 5 years after removal of the primary tumor. The size of the primary lesion itself is not predictive of survival, but nodal involvement, depth of penetration, and histologic differentiation are important also. Other poor prognostic signs include preoperative elevation of the carcinoembryonic antigen (CEA), hyperdiploid DNA content of the proliferating cells, more than five involved lymph nodes, tumor adherence to other organs, and colonic obstruction at diagnosis.

Metastatic colorectal cancer is not curable, and patients have a median survival of approximately 12 months. Over the last few years, however, several new compounds with activity against this malignancy have become available and will probably have a positive impact on the survival of these patients. Chemotherapeutic agents used in the metastatic setting include 5-fluorouracil with leucovorin, irinotecan, capecitabine, and oxaliplatin.

Chapter 68

ESOPHAGEAL CANCER

Michael A. Nelson

OVERVIEW

Esophageal cancer is a highly lethal malignancy with a 5-year survival of 14%. It occurs in approximately 12,000 Americans a year, with higher incidence reported in other areas of the world, such as parts of Asia. In North America, the disease is more common in men than in women, most often occurs in those older than 50 years of age, and is correlated with lower socioeconomic status. Two major subtypes of esophageal cancer account for 95% of all esophageal malignancies: squamous cell carcinoma and adenocarcinoma. Small-cell carcinoma, malignant melanoma, lymphoma, and mesenchymal tumors account for the small remainder of esophageal tumors.

Squamous cell carcinoma occurs more in blacks than in whites and is usually found in the upper and mid-esophagus, whereas adenocarcinoma is more common in whites than in blacks and occurs in the distal esophagus or at the gastroesophageal junction. Smoking and alcohol predispose toward the development of squamous cell carcinoma, whereas Barrett's esophagus and chronic reflux have been associated with adenocarcinoma. Ingested carcinogens, such as nitrates and lye, as well as ingestion of hot substances causing chronic mucosal irritation are other etiologic factors thought to be associated

TABLE 68-1 Tumor, Node, Metastasis Classification

Tumor (T)	Nodes (N)	(Distant) Metastasis (M)
T0: No evidence of tumor	N0: No regional lymph node involvement	M0: No distant metastasis present
Tis: Carcinoma *in situ*	N1: Regional lymph node metastasis	M1: Distant metastasis present
T1: Tumor invasion into the lamina propria or submucosa		
T2: Tumor invasion into the muscularis propria		
T3: Tumor invasion into the adventitia		
T4: Tumor invasion into adjacent structures		

with development of esophageal malignancy. Although squamous cell carcinoma had occurred far more frequently than adenocarcinoma until two decades ago, the two now occur with approximately equal frequency. Overall prognosis is correlated with staging and does not seem to significantly differ with the histology of the esophageal malignancy (Tables 68–1 and 68–2).

PATHOPHYSIOLOGY

Esophageal adenocarcinoma appears to result from Barrett's esophagus, the metaplastic process in which columnar epithelium replaces the stratified squamous epithelium that normally lines the distal esophagus. This transformation is thought to be an adaptive process brought about by chronic gastroesophageal reflux, in which the replacement columnar cells appear better able to resist chronic acid irritation than does the original squamous epithelium. The rate of progression of this metaplasia was initially thought to occur over years but now is thought to occur much more rapidly.

Three types of columnar epithelia are seen in Barrett's: junctional-type epithelium, gastric fundic-type epithelium, and specialized intestinal metaplasia, of which only the last is believed to be premalignant. The specialized intestinal metaplasia can become dysplastic with low-grade dysplasia, showing only mild architectural changes, or with high-grade dysplasia, in which markedly abnormal architectural changes occur. Dysplasia can then progress to frank adenocarcinoma, a process that, in Barrett's, appears to include alteration in the tumor-suppressor genes p53 and p16 and nonrandom losses of

TABLE 68-2 Tumor, Node, Metastasis Staging

Stage	Tumor (T)	Node (N)	Metastasis (M)
I	T1	N0	M0
IIA	T2 or T3	N0	M0
IIB	T1 or T2	N1	M0
III	T3	N1	M0
	T4	N0 or N1	M0
IV	Any T	N0 or N1	M1

heterozygosity. In addition, 90% of these adenocarcinomas have aneuploid or tetraploid populations. These changes lead to abnormal proliferation and, with subsequent accumulation of other mutations, can lead to monoclonal malignant proliferation. Similar abnormal accumulation of genetic mutations underlies the mechanism of transformation from normal squamous epithelium to malignant squamous cell carcinoma.

CLINICAL PRESENTATION

Most patients initially complain of progressive dysphagia and rapid weight loss. Classically, dysphagia first occurs with solid foods and gradually progresses as the tumor further blocks the esophageal lumen to include semisolids and liquids. These difficulties with swallowing usually do not occur until there is 60% occlusion of the lumen, a time at which the disease process is usually incurable. Dysphagia may also be associated with odynophagia, regurgitation, or vomiting, or various nonspecific pains of the back and chest. Esophageal cancer most commonly spreads to adjacent and supraclavicular lymph nodes, and distally to the liver, lungs, and pleura. In late disease, tracheoesophageal fistulas may develop. Squamous cell carcinomas can be associated with hypercalcemia via parathyroid hormone–related peptide secreted by tumor cells.

DIAGNOSIS

The diagnosis of esophageal cancer may be suggested by barium studies but is usually established via endoscopy. Analysis of the fundus of the stomach by retroflexing the endoscope is imperative during the evaluative process. Although lesions grossly often look malignant, frequently appearing as plaques, ulcerations, strictures, or circumferential masses, the diagnosis must be confirmed by biopsy. Studies have shown that increasing the number of biopsies from one to seven increases accuracy of diagnosis from 93% to 98%. Adding brush cytology to the seven biopsies increases accuracy to 100%. *In vivo* mucosal staining to help determine which area to biopsy is also helpful.

Staging (Tables 68–1 and 68–2), which determines outcome and prognosis, usually involves a computed tomography (CT) scan to detect metastatic disease and endoscopic ultrasound to determine the degree of invasion of the esophageal wall and presence of enlarged lymph nodes. Five-year survivals for stages I to IV are 60%, 31%, 20%, and 4%, respectively. Studies have shown that CT scan is better than endoscopic ultrasound for detecting lymph node metastases. Positron emission tomography in preliminary studies appears to be more sensitive than CT scan for the detection of distant metastases.

MANAGEMENT

Given the overall grim prognosis, most treatment modalities focus on palliation and symptom relief rather than cure. The various surgical interventions with bulk tumor resection are often associated with postoperative complications and rarely lead to tumor-free margins. Surgery may provide better palliative relief of dysphagia than primary radiation therapy, although radiation spares the patient the perioperative morbidity associated with surgery. The current approach to potentially resectable esophageal cancer involves combination chemotherapy and radiation followed by surgery, with some improvement in outcomes compared with historical controls. Unresectable, locally advanced cancer is treated with combined chemotherapy and radiation. Cisplatin plus infusion 5-fluorouracil is the combination chemotherapy most frequently used. The taxanes also have activity in this malignancy. Radiotherapy alone is usually only palliative, although it can be curative in selected patients.

Palliative approaches to esophageal obstruction include laser therapy, photodynamic therapy, and, most commonly, endoscopic stenting. Endoscopic stenting with self-expanding metal stents now plays a major role in palliation from dysphagia, with 95% success rates and relatively low rates of complication. Major disadvantages include high stent cost, hemorrhage, fistula formation, stent migration, and tissue ingrowth. Tumor ingrowth has been markedly reduced in stents coated with various materials, such as polyethylene. Stent migration has also been reduced with improved stents. Coated stents are the palliative treatment of choice in those patients who have developed a tracheo-esophageal fistula, with an 80% success rate in these cases.

Chapter 69

GASTRIC CANCER

Avlin B. Imaeda

OVERVIEW

Gastric cancer is the tenth leading cause of cancer death in the United States. The incidence in the United States, however, is much lower than it is in Japan, Costa Rica, China, and parts of Eastern Europe. Throughout the world, gastric cancer is associated with lower socioeconomic conditions; thus, it is not surprising that the overall incidence of gastric cancer has markedly decreased in the United States over the last 50 years. Interestingly, the decline in the incidence of gastric cancer is due to a decline in incidence of cancers of the distal stomach body and antrum. The incidence of cancers involving the proximal stomach and esophagogastric junction, cancers that more commonly affect higher socioeconomic classes, has continuously increased over time.

PATHOPHYSIOLOGY

Epidemiologic data suggest a separate etiology for distal versus proximal gastric cancer. Numerous conditions have been associated with gastric cancer. These include adenomatous gastric polyps, hereditary nonpolyposis colorectal cancer, familial polyposis coli, hypertrophic gastropathy, immunodeficiency syndromes, Barrett's esophagus, and achlorhydria or chronic atrophic gastritis (with intestinal metaplasia) caused by pernicious anemia, gastric resection, or childhood *Helicobacter pylori* infection. Chronic use of proton-pump inhibitors has not been found to lead to gastric cancer in humans. A model for the pathogenesis of gastric cancer has been suggested, in which a chlorhydria or bile reflux, or both, leads to hypergastrinemia and elevated gastric pH. Gastrin is a potent stimulus of cell proliferation, and the increase in pH allows colonization with bacteria. This leads to inflammation with free-radical release by inflammatory cells and further stimulus for proliferation by inflammatory mediators. The colonizing bacteria may interact with dietary elements known to be associated with gastric cancer, such as nitrates from smoked, salted, and pickled foods, to produce potent mutagens. Other host factors likely speed the acquisition of the threshold number of oncogenes needed for the tissue to behave as a cancer or, alternatively, influence *H. pylori* infection. These include environmental factors, such as use of tobacco, and low consumption of antioxidants found in fresh fruits and vegetables. Associated genetic factors include blood type A, loss of expression of the intracellular adhesion molecule E-cadherin, polymorphisms of the inflammatory mediator interleukin-1 beta, and the protooncogene-related syndromes listed above, nonpolyposis colorectal cancer and familial polyposis coli.

Gastric cancer initially spreads through lymphatics and local spread. Thus, metastases are initially found in local lymph nodes and other structures. Eventually, gastric cancer may disseminate, with the most common sites of metastasis being omentum, liver, and lung.

CLINICAL PRESENTATION

The most common presenting symptoms of gastric cancer are weight loss and abdominal pain. Others include dysphasia, nausea, and early satiety. Hematemesis and melena occur in 20% of cases. Physical examination findings are rare, but patients may present with an abdominal mass. Although rare, the paraneoplastic phenomena of diffuse seborrheic keratosis (sign of Leser-Trélat) and acanthosis nigricans can be seen. Other findings, found with disseminated disease, include periumbilical nodules (Sister Mary Joseph nodes), left supraclavicular adenopathy (Virchow's node), a mass in the cul-de-sac on rectal examination (Blumer's shelf), an enlarged ovary (Krukenberg's tumor), ascites with peritoneal carcinomatosis, and hepatomegaly with masses. The most common laboratory abnormality associated with gastric cancer is iron-deficiency anemia. Rare paraneoplastic manifestations that may be seen on laboratory evaluation or clinical presentation include microangiopathic hemolytic anemia and membranous nephropathy.

DIAGNOSIS

The most sensitive and specific means of diagnosing gastric cancer is endoscopy. A single biopsy has only 70% sensitivity. This sensitivity can be increased to higher than 98% by performing seven biopsies. *Linitis plastica*, or the diffuse type of gastric cancer, can be difficult to diagnose by biopsy, as it is often located deep, within the submucosa. In this case, a barium study may show a stiff, "leather-flask" stomach.

The gold standard for staging is laparoscopy; however, noninvasive methods are usually used first. Endoscopic ultrasound is most accurate for local staging. Computed tomography scanning is used for evaluation of spread outside the stomach. These methods should be used before laparotomy to make a preliminary decision regarding whether surgery is indicated.

Screening for gastric cancer is not indicated in the United States, owing to its relatively low incidence. Associated conditions in which screening is indicated include the presence of known gastric adenomas, familial polyposis coli, and Barrett's esophagus.

MANAGEMENT

Patients initially should be staged. On occasion, patients who cannot be resected for cure may benefit from palliative resection to treat obstructive or bleeding lesions. Subtotal resections rather than complete gastric resection and gastric bypass are recommended, as more aggressive surgery tends to shorten survival. There may be a benefit for adjuvant combined chemoradiotherapy in patients who have undergone a potentially curative resection. The chemotherapy should include 5-fluorouracil with leucovorin. The median survival of patients with metastatic disease is less than 12 months, and palliative chemotherapy may benefit selected patients in this setting. Studies of various types of immunotherapy have not consistently shown benefit.

Chapter 70

PANCREATIC CANCER

Richard Mark White

OVERVIEW

Pancreatic cancer remains one of the most aggressive malignancies, with a mortality of more than 96%. It is the fourth most common cause of cancer deaths in the United States. The incidence increases with age, and men and women are affected equally. It has been difficult to document clear risk factors for pancreatic cancer. The most closely linked is cigarette smoking, which confers a twofold to threefold increased risk in heavy smokers. Other risk factors are more controversial and include chronic pancreatitis and perhaps long-standing diabetes. Alcohol and coffee have long been touted as potential risk factors, but few studies have substantiated these claims. Diet has also been implicated, with high fat and high meat intake usually implicated. A variety of genetic predispositions has also been implicated, including associations with p16, BRCA2 mutations, hereditary nonpolyposis colorectal cancer and familial polyposis coli, multiple endocrine neoplasia type I, and ataxia-telangiectasia, and familial forms of pancreatic cancer exist.

PATHOPHYSIOLOGY

It is likely that the development of pancreatic cancer is similar to other forms of tumorigenesis in that a multitude of genetic alterations leads to the clinical expression of malignant disease. The mutation that has been most consistently linked to the pancreas has been the K-ras protooncogene. More than 90% of pancreatic tumors contain mutations in K-ras, usually at codon 12. This mutation occurs early in transformation and appears somewhat specific for pancreatic cancer (biliary, hepatic, gastric, and esophageal cancers do not usually harbor this mutation), thus raising the possibility of its being useful as a screening tool for early cancer. Most tumors of the pancreas are adenocarcinomas arising from the ductal epithelium. Approximately two-thirds arise in the head of the pancreas, which allows for somewhat earlier detection, because they cause common bile duct obstruction and jaundice. Tumors in the tail rarely present early and are often larger than 5 cm at presentation, which is highly associated with invasive and metastatic disease.

CLINICAL PRESENTATION

Most symptoms related to this cancer are insidious and somewhat nonspecific. The initial symptoms often consist of pain (visceral-type pain that commonly involves the back) and weight loss (present in 75% of patients). Eventually, most patients with tumors in the head of the pancreas develop obstructive jaundice, with attendant darkening of the urine and abnormal stool color. There is a striking incidence of depression in patients with pancreatic cancer, far above what would be expected when compared to other intraabdominal tumors. The reasons for this high incidence are not known. Trousseau's sign (migratory thrombophlebitis) is actually an unusual finding in pancreatic cancer (5% of patients), although it was originally described in a patient with this cancer. New-onset diabetes is often a clue to this diagnosis, and in a recent Mayo Clinic report, 40% of patients had diabetes diagnosed at the time of pancreatic cancer. There is a suggestion that adults presenting with new-onset diabetes with any upper gastrointestinal symptomatology should be screened for pancreatic cancer. The majority of patients with pancreatic cancer are diagnosed when symptoms have been present for more than 2 months and with advanced disease.

DIAGNOSIS

Suspicion for pancreatic cancer should be raised in patients presenting with nonspecific upper gastrointestinal complaints and weight loss, especially if associated with new-onset diabetes. Computed tomography scan of the abdomen with oral and intravenous contrast is considered the imaging modality of choice for the diagnosis of pancreatic cancer. It has excellent resolution and also allows for precise localization of level of obstruction, extent of tumor invasion, metastatic disease, and assessment of lymph nodes. Computed tomography also can help determine whether tumor is resectable based on its local invasion into nearby vascular structures.

The tumor antigen CA19-9 is often elevated in patients with advanced disease but may be low in patients with early disease, and thus not suitable for screening. Studies examining the use of other tumor markers, particularly alterations in K-ras, as a means of early detection are ongoing. At present, however, there remains no clinically reliable method for early detection and screening for pancreatic cancer.

Staging is based on the standard tumor, node, metastasis (TNM) classification (Table 70–1). Stage correlates with survival.

MANAGEMENT

Complete resection is the only known curative modality; however, only 10% to 15% of patients have resectable tumor at time of diagnosis, either because of metastatic disease or because of invasion of vascular structures. The majority of patients who are candidates for surgery have tumors confined to the head of the pancreas and present with obstructive jaundice (because their tumors are in a strategic location that allows for early clinical expression). The two standard operations are the Whipple procedure (pancreaticoduodenectomy) and complete pancreatectomy. There does not appear to be a differential survival benefit, and each has its own complications. Patients undergoing a Whipple procedure are prone to anastomotic leaks, whereas complete resection leads to

TABLE 70-1 American Joint Committee on Cancer (AJCC) Tumor, Node, Metastasis (TNM) Classification of Pancreatic Cancer

Classification		Description	
T1		Primary tumor limited to pancreas and ≤2 cm	
T2		Primary tumor limited to pancreas and >2 cm	
T3		Tumor extends beyond the pancreas but does not invade the celiac axis or superior mesenteric artery	
T4		Tumor extends beyond the pancreas and involves either the celiac axis or the superior mesenteric artery, or both	
N0		No regional lymph node metastases	
N1		Regional lymph node metastases	
Nx		Regional lymph node metastases cannot be assessed	
M0		No distant metastases	
M1		Distant metastasis	
Stage			
IA	T1	N0	M0
IB	T2	N0	M0
IIA	T3	N0	M0
IIB	T1–3	N1	M0
III	T4	N0–1	M0
IV	T1-4	N0–1	M1

diabetes and malabsorption. Five-year survival rates of 10% have been seen in large series.

Postoperative radiation plus chemotherapy with 5-fluorouracil has been shown to significantly enhance survival. Newer studies examining the role of alternative regimens using newer agents, such as gemcitabine, are ongoing.

For jaundiced patients, biliary decompression through endoscopic retrograde cholangiopancreatography, percutaneous drainage, stents, or surgical diversions should be considered. Although these procedures are palliative, they may have a significant impact on patients' quality of life. Some surgeons perform a chemical ablation of the splanchnic nerve plexus during a palliative bypass procedure to help reduce the pain from progressive pancreatic cancer.

Chemotherapy and radiation have proven disappointing in the treatment of pancreatic cancer. Single-agent studies of 5-fluorouracil yield a response rate of only 5% to 10%, and newer studies using gemcitabine likely are only slightly improved. Gemcitabine may have improved efficacy in terms of palliation, however, with improvements in pain, analgesic use, weight, and performance status.

The median survival for unresectable pancreatic cancer is approximately 6 months. Those with fully resectable tumors have a 5-year survival rate of approximately 10%. These numbers indicate the pressing need for newer approaches to this almost uniformly fatal disease.

Chapter 71

RENAL CANCER

Kathleen Stergiopoulos

OVERVIEW

Renal cell carcinoma is characterized by a lack of early warning signs, which results in a high proportion of patients with metastases at diagnosis, diverse clinical manifestations, and resistance to radiotherapy and chemotherapy. Renal cell carcinoma accounts for 2% of all cancers and for 80% to 85% of malignant kidney tumors. Other histologic types include transitional cell carcinoma of the renal pelvis, making up 15% to 20% of kidney cancers in adults. Renal cell carcinoma occurs nearly twice as often in men as in women, and in the United States its incidence is equivalent among whites and blacks. Patients are generally older than 40 years of age at diagnosis, and the disease occurs predominantly in the seventh and eighth decades of life. The incidence of renal cell carcinoma has been rising steadily, most likely owing to improved capability of diagnosis. Kidney tumors are detected more frequently by the newer radiologic techniques, often at lower stages, when they can be resected for cure. Environmental factors associated with renal cell carcinoma are cigarette smoking (accounting for 20–30% of cases), obesity, hypertension, unopposed estrogen therapy, and occupational exposure to petroleum products, heavy metals, or asbestos. The risk is increased in patients with acquired cystic kidney disease associated with end-stage renal disease and tuberous sclerosis. There are at least four forms of hereditary renal cancer.

PATHOPHYSIOLOGY

A current classification scheme based on the histologic classification distinguishes five types of carcinomas: clear cell (75–85% of tumors), chromophilic (papillary), chromophobic, oncocytic, and collecting-duct (Bellini's duct) tumors. A higher nuclear grade or the presence of a sarcomatoid pattern correlates with a poorer prognosis.

CLINICAL PRESENTATION

Small, localized tumors rarely produce symptoms, and for this reason the diagnosis is often delayed until after the disease is advanced. The most common presentations are hematuria (in 50–60% of patients), abdominal or flank pain (in 40%), and a palpable mass in the flank or abdomen (in 30–40%). These three symptoms occur in combination (i.e., "classic triad") in fewer than 10% of patients. Other signs and symptoms are relatively nonspecific, such as fever, night sweats, malaise, and weight loss. Two percent of male patients present with varicocele, usually left sided, due to obstruction of the testicular vein. Gross hematuria (31–76% incidence) is a late manifestation that represents erosion of the tumor into the collecting system. A palpable mass is more frequently present if the tumor involves the lower pole of the right kidney. Pain has been related to stretching of the renal capsule, in which instance it is usually mild but persistent. Sudden, severe flank pain may accompany bleeding into the tumor. The passage of blood clots mimics colic from a ureteral stone. Fever is likely secondary to necrosis of the tumor. Hypertension may be related to compression of the renal artery, with resultant renal ischemia.

One percent to 3% of tumors are bilateral. Twenty-five percent to 30% of patients have overt metastases at initial presentation. Frequent sites include the lung parenchyma (in 50–60% of patients with metastases), bone (in 30–40%), liver (in 30–40%), and brain (in 5%). Unusual sites of metastases are characteristic of renal cancer, however, and virtually any organ site can be involved, including the thyroid, pancreas, skeletal muscle, and skin or underlying soft tissue (i.e., skull metastases). A broad range of paraneoplastic syndromes, found in less than 5% of patients, has been reported, including erythrocytosis (secondary to increased erythropoietin), hypercalcemia (increased parathyroid hormone–related protein), hepatic dysfunction (Stauffer's syndrome), and amyloidosis (via the formation of immune complexes). The presence of paraneoplastic syndromes does not necessarily imply that there is metastatic disease or a contraindication to the resection of a localized tumor.

DIAGNOSIS

In recent years, the widespread application of computed tomography (CT) and ultrasound for other indications has led to increased detection of renal cell carcinoma as an incidental finding. At present, 25% to 40% of diagnoses are made after the detection of an incidental renal mass. Ultrasound and intravenous contrast-enhanced CT are more accurate in detecting and characterizing renal masses. For tumors 3 cm in diameter or smaller, the sensitivity of ultrasound and CT are 79% and 94%, respectively. CT is approximately 90% accurate in defining the extent of tumor (i.e., stage). Limitations include defining the extent of tumor invasion into the vena cava and evaluation of minimally enlarged lymph nodes. Magnetic resonance imaging with intravenous gadolinium is superior to CT in evaluating the inferior vena cava when tumor involvement is suspected.

MANAGEMENT

The most important determinant of survival is the anatomic extent of the tumor. A widely used staging system, developed by Robson, defines stage I tumors as being confined to the kidney, stage II tumors as extending through the renal capsule but being confined to Gerota's fascia, stage III tumors as involving the renal vein or vena cava (stage IIIA) or the hilar lymph nodes (stage IIIB), and stage IV as locally invasive to adjacent organs (excluding the adrenal gland) or distant metastases. Five-year survival varies by stage: 66% for stage I, 64% for stage II, 42% for stage III, and less than 10% for stage IV. The prognosis for resected stage IIIA is similar to that for I or II; however, for stage IIIB, the 5-year survival is only 20%. A TNM (tumor, node, metastasis) system also exists and is used for the staging of renal cell cancer.

Surgical resection remains the cornerstone of treatment for localized renal cell carcinoma. Radical nephrectomy with removal of the ipsilateral adrenal and hilar nodes is the standard operation for unilateral renal neoplasms. The kidney is removed en bloc with the surrounding Gerota's fascia and perinephric fat. Involvement of the ipsilateral adrenal gland has an overall incidence of approximately 4% and, in most cases, is a result of direct extension of an upper pole lesion or in association with advanced regional or metastatic disease. Adrenalectomy may be reserved for patients with large upper pole lesions or abnormal-appearing adrenal glands on a preoperative CT scan. The extent and benefit of lymphadenectomy remains controversial, given that the presence of nodal involvement is associated with relapse with distant metastases in virtually all patients, despite lymphadenectomy. Partial nephrectomy should be attempted in patients with bilateral tumors or cancer of an anatomically or functionally solitary kidney and in patients in whom the contralateral kidney is threatened by an associated disease. Vena cava involvement in the absence of distant metastases is treated with surgical resection using cardiopulmonary bypass, if needed. In these cases, approximately one-half of patients have prolonged survival. Nephrectomy in patients with metastatic disease may be justified in selected patients when the intention is to improve quality of life, as by alleviating local symptoms. Twenty percent to 30% of patients with localized tumors relapse after radical nephrectomy, most commonly as lung metastases. Local recurrences occur less than 5% of the time. The median time before a relapse after nephrectomy is 15 to 18 months, and 85% of relapses occur within 3 years.

Metastatic renal cell carcinoma is resistant to chemotherapeutic agents and to hormonal therapy. Immunotherapy, mainly interleukin-2 and interferon, has been studied extensively and is shown to produce low response rates, ranging from 10% to 20%. Toxic effects associated with interleukin-2 are related to increased vascular permeability (i.e., capillary leak syndrome), fever, chills, fatigue, and hypotension. Another option for patients with metastatic disease is close surveillance, with systemic treatment delayed (and thus toxicity avoided) until symptoms appear or there is evidence of progression.

Chapter 72

PROSTATE CANCER

John Toksoy

OVERVIEW

Prostate cancer is the most commonly diagnosed male malignancy and the second leading cause of cancer death in men in the United States. The risk of a 50-year-old American man with a 25-year life expectancy of having microscopic cancer is 42%; of clinically apparent cancer, 9.5%; and of dying from prostate cancer, 2.9%. Risk factors include older age, black race (1.5 times the average risk), family history of prostate cancer (2–3 times the average risk if a first-degree relative was affected), and possibly a high-fat Western diet. The natural history of prostate cancer is poorly understood. Its severity ranges from fast-growing fatal tumors to slow-growing occult cancers that are discovered only on autopsies. The screening methods currently available include digital rectal examination (DRE) and serum prostate-specific antigen (PSA). In combination, an abnormal PSA (>4 ng/mL) or DRE, or both, has a sensitivity of approximately 84% and specificity of 92%. DRE and PSA testing are indicated annually for patients in whom screening is chosen. The American Cancer Society and the American Urological Association recommend screening beginning at age 50 years for white men without a family history of prostate cancer and with a life expectancy of at least 10 years. For African-American men and those with a family history of the disease, screening is recommended beginning at age 40 years. Whether early detection of prostate cancer by screening improves survival and decreases morbidity is not yet known. The optimal form of treatment for various stages of prostate cancer remains controversial and is discussed in this chapter.

PATHOPHYSIOLOGY

More than 95% of prostate cancers are adenocarcinomas and arise in the prostate acini. They are frequently multifocal and have a predilection for the periphery. These characteristics are in contrast to benign prostatic hyperplasia (BPH), which occurs commonly in the periurethral region. Other prostatic cancers include squamous cell and transitional cell carcinomas, carcinosarcomas of the mesenchymal elements, and metastases from bronchogenic carcinoma, melanoma, or lymphoma. The foregoing discussion focuses on adenocarcinoma.

Serum PSA is a serine protease secreted by the epithelial cells that line the prostatic ducts. A small proportion of the PSA is absorbed into the systemic circulation, where it predominantly complexes with either the $alpha_1$ subunit of antichymotrypsin or the $alpha_2$ subunit of macroglobulin. A small proportion of PSA in the serum remains unbound. For incompletely understood reasons, the percentage of total PSA that is free (unbound) is lower in men with prostate cancer than in men with BPH.

There are three routes of spread for prostate cancer: direct extension, the lymphatics, and the bloodstream. Direct extension may involve the seminal vesicles and the bladder floor. Lymphatic spread usually occurs to the obturator, internal iliac, common iliac, presacral, and then paraaortic nodes. Hematogenous spread occurs more commonly to bone than to viscera. Bony metastases involve the pelvis, lumbar vertebrae, thoracic vertebrae, and ribs. Visceral metastases involve the lungs, liver, and adrenal glands.

CLINICAL PRESENTATION

Most patients are asymptomatic at the time of diagnosis. Obstructive voiding symptoms are most commonly due to BPH, not cancer. Nevertheless, common symptoms of cancer include dysuria, difficulty voiding, increased urinary frequency, urinary retention, back pain, pathologic fractures, and hematuria. Complications of advanced disease also include spinal cord compression from intradural metastases, deep venous thrombosis and pulmonary embolism, and myelophthisis.

DIAGNOSIS

The serum PSA and DRE are used in combination for early detection of prostate cancer. PSA has a 35% false-negative rate and lacks specificity, however. It can be elevated in other conditions, such as BPH, prostatitis, prostatic infarctions, urinary retention, and catheterization. DRE and ejaculation may cause a slight elevation in PSA, which usually returns to baseline level within 24 hours. Finasteride, a 5-alpha reductase inhibitor, may lower the PSA by 50% in men without cancer who have received this medication for more than 6 months. If the DRE is abnormal or if the PSA level is higher than 10 ng per mL, a transrectal ultrasound (TRUS)–guided biopsy is usually indicated. If the DRE is normal and the PSA is between 4 and 10 ng per mL, three options are available: biopsy, biopsy if TRUS is abnormal, or to increase the specificity of PSA in alternative ways to help decide on biopsy. The third option involves such measurements as PSA, density (ratio of PSA to prostate volume using TRUS), age-specific PSA (using higher PSA thresholds for biopsy with increasing age), PSA velocity (a rise >0.75 ng/mL per year being more suggestive of prostate cancer), or percent free PSA (using a ratio of <25% as a cutoff for biopsy). Of note, approximately 75% of men with PSA levels of 4 to 10 ng per mL do not have cancer on biopsy. Also of note, nevertheless, the traditional use of a set of six biopsy specimens in sextant pattern results in a false-negative rate of at least 10%.

Pathologic grading of prostate cancer is based on the Gleason system, whereby a primary and a secondary score from 1 to 5 (well to least differentiated) are assigned to the architectural pattern of cancerous glands in the largest and the next largest areas of cancerous growth, respectively. The Gleason sum (range, 2–10) can then be used along with staging to evaluate prognosis and treatment. The tumor, node, metastasis (TNM) staging scheme has replaced the Whitmore-Jewett system and involves assessment of the primary tumor, nodes, and metastases. Stages T1 and T2 are both confined to the prostate, but only stage T2 cancers are palpable by DRE. Stage T3 disease represents palpable tumor extending beyond the prostatic capsule but not to the pelvic nodes. Stage M1-2 refers to involvement of pelvic nodes alone, whereas stage M2+ refers to widespread metastatic disease. Any of the stages T1 through T3 can have simultaneous metastatic involvement. Magnetic resonance imaging and computed tomography may be helpful in clinical staging. Bone metastases are rare if the PSA is less than 10 ng per mL. For patients with higher PSA levels, bone scans should also be used in initial staging, although they are not specific.

TREATMENT

Most patients with clinically localized (stages T1 and T2) cancers and anticipated survival in excess of 10 years are treated with radical prostatectomy or radiation therapy. In radical prostatectomy, the seminal vesicles, prostate, and ampullae of the vas deferens are removed. Radiation therapy can be given either as external beam radiotherapy or by implantation of radioisotopes (brachytherapy). Almost all patients who elect radiotherapy also receive neoadjuvant androgen deprivation. In contrast, androgen deprivation does not have a clearly established role in patients undergoing radical prostatectomy. Androgen deprivation can be achieved in several ways: (i) estrogen therapy (diethylstilbestrol); (ii) steroidal antiandrogens (progestins, e.g., megestrol acetate, cyproterone acetate, medroxyprogesterone acetate); (iii) nonsteroidal antiandrogens (flutamide, bicalutamide, and nilutamide); (iv) luteinizing hormone–releasing hormone (LHRH) analogs (leuprolide and buserelin); (v) ketoconazole (usually combined with hydrocortisone); and (vi) bilateral orchiectomy. The current first-line androgen deprivation therapy includes an LHRH analog combined with one of the nonsteroidal antiandrogens.

Patients with locally advanced disease (stage T3) can also be treated with radical prostatectomy or radiotherapy, but single-modality treatment is less successful in curing this stage. Combination therapy (using androgen deprivation with surgery or radiotherapy) and hormonal therapy alone are being used. Treatment for metastatic disease is regarded as palliative and consists primarily of hormonal therapy. Primary androgen blockade usually consists of orchiectomy or the administration of an LHRH analog. Diethylstilbestrol is now infrequently used owing to increased risk of death from cardiovascular disease. Complete androgen blockade by combining an LHRH agonist (but not orchiectomy) with an antiandrogen may improve survival in those with limited metastases. Chemotherapy or withdrawal of androgen deprivation can be tried in relapses. Adequate use of analgesics, focal irradiation, or bisphosphonates for symptomatic bone involvement is essential in the supportive care of these patients.

Chapter 73

TESTICULAR CANCER

Joseph V. Agostini

OVERVIEW

Testicular cancer is the most common solid tumor in men between the ages of 20 and 35 years. These germ cell neoplasms are potentially curable if found early, and thus the etiology of a new scrotal mass in a young man must be definitively worked up. Nonmalignant causes of testicular mass include hydrocele, epididymitis, orchitis, and spermatocele. Risk factors for the development of testicular cancer include cryptorchid (undescended) testes, Klinefelter's syndrome (47,XXY karyotype), and testicular cancer in the contralateral testis.

PATHOPHYSIOLOGY

Ninety-five percent of testicular tumors arise from germinal cells, usually divided into seminomas and nonseminomas (teratomas, embryonal cell tumors, and choriocarcinomas). Seminomas usually spread via lymphatics and are highly responsive to radiation therapy, whereas the nonseminomas often spread hematogenously and are less radiosensitive. Stromal cell tumors, arising from the Leydig and Sertoli cells, are rare.

Rarely, extragonadal germ cell tumors develop in the retroperitoneum or in the mediastinum, without evidence of primary disease in the testis. It is presumed that these tumors arise from malignant transformation of residual germ cells from the embryonic period.

CLINICAL PRESENTATION

A testicular swelling or mass, sometimes painful, most commonly leads to patient or physician detection. Patients with advanced disease may present with dyspnea due to pulmonary metastases, back pain due to retroperitoneal lymphadenopathy, urinary obstruction, or neurologic symptoms due to brain metastasis.

DIAGNOSIS

Physical examination and ultrasound imaging help to identify a lesion arising from the testis. Diagnosis is established with surgical exploration through an inguinal incision. Further staging workup includes chest and abdominal computed tomography scans. Human chorionic gonadotropin levels are elevated in some patients with testicular cancer, and alpha-fetoprotein may be elevated in patients with nonseminomatous testicular cancer. Lactate dehydrogenase is elevated in patients with advanced testicular cancer, and, like human chorionic gonadotropin and alpha-fetoprotein, has prognostic significance, with higher levels correlating with a larger tumor burden.

MANAGEMENT

High inguinal orchiectomy is required. Early stage seminomas are usually managed with retroperitoneal nodal irradiation; late-stage disease requires chemotherapeutic regimens based on cisplatin. Early stage nonseminoma management entails retroperitoneal lymph node dissection or chemotherapy, or both. Patients with advanced disease are treated with combination chemotherapy. The follow-up of patients with treated testicular cancer includes regularly scheduled physical examinations, tumor marker measurement, and radiologic imaging. Early stage cure rates approach 97%, versus 80% to 85% for advanced stages. The potential to cure even metastatic disease demonstrates the significant advances made in the treatment of testicular cancer in the last quarter-century.

Chapter 74

OVARIAN CANCER

Melissa A. Simon

OVERVIEW

There are many varieties of tumors of the ovaries, both benign and malignant, with 80% of ovarian tumors being benign. Ovarian cancer is the fifth most common cancer in women in the United States, and the third most common cancer of the female genital tract after cervical and endometrial cancer. It is responsible for more than one-half of all deaths from cancer of the female genital tract, however. This high mortality is due mostly to the lack of effective screening tools for early diagnosis and partially to the cancer's spread by direct invasion into the peritoneal cavity. The 5-year survival rate for women with ovarian cancer is only 25% to 30%.

PATHOPHYSIOLOGY

Ovarian tumors are derived from one of the three components of the ovary: the surface coelomic epithelium, the stroma, and the germ cells. Ninety percent of ovarian cancers are from the coelomic epithelium. Approximately 5% to 10% of ovarian cancers are metastatic from other primary tumors in the body—usually from the gastrointestinal tract, breast, or endometrium—and are known as *Krukenberg tumors.*

The cause of ovarian cancer is unclear. It is thought that prolonged periods of chronic, uninterrupted ovulation cause malignant transformation of ovarian tissue via somatic gene deletions and mutations. Other proposed etiologic agents have been high dietary fat, asbestos, talc, and the mumps virus.

Women at highest risk for ovarian cancer are those with a family history of ovarian cancer and those with a history of uninterrupted ovulation—those who are nulliparous or have decreased fertility, delayed childbearing, or late-onset menopause. Women with breast cancer have a twofold increase in the incidence of ovarian cancer. Oral contraceptive pills have been found to have a modest protective effect, likely due to the suppression of ovulation. Women carrying mutations of the BRCA1 and 2 genes have a lifetime risk of developing ovarian cancer of 15% to 65%.

Ovarian cancer is spread by direct exfoliation of the malignant cells. Metastasis often follows the circulatory path of the peritoneal fluid, and, as such, the regional lymph nodes are usually involved.

CLINICAL PRESENTATION

Patients with ovarian cancer are often asymptomatic until the late stages of the disease. Approximately 75% of patients present with stage III or IV disease (Table 74–1). Some patients present with weight loss or vague lower abdominal pain and abdominal enlargement. As the tumors progress, other symptoms may develop, such as gastrointestinal complaints, urinary frequency, dysuria, and pelvic pressure. In later stages, ascites may develop. On physical examination, the primary finding is a solid, fixed pelvic mass that may extend into the upper abdomen (Table 74–2).

DIAGNOSIS

Pelvic ultrasound is the primary diagnostic tool for investigating an adnexal mass (Table 74–3). Computed tomography and magnetic resonance imaging of the pelvis and abdomen are valuable for staging and sometimes help in establishing the diagnosis of ovarian cancer. Levels of alpha-fetoprotein and human chorionic gonadotropin are elevated in some women with germ cell tumors. CA-125 is often elevated in patients with advanced epithelial ovarian cancer but is used mainly for monitoring response to therapy and not for establishing the diagnosis. Screening for ovarian cancer with measurement of blood CA-125 and annual pelvic ultrasounds are recommended for patients

TABLE 74–1 Abbreviated Staging of Ovarian Carcinoma	
Stage I	Growth limited to the ovaries
IA	Limited to one ovary; no ascites
IB	Limited to both ovaries; no ascites
IC	Tumor IA or IB with ascites or positive peritoneal washings
Stage II	Extension of the neoplasm from the ovary to the pelvis
IIA	Extension and/or metastases to the uterus and/or tubes
IIB	Extension to other pelvic tissues
IIC	Tumor stage IIA or IIB with ascites or positive peritoneal washings
Stage III	Growth involving one or both ovaries with disease extension outside of the pelvis and/or positive retroperitoneal nodes; or histologic proof of extension of tumor to omentum or small bowel
Stage IV	Growth involving one or both ovaries with distant metastatic disease; pleural effusion with positive cytology; parenchymal liver metastases

TABLE 74-2 Characteristics of Pelvic Mass on Physical Examination

	Benign	Malignant
Mobility	Mobile	Fixed
Consistency	Cystic	Solid or firm
Bilateral or unilateral	Unilateral	Bilateral
Cul-de-sac involvement	Smooth	Nodular

with a family history of ovarian cancer, although this approach has not been shown to reduce mortality from this malignancy.

Once the diagnosis has been made, abdominal and pelvic computed tomography scans, pelvic ultrasound, chest x-ray, intravenous pyelography, barium enema, cystoscopy, and flexible sigmoidoscopy are often used to look for metastases to complete the staging and to plan surgery.

MANAGEMENT

Ovarian cancer is staged surgically. Exploratory laparotomy through a vertical abdominal incision with thorough evaluation of the abdomen is performed. Ascitic fluid and peritoneal washings are collected. Regional lymph nodes (pelvic and paraaortic) are sampled, and a partial omentectomy is performed. Most patients undergo a transabdominal hysterectomy and bilateral salpingo-oophorectomy. All gross residual disease is resected, if possible.

Patients with stage IA or IB disease with well or moderately differentiated tumors require no additional therapy post surgery. All other patients usually receive therapy after surgery, which may include intraperitoneal chemotherapy or systemic chemotherapy. In some cases, second-look surgery is performed to evaluate for remission, assess response, and allow further cytoreductive surgery in an attempt to prolong survival. In young women with early-stage disease who desire fertility, a conservative approach with uterine and contralateral adnexal preservation may be considered.

The most commonly used systemic chemotherapy agents are cyclophosphamide, cisplatin, carboplatin, and paclitaxel. Paclitaxel with cisplatin or carboplatin is the most popular. Intraperitoneal chemotherapy enables the exposure of malignant cells to higher doses of chemotherapy over time with less toxicity than systemic chemotherapy.

Ovarian cancer is a chemotherapy-sensitive disease; however, no more than 1% to 5% of patients with advanced disease are cured with combination chemotherapy. The median survival of patients with advanced ovarian cancer is approximately 3 years.

TABLE 74-3 Radiographic Characteristics of Adnexal Masses

	Benign	Malignant
Size	<8 cm	>8 cm
Consistency	Cystic	Solid or cystic and solid
Septation	Unilocular	Multilocular
Bilateral or unilateral	Unilateral	Bilateral
Other	Calcification (especially teeth)	Ascites

Chapter 75

PRIMARY BRAIN TUMORS

Vinni Juneja

OVERVIEW

Primary brain tumors account for only 2% of all neoplasms, with an incidence of 17,400 tumors reported in 1998, but result in a relatively high share of mortality, with a 5-year survival rate the third lowest among all cancers, after lung and pancreatic tumors. The most common adult primary tumors are high-grade glioblastomas and anaplastic astrocytomas, meningiomas, and low-grade astrocytomas, accounting for approximately 50%, 20%, and 10%, respectively, of all adult primary brain cancer. These tumors are more common in men, with the exception of meningioma. Meningiomas are benign in 90% of cases but can cause symptoms from compression of other brain structures. Medulloblastomas, ependymomas and other embryonal tumors are rarely seen after the age of 20 years. Favorable prognostic factors in any primary central nervous system (CNS) tumor include high performance status, lower pathologic grade, and age younger than 55 years. Metastatic tumors to the CNS, which are not discussed here, are more prevalent than are primary brain tumors.

Since 1950, the incidence of brain tumors has been on the rise (by approximately 80% in whites), as has the mortality from these malignancies (by approximately 45%) in industrialized nations, regardless of ethnicity, gender, or geography. Especially notable is primary CNS lymphoma, which has tripled in incidence over the past 20 years (although still only accounting for 3–5% of all primary CNS tumors), only in part because of the rising number of immunocompromised (human immunodeficiency virus and transplant) patients. The rise in incidence of all brain neoplasms may partially be accounted for by better diagnostic techniques.

Risk factors for brain tumors have been difficult to specify owing to the low overall incidence of brain cancer. Ionizing radiation, working in the rubber industry, and certain genetic syndromes (neurofibromatosis 1 and 2, von Hippel-Lindau syndrome, Li-Fraumeni syndrome, Turcot's syndrome, tuberous sclerosis) have been elicited as definite risk factors. The role of nonionizing radiation, dietary nitrosamines, viral infections, and physical and acoustic trauma as possible risk factors remains to be defined.

PATHOPHYSIOLOGY

The pathogenesis of brain tumors is similar to that of other cancers. Inactivation of tumor-suppressor genes or activation of oncogenes in brain cells, such as the astrocytes, oligodendrocytes, and meningeal cells, occurs, and such mutations may sequentially add up to the development of neoplasia. Common chromosomal locations of tumor-suppressor genes lost in the development of these cancers include the long arm of chromosome 22 in meningiomas, 14q in malignant meningiomas, 6 and 13 in low-grade astrocytomas, 10q and 22 in glioblastoma, and 19q in anaplastic astrocytomas.

Common oncogenes activated in the development of brain tumors include p53 in meningiomas, EGFR in anaplastic astrocytomas, and PDGFR in astrocytomas. Almost all of the cases of primary CNS lymphoma seen in immunocompromised individuals are associated with Epstein-Barr virus infection; however, in immunocompetent patients with this tumor, the association with Epstein-Barr virus is much less common.

The classification of primary CNS tumors is based on the World Health Organization classification system that combines tumor names, based on histologic features of mitotic activity, proliferation, and necrosis, with a grading system. In this system, such tumors as astrocytomas (including juvenile pilocytic astrocytomas), oligodendrogliomas, and meningiomas are given a grade of 1 to 2 and have a relatively benign prognosis, whereas anaplastic astrocytoma, glioblastoma multiforme, anaplastic oligodendroglioma, and anaplastic meningiomas are given a grade of 3 to 4 and have a poorer prognosis. Meningiomas are graded on a scale of 1 to 3 rather than 1 to 4.

CLINICAL PRESENTATION

Primary brain tumors have a variety of presentations owing to the functional segmentation of the different areas of the brain, the variety of histologic types, and differences in tumor growth rates. They produce generalized symptoms because of their expanding mass effect and can produce focal symptoms by direct compression on, or infiltration into, the surrounding tissue. Symptoms can be subtle, such as gradual onset of depression or of personality changes, or acute, such as seizures or focal or generalized weakness and sensory deficits. Meningiomas and low-grade gliomas may not cause any symptoms and may be discovered incidentally. Headaches are the most common initial symptom and can vary from tension type to migraines, diffuse or focal. In fact, the traditional brain tumor headache of an early morning headache is quite uncommon. Features of the headache that may suggest a possibility of tumor presence include change in pattern of chronic headaches, focal neurologic signs, and worsening of headache with maneuvers that increase intracranial pressure (ICP), such as Valsalva, coughing or sneezing, or bending over. Sleeping may actually worsen the headache secondary to elevated ICP, decreased venous blood return, and increased PCO_2, which leads to vasodilation. Seizures are present in 25% to 50% of primary brain tumors, are more commonly seen in primary tumors than in metastatic tumors, and are most often seen in slower-growing tumors, such as low-grade gliomas. Primary brain tumors have been found to have a higher incidence of inducing hypercoagulable states relative to other systemic tumors. Juvenile pilocytic astrocytomas tend to present in patients younger than 25 years of age and have a much better prognosis than other low-grade gliomas.

DIAGNOSIS

In terms of radiologic diagnosis, several options are available. Computed tomography (CT) is the most appropriate test in an emergency situation, and it is also the test of choice for detecting metastasis to the skull base. Magnetic resonance imaging (MRI) is preferred over CT in other situations, as it permits better evaluation of the meninges, vascularity, and subarachnoid space. Magnetic resonance spectroscopy analyzes chemical composition of areas of abnormality seen on MRI and can thus be used to differentiate between tumor and other CNS processes. Functional MRI scanning examines blood flow to different areas of the brain and is especially useful in the planning of operative technique in patients with tumors located in higher cortical levels.

It also can be done faster than standard MRI, so it is useful in patients with claustrophobia. Positron emission tomography scanning examines the uptake of glucose within brain tissue, with more metabolically active, higher grade tumors tending to uptake more glucose. Positron emission tomography may be used with functional MRI for preoperative planning of tumors located in higher cortical levels. It also has a role in differentiating tumor from changes due to radiation necrosis, as the latter does not metabolize glucose. The traditional means of differentiating low from high-grade neoplasms is by looking for enhancement on CT or MRI, although it is ultimately histology that makes the final diagnosis of tumor subtype; however, the results of histology slides from operating room specimens are subject to sampling error, especially in heterogeneous tumors. All primary brain tumors necessitate either stereotactic or open biopsy to make the histologic diagnosis.

MANAGEMENT

Only certain tumors have been shown to have an enhanced survival when surgical resection is performed at the time of biopsy. The decision to debulk a tumor is made after preliminary results of histology specimens are available post biopsy. Tumors that have been shown to improve prognosis with resection include glioblastoma multiforme, anaplastic astrocytomas, and oligodendrogliomas. Malignant glioblastomas (glioblastoma multiforme and anaplastic astrocytoma) have a particularly poor prognosis, with median survival extended from 14 weeks without therapy to 40 to 50 weeks with a combination of surgery, postoperative irradiation, and chemotherapy. Active chemotherapeutic agents that penetrate the blood–brain barrier include carmustine (BCNU, or bischloroethylnitrosourea), procarbazine, lomustine (CCNU, or cyclohexylchloroethylnitrosurea), vincristine [PCV, or procarbazine, CCNU (or lomustine), vincristine regimen], and temozolomide, an oral agent. A survival benefit of adding chemotherapy to surgery and radiation has been demonstrated in patients who are younger than 65 years. Glioblastoma multiforme and anaplastic astrocytoma are difficult to treat surgically, as their actual infiltrative margins often extend outside the margin visualized on CT or MRI. Most tumors recur within 2 cm of the original site of resection.

A variety of new approaches is currently being investigated for the treatment of brain lesions. Radiosurgery (gamma knife) uses a stereotactic device for precise localization of high-dose radiation to brain tumors. It can be used to treat both primary brain tumors and metastatic disease, as long as the tumor mass is less than 3 to 4 cm in diameter. Also being studied are agents that increase the permeability of the blood–brain barrier, such as the bradykinin analog RMP-7, possible immunomodulation with interferon or monoclonal antibodies, and gene therapy.

Controversy exists regarding low-grade astrocytomas, low-grade oligodendrogliomas, and juvenile pilocytic astrocytoma as to whether debulking and radiation therapy should be performed versus solely observation. Thirty percent of low-grade astrocytomas and oligodendrogliomas tend to eventually evolve into anaplastic astrocytoma or glioblastoma, with tumors enhancing on CT scan having a greater probability of degeneration. CNS lymphomas are treated with radiation and chemotherapy rather than resection; at present, this tumor has a poor prognosis of a 12-month to 24-month median survival. New approaches using predominantly chemotherapy to treat these lymphomas are showing promising results, however, with some patients surviving several years from their diagnosis. Asymptomatic meningiomas may be managed with simply observation, whereas meningeal tumors causing symptoms related to compression or edema should be resected.

In patients with symptoms due to increased ICP, neurosurgical intervention is required immediately. Furosemide, fluid restriction, elevation of the head of the bed, hyperventilation, corticosteroids, and mannitol should all be considered in the medical management of acutely increased ICP. In patients with nonacute tumor-induced vasogenic edema, corticosteroids are indicated.

Seizures should be treated with phenytoin, valproic acid, or carbamazepine; none of these agents has been shown to be superior to the others. Surgical resection of the tumor should be considered in patients who have seizures refractory to medical therapy. Antiepileptics are not recommended for prophylactic use in patients with brain tumors who have never had a seizure or for patients with brain metastases.

For patients who have experienced deep venous thromboses or pulmonary emboli secondary to tumor-induced hypercoagulability or other extrinsic factors, such as immobility, management remains controversial. Inferior vena cava filters are the intuitive choice rather than anticoagulation in a patient with brain tumors, but they cause filter thrombosis and the development of collateral veins, leading to recurrent deep venous thromboses and pulmonary emboli. The risks of bleeding with the use of warfarin anticoagulation to a therapeutic international normalized ratio of 2.0 to 3.0 may be exaggerated, as suggested by several retrospective studies. Consideration of anticoagulation should be made in patients with primary brain tumors and nonvascular metastatic brain tumors who have experienced thromboembolic disease. Prophylactic anticoagulation should be considered in patients with high-grade gliomas, as they have been found to have the highest risk of clotting among the brain tumors.

Section 6

Neurology and Psychiatry

Chapter 76

UNRESPONSIVE PATIENT

David S. Smith

OVERVIEW

Unresponsiveness may be a presentation in the field, or it may arise as a result of medical illness and treatment in a hospitalized patient. Development of a diagnostic approach based on careful history, directed examination, and neuroimaging is the key to identifying and promptly treating reversible causes.

PATHOPHYSIOLOGY

Stupor implies a state from which the patient can be aroused with vigorous stimuli, whereas *coma* describes a state from which arousal does not occur, even to painful stimuli. Coma is often preceded by *delirium*, which is confusion associated with agitation, and a hypersympathotonic state. Wakefulness requires activation of the cerebral hemispheres by the brainstem reticular activating system, so coma may be caused by widespread damage to both hemispheres, usually owing to anoxia or trauma; suppression by drugs, toxins, or metabolic derangements (e.g., hypoglycemia, hepatic failure, hypercalcemia); or brainstem lesions in the rostral pons to the caudal diencephalon. Brainstem lesions that produce coma also affect pupillary function and eye movement. Hemispheric lesions cause coma indirectly, by secondary compression of the upper brainstem due to transtentorial herniation, accompanied by dilated pupils. Brain stores of glucose provide energy for 2 minutes after blood flow is interrupted. Consciousness is lost within 8 to 10 seconds.

CLINICAL PRESENTATION

Unresponsiveness often presents in a continuum with or as a progression of delirium. Recognizing the signatures of common intracerebral catastrophes is helpful for diagnosis. Basal ganglia and thalamic hemorrhage produces acute to subacute onset of vomiting, headache, and eye signs. Subarachnoid hemorrhage has an instantaneous onset of a severe headache, stiff neck, third and sixth nerve palsies, and extensor posturing. Pontine hemorrhage produces pinpoint pupils, loss of corneal responses, eye bobbing, posturing, hyperventilation, and sweating. Cerebellar hemorrhage is accompanied by occipital headache, vomiting, gaze paresis, and inability to stand. Basilar artery thrombosis has a prodrome of transient ischemic attacks, dysarthria, diplopia, vomiting, and asymmetric limb paresis. Loss of consciousness is common with head trauma, but if it persists, it is usually due to subdural, epidural, or deep cerebral hemorrhage, or bilateral frontotemporal contusions.

DIAGNOSIS

Every patient presenting to the emergency department with coma should receive a computed tomography scan of the brain, which usually reveals any structural lesion, although unresponsiveness is often due to toxic or metabolic derangements, so the clinician is well advised to formulate a plan based on history and physical signs. It is important to note that the computed tomography scan may miss important conditions, such as isodense subdural hematoma, early bilateral hemispheric infarction, encephalitis, absent cerebral perfusion, axonal shearing due to closed head trauma, and saggital sinus thrombosis; therefore, magnetic resonance imagine or magnetic resonance angiography usually is indicated. History from family and witnesses provides important clues about the circumstances and temporal profile of onset, preceding neurologic symptoms, medical problems, and medication or drug use. General physical examination can reveal clues. Fever suggests meningitis, encephalitis, or disturbance of thermoregulatory centers of the brain. Very high fever (>42°C) and dry skin suggest heat stroke or anticholinergic intoxication. Hypothermia suggests environmental exposure, alcohol, barbiturate or phenothiazine overdose, hypoglycemia, or hypothyroidism. Marked hypertension occurs with hypertensive encephalopathy or cerebral hemorrhage. Hypotension results from hemorrhage, sepsis, myocardial infarction, or adrenal crisis. Funduscopy can be used to detect subhyaloid hemorrhages, seen with subarachnoid hemorrhage, and papilledema, seen with increased intracranial pressure.

Decorticate posturing is upper-extremity flexion and lower-extremity extension in response to noxious stimuli, suggesting bilateral damage to the hemispheres above the midbrain. *Decerebrate* posturing is upper-extremity extension, adduction, and pronation, along with lower-extremity extension, suggesting damage to the corticospinal tracts in the midbrain or caudal diencephalons, and portends a poorer prognosis. Myoclonus is found in metabolic disorders, particularly azotemia, anoxia, or drug overdose.

Brainstem responses provide key clues to localization. Symmetric, round, reactive pupils exclude midbrain damage as the cause of the coma. A unilateral dilated (>5 mm) pupil results from an ipsilateral midbrain lesion or from herniation with pressure on the third cranial nerve. Bilateral dilated unreactive pupils indicate severe midbrain damage. Bilateral reactive small (but not pinpoint) pupils are seen in metabolic encephalopathy or thalamic hemorrhage. Bilateral pinpoint pupils are characteristic of narcotic or barbiturate overdose, or bilateral pontine hemorrhage. Bilateral adducted eyes are due to sixth nerve injury with elevated intracranial pressure. Vertical separation of ocular axes is due to pontine or cerebellar lesions. Conjugate horizontal roving eye movements exclude a midbrain or pontine lesion. Ocular bobbing (brisk downward and slow upward movement) is characteristic of a bilateral pontine lesion. The oculocephalic "doll's eye" reflex is elicited by moving the head side to side. In metabolic or drug-induced coma, the eyes move loosely in the opposite direction of the head owing to disinhibition of the hemispheric input into the brainstem reflexes. By the same mechanism, the oculovestibular reflex produces tonic deviation toward the side of instillation of cold water, without nystagmus. With conjugate horizontal ocular deviation, the eyes look toward the side of a hemispheric lesion and away from a brainstem lesion.

Anoxic brain injury occurs after such events as cardiac arrest or near drowning. A metaanalysis found that four clinical signs predicted a poor clinical outcome with nearly 100% specificity: (i) absence of papillary light

TABLE 76-1 Glasgow Coma Scale for Head Injury

Finding	Score
Eye opening:	
Spontaneous	4
To loud voice	3
To pain	2
None	1
Best motor response:	
Obeys	6
Localizes	5
Withdraws (flexion)	4
Abnormal flexion posturing	3
Extension posturing	2
None	1
Verbal response:	
Oriented	5
Confused, disoriented	4
Inappropriate words	3
Incomprehensible sounds	2
None	1

reflexes after 72 hours, (ii) absent motor responses to pain after 72 hours, (iii) bilateral absence of early cortical response to median nerve somatosensory evoked potentials within the first week, and (iv) burst suppression or isoelectric pattern on the electroencephalogram within the first week.

The Glasgow Coma Scale (Table 76-1) was developed for prognosis in traumatic brain injury and is often used to grade level of consciousness and follow progress. A combined score of 3 to 4 is associated with an 85% chance of dying or remaining in a vegetative state. Scores above 11 indicate an 85% chance of recovery with moderate or no disability.

MANAGEMENT

Intubation to protect the airway is a high priority. Mechanical ventilation is often necessary. Prompt identification and reversal of precipitating causes, such as hypotension, hypoglycemia, hypercalcemia, hypoxia, CO_2 retention, or hyperthermia, minimizes further brain injury. Naltrexone and intravenous 50% dextrose should be given immediately if opiate overdose or hypoglycemia is at all suspected. In traumatic coma, the neck must be secured until cervical spine injury is ruled out. If meningitis is suspected, immediate lumbar puncture and an intravenous dose of ceftriaxone are indicated. A unilateral "blown pupil" mandates an attempt to lower intracranial pressure by evacuation of a hematoma, use of hyperosmolar mannitol, or hyperventilation, depending on the cause.

Chapter 77

SEIZURE AND STATUS EPILEPTICUS

Stephanie Rosborough

OVERVIEW

Seizure is a common presenting problem, accounting for up to 1% of all emergency department visits. As many as 10% of people will have a seizure in their lifetime. Status epilepticus has a frequency of 100,000 to 150,000 cases per year, roughly 55,000 of which prove fatal.

Head trauma and low levels of anticonvulsant drugs are the most frequent causes of seizure in young adults. In adults aged 30 to 60 years, alcohol withdrawal is the leading cause. Stroke is by far the most common precipitant in adults older than age 60 years, accounting for 40% of seizures in this group. Other causes of seizure include drug overdose, metabolic disorders, central nervous system (CNS) infections, brain tumors, and trauma; a summary of their etiology follows:

- CNS infections (meningitis, abscess, encephalitis)
- Metabolic disorders (hypernatremia, hyponatremia, hyperglycemia, hypoglycemia, hypocalcemia, hypomagnesemia, renal failure, hepatic failure, hyperosmolar states)
- Vascular causes (cerebrovascular accident, intracranial hemorrhage)
- Drugs (including cocaine, lidocaine, antidepressants, theophylline) and drug withdrawal (alcohol, benzodiazepines, barbiturates)
- CNS tumor
- Trauma
- Eclampsia (prepartum or postpartum)
- Hypertensive encephalopathy
- Hypoxemia

PATHOPHYSIOLOGY

A seizure results from prolonged firing of neurons and failure of inhibitory mechanisms. The origin of abnormal discharges is sometimes a structural defect in the brain, such as a scar from a previous stroke or head injury. Metabolic disturbances, such as hypoglycemia, hyponatremia, alcohol withdrawal, eclampsia, and sleep deprivation, also can contribute to the onset of seizures. Hypoglycemia is usually due to excessive insulin or oral hypoglycemics; islet cell tumors are rare but may present with seizure. A precipitous fall in the serum sodium level can initiate a seizure. Hypomagnesemia, but rarely hypocalcemia, is associated with seizures. Syncope with transient cerebral hypoxia can produce brief tonic-clonic movements.

Patients with epilepsy have recurrent seizures due to presumably irreversible brain defects. If abnormal neuronal firing and inhibitory failure persist, patients can enter a state of prolonged seizures called *status epilepticus*. Status epilepticus often has been defined as seizures that persist for 20 to 30 minutes; however, because treatment for status epilepticus must begin well before 20 minutes to avoid further CNS damage, this definition is impractical. Isolated convulsive seizures rarely last more than 120 seconds. Therefore, a functional definition of status epilepticus is either (i) continuous seizures lasting more than 5 minutes or (ii) two or more seizures between which there is incomplete recovery of consciousness. Status epilepticus should be considered in any patient who is seizing on arrival to the emergency department.

CLINICAL PRESENTATION

The clinical presentation of a seizure depends on the type of seizure. Seizures fall into one of two main types: generalized, in which consciousness is always lost, and partial (focal), in which consciousness is retained fully or partially. Generalized seizures include the familiar tonic-clonic or *grand mal* seizure (sudden muscular rigidity, then jerking) and the absence or *petit mal* seizure (brief loss of consciousness with retention of muscular tone; "blank stare"). Other types of generalized seizures are the myoclonic (brief, often generalized, muscular jerk), clonic (repetitive jerks), tonic (rigid), and atonic (flaccid) seizures.

Partial (focal) seizures are classified as either simple partial (localized motor or sensory disturbances with full consciousness) or complex partial (localized, often bizarre, motor automatisms, or sensory or emotional disturbances with impaired consciousness). Partial (focal) seizures sometimes spread to both cerebral hemispheres and mimic a generalized seizure (secondary generalization). All seizures except absence and simple partial seizures are associated with a postictal state of lethargy and confusion that can last from minutes to hours as consciousness returns. If a patient appears to be in a prolonged postictal state, however, check for signs of continued seizure (e.g., nystagmus or finger twitching) that may indicate status epilepticus.

DIAGNOSIS

A detailed history should be taken from the patient and witnesses to determine whether the attack was indeed a seizure. Seizures typically are unprovoked and abrupt in onset; last less than 2 minutes; involve some loss of consciousness; have bilateral, purposeless movements; and are followed by a postictal state. Seizures occasionally may be preceded by a prodrome, such as a sense of foreboding, or by a sensory aura lasting only a few seconds. Alternate diagnoses to consider include syncope, hyperventilation syndrome, psychogenic seizures, panic attacks, migraine, transient ischemic attacks, and narcolepsy. The history should also inquire about past seizures, medications and drug use, past head trauma or stroke, and possible acute precipitants.

Physical examination should include temperature, bedside glucose, and a search for signs of systemic or CNS infection. The patient should be evaluated thoroughly for injuries, including posterior shoulder dislocations and tongue lacerations. Serial neurologic examinations allow for confirmation of returning consciousness and neurologic status. Patients occasionally experience Todd's paralysis, a temporary postictal focal neurologic deficit that usually resolves within 48 hours.

Laboratory tests are often helpful in isolating the cause of a seizure. Known epileptics may require only a serum anticonvulsant drug level. All others should have glucose; electrolytes; chemistry panel, including calcium and magnesium; complete blood count; prothrombin time; pregnancy test; and toxicology screen. Postictal patients can experience lactic acidosis that typically clears within 1 hour. Lumbar puncture is occasionally helpful when CNS infection is suspected, although seizures themselves can cause fever and pleocytosis. Head computed tomography should be ordered for patients with a first seizure or with a history of cancer, fever, human immunodeficiency virus, severe headache, recent head trauma, and new focal deficits or a change in seizure pattern. Reliable, fully recovered patients with nonfocal examinations who have no risk factors for intracranial abnormalities can be referred for outpatient magnetic resonance imaging.

MANAGEMENT

All patients should be assessed for an adequate airway and receive oxygen, pulse oximetry, intravenous normal saline (phenytoin is not compatible with glucose), and cardiac monitor, if indicated. If a patient is actively seizing, protect him or her from injury, using gentle restraint if necessary. There is no need to insert a bite block, because doing so may result in injury to the teeth.

If the patient has a known history of seizures, and anticonvulsant levels are low, a loading dose of medication should be given and the patient restarted on his or her regular regimen. The loading dose of phenytoin is 18 mg per kg PO (sometimes divided into 3 doses q2h; therapeutic in 2–24 hours) or 50 mg per minute IV (therapeutic in 1–2 hours). Carbamazepine can be loaded at a dose of 8 mg per kg oral suspension.

Patients with an apparent first seizure generally require neurologic consultation for outpatient electroencephalography (EEG). The decision to start the patient on anticonvulsant therapy is based on the risk of seizure recurrence, and no clear guidelines exist. Two-year recurrence rates range from 20% to 70% and increase with abnormal EEG examinations (50%), neurologic injury or illness (50%), or both (65%). Recurrence does not appear to be related to age, gender, family history of seizures, or status epilepticus on presentation. Because anticonvulsants can cause significant side effects, inconvenience, and expense for patients, patients should be involved in any decision to begin anticonvulsant therapy. In general, anticonvulsant therapy can be started from the emergency department in patients with seizures due to an identifiable neurologic injury or illness. If anticonvulsant therapy is chosen, a loading dose (see previous details) and then an initiation regimen of phenytoin (start 300 mg qd) or carbamazepine (start 200 mg b.i.d.) should be given for generalized tonic-clonic or partial seizures.

Status epilepticus is a medical emergency, and patients need quick therapy to avoid the neurologic damage that begins 30 to 60 minutes into the seizure. Initial evaluation and management should proceed as discussed previously, with special attention to airway management, temperature, and arterial blood gas monitoring. These patients may have severe metabolic acidosis that corrects itself when seizures have stopped; treatment with sodium bicarbonate should be reserved for extreme cases. If there is laboratory or clinical evidence of respiratory distress, bag-valve-mask ventilation or intubation with short-acting neuromuscular blockade (e.g., vecuronium, 0.1 mg/kg) may be necessary. Note that any patient with status epilepticus who has been administered long-acting paralytics should have emergent EEG monitoring to track seizure progress. Thiamine (100 mg IV) and glucose (25–50 g IV) should be given if malnourishment or hypoglycemia is suspected.

Treatment of status epilepticus should begin immediately after diagnosis with lorazepam (0.1 mg/kg IV at 2 mg/minute). If seizures continue, give phenytoin (20 mg/kg IV at 50 mg/minute), followed by an additional dose of phenytoin (5–10 mg/kg) if seizures persist. If the patient continues to seize, give phenobarbital (20 mg/kg IV at 50–75 mg/minute) followed by more phenobarbital (5–10 mg/kg) if the first dose is not effective. If this treatment regimen fails, or if the seizure has persisted for 60 minutes, proceed immediately to anesthesia with midazolam (0.2 mg/kg slow IV bolus, then 0.75–10.00 mg/kg/minute) or propofol (1–2 mg/kg, then 2–10 mg/kg/hour). With anesthesia infusion, the patient should be intubated and placed on continuous EEG monitoring. The infusion is typically continued for 12 to 24 hours, and when gradually withdrawn, the patient is monitored for seizure recurrence. Therapy is stopped if EEG spikes are suppressed or EEG shows a burst-suppression pattern with less than 1-second intervals between bursts. Hypotension that occurs during infusion should be treated with intravenous fluids and dopamine; if necessary, add dobutamine. If signs of cardiovascular compromise appear, decrease the dose of midazolam or propofol.

Admission is indicated for patients with seizures due to head trauma, CNS infection or lesions, eclampsia, hyponatremia, hypoglycemia, dysrhythmia, significant hypoxia or alcohol withdrawal, or status epilepticus. A patient with a persistent change in mental status or a persistent metabolic disturbance should also be admitted. Patients who are discharged should be accompanied by a responsible adult and receive neurologic follow-up. Discharged patients should be reminded not to swim, drive, operate heavy machinery, or engage in other potentially dangerous activities until they have been further evaluated.

Chapter 78

STROKE AND TRANSIENT ISCHEMIC ATTACK

Stephanie Rosborough

OVERVIEW

Stroke is the third leading cause of death and the third most common admission diagnosis in the United States. A stroke results from blockage of blood flow or bleeding into the brain that causes neurologic deficits referable to the involved areas of the central nervous system. Transient ischemic attack (TIA) has the same etiology as ischemic stroke, but the symptoms of TIA resolve within 24 hours. New developments in thrombolytic therapy emphasize the need for timely diagnosis and treatment.

PATHOPHYSIOLOGY

Stroke is divided into two broad types based on mechanism: ischemic and hemorrhagic. Ischemic stroke represents 75% of all cases and is usually the result of emboli, especially from cardiac sources, particularly atrial fibrillation and myocardial infarction. Atherosclerotic large-vessel thrombosis and hemorrhagic strokes each are responsible for 10% to 15%. Roughly 30% to 50% of hemorrhagic stroke patients die within a month of the event. There are two types of hemorrhagic stroke: subarachnoid hemorrhage and intracerebral hemorrhage. Subarachnoid hemorrhage is commonly the result of a ruptured berry aneurysm or arteriovenous malformation. Causes of intracerebral hemorrhage include hypertension, cocaine use, bleeding diatheses, vascular malformations, anticoagulant medications, and hemorrhagic conversion of a thrombotic stroke.

On the cellular level, the effects of acute ischemia follow a time-dependent course of decreased energy production, hyperstimulation of glutamate receptors due to lack of reuptake, accumulation of ions (Na^+, Cl^-, Ca^{2+}), mitochondrial injury, and cell death. Focal ischemia quickly produces a core lesion of infarcted brain tissue surrounded by an ischemic penumbra. The goal of rapid treatment of ischemic stroke is to quickly restore normal blood circulation to interrupt the ischemic cascade and protect the potentially salvageable area of hypoxic tissue.

CLINICAL PRESENTATION

The sudden onset of symptoms, in association with a focal neurologic deficit and no history of trauma, is highly suggestive of stroke. Patients may demonstrate motor dysfunction, including weakness, dysphagia, ataxia, and dysarthria. Numbness and paresthesias in the extremities or face, vertigo, loss of vision or diplopia, visual field changes, and aphasia can also occur. The signs and symptoms of stroke can be subtle, but combinations suggest regional brain involvement. For example, diplopia alone is seldom due to stroke, but when occurring in combination with facial weakness and hemiataxia, it suggests brainstem ischemia. Early diagnosis of subarachnoid hemorrhage, suggested by the presence of headache, vomiting, and nuchal rigidity, can be life saving.

On physical examination, vascular bruits in the carotid and retro-orbital regions should be sought and the heart examined for murmurs and arrhythmia. Skin or retinal signs of emboli and papilledema or subhyaloid hemorrhages on funduscopy are also helpful findings to determine cause.

DIAGNOSIS

Initial history taking should focus on assessing the time of onset of symptoms to determine the patient's eligibility for thrombolytic therapy. The patient or a witness should describe the onset of the stroke itself and note whether nausea, vomiting, headache, recent head or neck trauma, or recent TIA-type symptoms preceded the onset. The neurologic examination should include an assessment of level of consciousness, cranial nerves, vision and fundi, sensation and neglect, motor and cerebellar function, and speech; carefully documenting deficits in a quantifiable way that can be followed over time is helpful.

Laboratory tests should be initiated quickly. Obtain a bedside blood glucose measurement, electrocardiogram, chest x-ray, and oxygen saturation. Blood should be sent for a complete blood count, including platelets, coagulation studies, cardiac enzymes, and routine chemical analysis. The patient should be sent for early noncontrast head computed tomography (CT), which may provide evidence of early ischemia, including subtle parenchymal hypodensity, focal brain swelling, or a hyperdense middle cerebral artery. The most important reason to get an emergent CT is to diagnose nonischemic causes of symptoms, including hemorrhage, cerebral edema, or tumor.

The differential diagnosis of acute stroke includes hypoglycemia, Bell's palsy, Todd's (postictal) paralysis, focal seizure, brain tumor or abscess, subdural or epidural hematoma, encephalitis (especially herpes), hypertensive encephalopathy, diabetic ketoacidosis, hyperosmotic coma, and migraine.

MANAGEMENT

Treatment of acute stroke should begin as soon as possible. Stroke patients should initially have vital signs measured frequently and be placed on continuous cardiac and oxygen saturation monitoring. Patients with poor airway or respiratory status should be intubated and mechanically ventilated. Patients should usually have intravenous (IV) access and receive IV hydration. A patient's clinical presentation, CT scan results, and laboratory values determine whether immediate thrombolytic therapy or observation within a stroke unit is most appropriate.

If the diagnosis of ischemic stroke is made within 2 hours of the onset of symptoms, thrombolytics should be considered. For eligible patients, thrombolytic therapy with tissue plasminogen activator should begin at a dose of 0.9 mg per kg IV (maximum of 90 mg), with 10% of the total dose given as an initial bolus and the remainder infused over 1 hour. Eligible patients are those older than 18 years of age with a diagnosis of ischemic stroke associated with the onset of neurologic deficits within the past 3 hours who have none of the following contraindications to thrombolytic therapy: minor or rapidly improving signs and symptoms, CT signs of intracranial hemorrhage, head trauma within the past 3 months, gastrointestinal or urinary hemorrhage within the past 21 days, major surgery within the past 14 days, arterial puncture at a noncompressible site or lumbar puncture within the past 7 days, any past intracranial hemorrhage, seizure at the onset of stroke, symptoms suggesting subarachnoid hemorrhage, systolic blood pressure (BP) over 185 mm Hg, diastolic BP over 110 mm Hg at the time of initiation of therapy, current use of oral anticoagulants (prothrombin time >15 seconds or international normalized ratio >1.7), elevated partial thromboplastin time in association with heparin therapy within the past 48 hours, platelet count under 100,000 per mL, glucose lower than 50 mg per dL or higher than 400 mg per dL, or current pregnancy or lactation. After tissue plasminogen activator administration, BP should be kept under 180/105 mm Hg, and antithrombotic agents should be avoided for 24 hours. Patients should be admitted to a monitored bed, and frequent BP and neurologic checks should be performed. If acute hypertension, severe headache, or nausea and vomiting occur, stop the infusion and obtain an emergency CT scan, consulting neurosurgery if hemorrhage is present.

Patients with ischemic stroke who present more than 3 hours after the onset of symptoms or who are not candidates for thrombolytic therapy should receive supportive therapy. Both dehydration, which risks worsening infarction, and overhydration, which increases cerebral edema, should be avoided. Hypotension should be corrected with fluid, but only severe hypertension (systolic BP >220, diastolic BP >120) should be treated during the first 10 days, because cerebral perfusion pressure equals mean arterial pressure minus intracranial pressure. Hyperglycemia should be avoided, and early attention should be paid to prophylaxis of deep vein thrombosis with pneumatic compression devices in immobile patients. The risk of recurrent stroke within days to weeks of the initial event is 5% to 20%. Follow-up magnetic resonance imaging 24 hours after stroke onset can evaluate the extent of injury and help guide decisions regarding initiation of aspirin or other anticoagulant therapy, which may be warranted if the stroke is cardioembolic or is in a large artery distribution.

Patients with hemorrhagic strokes should be watched for signs of increasing intracranial pressure. Hyperventilation, mannitol, loop diuretics, and maintenance of BP below 200/120 mm Hg are initial medical treatments, but severely elevated intracranial pressure may require neurosurgical consult and craniotomy. Patients with subarachnoid hemorrhage, after an emergency neurosurgery consult is called, should receive prophylactic phenytoin (for seizure) and nimodipine (for vasospasm), and should have mean arterial pressure maintained at 110 mm Hg to prevent rebleeding. They should have an early angiogram to determine the need for neurosurgical intervention. Some other forms of intracerebral hemorrhage also benefit from surgery, such as cerebellar hemorrhage.

All stroke patients should receive follow-up studies, typically carotid ultrasound, transesophageal echocardiogram, and magnetic resonance imaging or magnetic resonance angiography, to find the cause of the stroke. Evaluations by physical and occupational therapy to determine the extent of functional deficits are helpful in developing an optimal rehabilitation plan. Preventing recurrent strokes is essential, and interventions may include warfarin treatment of atrial fibrillation, carotid endarterectomy, antiplatelet therapy, BP control, statin therapy, and smoking cessation.

Chapter 79

SYNCOPE

Craig G. Gunderson

OVERVIEW

Syncope is transient loss of consciousness and accompanying postural tone due to inadequate cerebral blood flow. Conditions that may mimic syncope include seizures, hypoglycemia, and vertigo. Syncope is relatively common, accounting for an estimated 3% of emergency room visits and 1% of hospital admissions. It can represent anything from a benign neurogenic dysfunction to a premonitory sign of sudden cardiac death.

PATHOPHYSIOLOGY

A recent prospective study found cardiac causes (usually bradyarrhythmia or tachyarrhythmia) in 23%, neurally mediated causes in 58%, neurologic or psychiatric causes in 1%, and unexplained syncope in 18%. Syncope is partly defined by its pathophysiologic mechanism, the transient disruption of cerebral blood flow. Beyond that, the precise mechanism varies with etiology. For example, with aortic stenosis, the mechanism is frequently a drop in vascular tone superimposed on a fixed cardiac output—for example, exercise-induced vasodilatation. With hypertrophic cardiomyopathy (HCM), dynamic obstruction occurs owing to systolic anterior motion of the mitral valve against the hypertrophied septum, although these patients are also at risk for arrhythmia. With pulmonary embolism, cardiac output drops owing to right-sided failure. With neurocardiogenic syncope (NCS), the mechanism is a combination of increased vagal tone with resulting bradycardia and decreased sympathetic tone with loss of vascular resistance. With situational syncope, the "situation" is really a Valsalva maneuver that leads to increased pressure in the carotid body and resultant increased vagal and decreased sympathetic tone. Carotid body hypersensitivity has a similar mechanism and occurs in situations in which external pressure is applied to a carotid sinus—for example, from a tight-neck collar or targeted shower spray.

DIAGNOSIS

The causes of syncope may be divided into two main categories: cardiac and noncardiac. The "can't miss" diagnoses are generally cardiac (because of a 24% risk of subsequent sudden death). The more common are the noncardiac. The younger the patient, the fewer the risk factors, and the more likely a noncardiac cause. Cardiac causes include
- Mechanical: aortic stenosis, other stenoses (e.g., HCM), atrial myxoma, pulmonary embolism, myocardial infarction, pulmonary hypertension, pericardial tamponade, aortic dissection, and subclavian steal
- Arrhythmia: ventricular tachycardia, ventricular fibrillation, supraventricular tachycardia, bradyarrhythmias, prolonged QT (congenital or acquired), and Wolff-Parkinson-White syndrome (WPW)

Noncardiac causes include
- Reflex mediated: NCS (i.e., vasovagal), situational syncope (e.g., posttussive, micturitional), carotid sinus hypersensitivity
- Orthostatic hypotension: either related to autonomic dysfunction (age, diabetics, Shy-Drager syndrome), dehydration, anemia (e.g., gastrointestinal bleed), or drug side effect
- Cerebrovascular insufficiency: including severe global cerebrovascular disease and subclavian steal

The differential also includes seizure, hypoglycemia, psychiatric causes, vertigo, disequilibrium, and head trauma.

The cause of an episode of syncope can be hard to uncover, because several of its more common causes are themselves potentially difficult to diagnose: arrhythmia because of its intermittency, orthostasis because of its ubiquity, and NCS because of the lack of a clearly reliable diagnostic test. Of patients who are diagnosed with a specific cause of syncope, 55% are diagnosed based on the history and physical, 21% based on prolonged cardiac monitoring, 12% based on the electrocardiogram, and only a few percent each for the remaining studies.

History and physical examination is the cornerstone of diagnosis. The basic approach is to review the events leading up to the episode. What was the patient doing at the time? Was the event exertional (aortic stenosis, HCM)? Was the patient exercising an arm (subclavian steal) or applying pressure or stretch to a carotid body (carotid hypersensitivity)? Was the patient doing a Valsalva maneuver (situational syncope)? Was the patient in a stressful situation (NCS)? Were there premonitory symptoms to suggest NCS, most commonly weakness, diaphoresis, nausea or vomiting? Did the event begin without warning, suggestive of arrhythmia? Was there any chest pain or palpitations? Did any seizure activity or an aura occur? How fast did the patient recover? The medical history should be reviewed, with attention toward coronary risk factors and resultant substrate for arrhythmia. Also, ask whether the patient has had previous syncopal episodes. Recurrent syncope is unlikely to be due to a dangerous arrhythmia. Medications should be reviewed, with attention to drugs that cause hypotension or arrhythmia. Drugs that prolong the QT interval include class 1A ("quinidine syncope") and class 3 antiarrhythmics, tricyclics, phenothiazides, terfenadine (Seldane), and azole antifungals. The family history should be explored for relatives with syncope or sudden cardiac death (prolonged QT syndrome, HCM, WPW).

The physical examination should be complete and include orthostatics, pulses, carotid examination, detailed cardiac and neurologic examinations, and stool guaiac. Orthostatic hypotension and carotid sinus hypersensitivity are common phenomena in the elderly and should be assigned etiologic significance only if they are symptomatic and there is no other apparent cause of the patient's syncope.

Basic laboratory tests should include a complete blood count, electrolytes, glucose, and cardiac enzymes if indicated. Electrocardiography should be the first study in a syncope evaluation, looking for arrhythmia, ischemia, left ventricular hypertrophy (of HCM), shortened PR interval and slurred upstroke (of WPW), and QT prolongation (favoring torsades de pointes). Prolonged monitoring should be done, either with telemetry if hospitalized or outpatient 24-hour Holter monitoring. Loop event recorders are available for outpatient monitoring for up to 1 month. Further studies are tailored to the specific patient. Echocardiography can be performed if a mechanical cause of syncope is suspected. Upright tilt table is a provocative test for NCS. A positive test is defined by symptomatic hypotension or bradycardia. Because there is no gold standard for NCS, the sensitivity and specificity of the test are unknown. Computed tomography or magnetic resonance imaging of the head is indicated if the patient has focal findings, or if head trauma is suspected as a consequence of the event. Carotid ultrasound should be done if the patient has findings consistent with severe cerebrovascular disease or bilateral carotid artery disease. Electroencephalography is performed if the history is suggestive of seizure. Electrophysiologic study should be considered in patients with known coronary artery disease, depressed left ventricular ejection fraction, or evidence of conduction disease without clear explanation. In patients with structural heart disease, electrophysiologic study can identify a cause of syncope in up to 70%, and inducible ventricular tachycardia is correlated with a high risk of sudden death.

MANAGEMENT

In general, the particular therapy for syncope depends on the specific cause. Cardiac syncope treatment again depends on the underlying cause and ranges from surgery for some mechanical causes, to pacemaker for sinus node or conduction disease, to implantable cardiac defibrillators or medication, or both, for ventricular dysrhythmias. Numerous treatments for NCS exist. Probably the most commonly used are beta-blockers (e.g., atenolol or metoprolol). Other drugs that have been used include ephedrine, disopyramide, and fluoxetine. In severe refractory cases, cardiac pacemakers have even been used.

Chapter 80

GUILLAIN-BARRÉ SYNDROME

Gaby Weissman

OVERVIEW

Guillain-Barré syndrome (GBS), or acute demyelinating polyradiculoneuropathy, is considered a postinfectious acute peripheral neuropathy. GBS is the most common cause of nontraumatic generalized paralysis in young adults, with an annual incidence of 1.2 cases per 100,000. This disease affects the young and old, with its first peak in young adults and a second, smaller peak in the fifth to seventh decades. There is also a slight predominance in men. GBS represents a medical emergency, and as such it is critical to recognize it early in its course.

PATHOPHYSIOLOGY

GBS is an inflammatory condition that leads to demyelination along the peripheral nerves and nerve roots. Its pathologic hallmark is a perivascular infiltration of lymphocytes, monocytes, and sometimes plasma cells in the endoneurium and myelin sheath. This infiltration is usually seen around the ventral nerve roots in the plexus and the proximal nerve trunks. Less common is a more distal involvement of the myelin sheath. In some patients, axonal degeneration may also be seen in addition to demyelination. There is an immune-mediated component in this syndrome, with some studies suggesting a role for antibodies against the myelin sheath.

GBS is often associated with a viral infection, most often upper respiratory, several weeks before presentation, perhaps triggering the immune response. In addition, some studies have reported that up to 38% of patients have had a recent *Campylobacter jejuni* infection, and a patient with a *C. jejuni* infection has a 100-fold increased risk of developing GBS. This heightened risk may be caused by cross-reacting antibodies to GM1 ganglioside (present in high concentrations in peripheral nerve myelin) formed in response to similar epitopes expressed by the *Campylobacter*. In addition, GBS has been associated with Epstein-Barr virus, cytomegalovirus, viral hepatitis, human immunodeficiency virus, mycoplasma, Lyme disease, and sarcoidosis. The symptoms of GBS often begin 1 to 2 weeks after the acute infection.

CLINICAL PRESENTATION

The initial symptoms are fine paresthesias of the toes and fingers, followed by ascending weakness. The legs are usually first affected, followed in a few days by arm weakness. The proximal and distal muscle groups are usually equally involved, and the weakness is bilaterally symmetric, with symmetric deep tendon reflex loss. Although GBS may present with a rapid course of paralysis that may reach its maximal levels within 1 or 2 days, the weakness more commonly progresses over 1 to 2 weeks. Fifty percent of patients have cranial muscle weakness, whereas one-third have respiratory muscle dysfunction. Fifty percent of patients have autonomic nerve involvement leading to such symptoms as blood pressure lability. The sensory system is usually very mildly affected, with few physical examination findings. Vibratory sensation is the most often affected of the senses. A form of GBS named the *Miller-Fisher variant* is characterized by ophthalmoplegia and ptosis followed by ataxia. Patients go on to develop absent reflexes and may have cranial nerve, limb muscle, and respiratory muscle weakness.

The disease is usually self-limiting, with the symptoms reaching a plateau in 2 to 4 weeks, followed by a slow recovery. Overall, one-half of patients have some residual neurologic abnormality, with 5% having significant disability. The mortality of GBS is reported to be between 2% and 5%, often secondary to complications, such as sepsis.

DIAGNOSIS

The diagnosis of GBS may be difficult to make, and a broad differential diagnosis should be kept in mind. The classical laboratory finding is an increase in cerebrospinal fluid protein. This elevation often begins 1 to 2 days after the start of symptoms but may be normal in up to 18% of patients as far out as the second week of the disease. In addition, a lymphocytic pleocytosis may be seen, usually up to 100 cells per mm^3. Electromyography may demonstrate a demyelinating peripheral neuropathy with slow conduction velocities, dispersed compound muscle action potentials, multifocal conduction block, and abnormal H-wave reflex. These abnormalities also develop over the first few days of the illness.

It is important to rule out other conditions that may cause similar symptoms. A list of conditions that may mimic GBS follows:
- Spinal cord compression
- Human immunodeficiency virus
- Transverse myelitis
- Carcinomatous meningitis
- Spinal cord infarction
- Sarcoidosis
- Critical illness polyneuropathy
- Paraneoplastic acute peripheral neuropathy
- Toxins (including arsenic, thallium, lead tetrodotoxin, organophosphates, hexacarbons)
- Hypokalemic periodic paralysis
- Diphtheria
- Drugs (dapsone, isoniazid, gold, nitrofurantoin, chloroquine)
- Myasthenia gravis
- Autoimmune systemic disease (systemic lupus, polyarteritis nodosa)
- Botulism
- Poliomyelitis
- Lyme disease

If there is evidence of a focal lesion, an emergent magnetic resonance image of the appropriate spinal level should be obtained. If the cerebrospinal fluid on initial presentation is normal, a repeat lumbar puncture in 1 to 2 weeks may be helpful. All patients should be screened for human immunodeficiency virus and autoimmune inflammatory diseases, in addition to getting a complete blood count, electrolytes, liver function, and renal function tests. A urine test for acute intermittent porphyria is indicated as well. Patients may be screened for the other diseases in the differential list as the clinical circumstances indicate. Tests for Epstein-Barr virus, cytomegalovirus, hepatitis viruses, and mycoplasma should be considered. Any patient with acute paralysis should be screened for myasthenia gravis or tick paralysis. Botulism should be considered in patients with primarily cranial nerve findings.

MANAGEMENT

GBS is always managed in an inpatient setting for close observation of the patient, as the primary aspect of treatment is aggressive medical support. Respiratory muscle compromise can be a significant part of GBS. It is therefore important to get baseline spirometry in all patients with GBS and to follow those values closely for a possible deterioration. The "20/30/40" rule applies: Patients with a vital capacity less than 20 mL per kg, maximal inspiratory pressure lower than 30 cm H_2O, or a maximal expiratory pressure below 40 cm H_2O are likely to progress to require mechanical ventilation. It is wise to maintain a low threshold for intubation and to consider intubating even if the patient does not meet objective criteria for intubation but clinically appears to be doing poorly. Patients often need to be in an intensive care setting for closer monitoring until it is clear that the symptoms have stabilized or are improving.

Both plasma exchange and intravenous immunoglobulin have been shown to decrease the time to clinical improvement; however, both need to be started early in the disease to have a significant benefit. Although both treatment modalities are more effective than no treatment, it is currently debatable whether one is superior to the other. Potential complications of plasmapheresis are associated with the venous access needed, such as line sepsis and obtaining the access. Intravenous immunoglobulin is considered relatively safe, with rare complications including acute renal failure, hepatitis C infection, myocardial infarction, and stroke. Corticosteroids have also been studied in the management of this disease; however, clear benefit has not been shown.

Chapter 81

HEADACHE

Seonaid F. Hay

OVERVIEW

Most adults experience headaches, with 80% to 90% of healthy adults reporting recurrent headaches. Of these, more than 90% are tension or migraine-type headaches; however, urgent causes of headache exist and are important to know so that diagnosis and treatment may be initiated promptly.

PATHOPHYSIOLOGY

Headache can be produced by any pain-sensitive structure in the head, from the skin down to the intracranial vessels. The brain parenchyma itself is not pain sensitive. Tension headaches are most likely caused by increased muscle and psychological stress and are also called "common" headaches. Migraines are thought to be vascular headaches caused by intracranial vasodilation's triggering pain neurons; they occur more commonly in women and are often related to decreases in estrogen at the beginning of the menstrual cycle. Subarachnoid hemorrhage is bleeding in the subarachnoid space often caused by trauma, aneurysmal rupture, or drugs, such as alcohol or cocaine. Temporal arteritis (a form of giant cell arteritis) causes temporal headaches secondary to inflammation of the temporal arteries. Meningitis causes headaches through inflammation of the meninges. Cluster headaches are also thought to be vascular but are not well understood. Tumors cause headaches by increasing intracranial pressure through mass effect or edema. Benign intracranial hypertension (pseudotumor cerebri) is an unusual cause of headache in young, obese, or pregnant women who have high intracranial pressures of unclear etiology.

CLINICAL PRESENTATION

Tension headaches present with bilateral bandlike, moderately severe pain, occasionally with concomitant visual "spots." Migraines may present with a prodrome of visual aura, such as a scintillating scotoma, but more commonly begin with premonitory symptoms but no real aura. The headache is usually unilateral, pulsatile, and associated with photophobia, phonophobia, nausea, vomiting, and sometimes focal neurologic signs (complex migraine). Subarachnoid hemorrhage is a "thunderclap" headache, sudden in onset and described as the worst headache in the patient's life. Patients often have a depressed mental status as well. Temporal arteritis presents in older patients with fever, generalized headache, tender temporal arteries, and associated polymyalgia rheumatica. Meningitis presents with fever, generalized headache, and stiff neck. Tumors present with headache on awakening that improves through the day but rarely presents without associated focal neurologic signs. Cluster headaches occur mostly in men and present as severe headaches lasting an hour, occurring many times in a day for weeks to months and then resolving completely. Benign intracranial hypertension presents with a generalized headache, which gradually and progressively worsens, with papilledema and occasionally cranial nerve VI dysfunction.

DIAGNOSIS

Tension headaches, migraines, and cluster headaches can be diagnosed by history and physical examination, with care given to doing a thorough neurologic and funduscopic examination to rule out a focal lesion or increased intracranial pressure. Subarachnoid hemorrhage can be diagnosed with computed tomography scan or lumbar puncture. Biopsy of the temporal artery, elevated sedimentation rate, and clinical features diagnose temporal arteritis. Meningitis is diagnosed by pleocytosis and positive Gram stain on the lumbar puncture. Tumors are diagnosed with computed tomography or magnetic resonance imaging of the brain and then biopsy for histology. Benign intracranial hypertension is diagnosed by the findings of papilledema and an increased opening pressure (>20 cm H_2O) on lumbar puncture.

Computed tomography scanning of patients with normal funduscopic and neurologic examinations rarely yields a diagnosis and should be reserved for cases in which subarachnoid hemorrhage, subdural hematoma, or brain tumor is strongly suspected. A magnetic resonance image or angiography is indicated when intracranial mass or vascular lesions are suspected.

MANAGEMENT

Tension headaches are treated with over-the-counter analgesics, low-dose tricyclics, and stress relief. Migraines can be aborted by triptans or nonsteroidal antiinflammatory drugs and prevented by daily use of beta-blockers, calcium channel blockers, tricyclics, gabapentin, and topiramate. Oxygen therapy at 5 L per minute, triptans, and analgesia treat cluster headaches. For these benign headaches, avoidance of triggers, such as alcohol and smoking for cluster headache and red wine, cheeses, and monosodium glutamate for migraines, also plays a major role in their management. Subarachnoid hemorrhage can be evacuated surgically if necessary but can reabsorb spontaneously depending on the size and associated symptoms. Temporal arteritis should be aggressively treated with corticosteroids when suspected to prevent vision loss. Meningitis is treated immediately with appropriate antibiotics and supportive therapy. Benign intracranial hypertension usually resolves spontaneously but can be treated with acetazolamide (Diamox) or serial lumbar punctures to decrease intracranial pressure or, infrequently, cerebrospinal fluid shunting.

Chapter 82

PERIPHERAL NEUROPATHY

Joseph V. Agostini

OVERVIEW

Peripheral neuropathy is typically characterized by symmetric distal sensory burning or weakness. It consists of peripheral nerve disorders involving one nerve (mononeuropathy) or multiple nerves (polyneuropathy). Disorders can be characterized by the degree of axonal degeneration or segmental demyelination, the degree of motor or sensory involvement, and the acuity of onset.

PATHOPHYSIOLOGY

Common etiologies of mononeuropathy include isolated trauma to a peripheral nerve and pressure or entrapment of a specific nerve, such as the radial nerve (resulting in "Saturday night palsy"), median nerve (carpal tunnel syndrome), or posterior tibial nerve (tarsal tunnel syndrome). Mononeuropathy multiplex is simultaneous involvement of noncontiguous nerve trunks due to infarcts in the vasa nervorum. It arises in patients with connective tissue disorders, vasculitis, and some infiltrative disorders, including primary amyloidosis and sarcoidosis. Polyneuropathies can be due to metabolic disease (renal insufficiency, diabetes mellitus), infection (human immunodeficiency virus), nutritional compromise (alcoholism, vitamin B_{12} deficiency, thiamine deficiency, and pyridoxine deficiency in those taking isoniazid for tuberculosis), inherited conditions (the porphyrias, Charcot-Marie-Tooth disease), malignancy (multiple myeloma), drugs (e.g., vincristine, cisplatin, and antiretrovirals, such as dideoxycytidine and didanosine), and toxins (inorganic lead and arsenic).

CLINICAL PRESENTATION

Clinical presentation for selected disorders is variable based on etiology. Symptoms common in the presentation include sensory changes or dysesthesias (numbness, tingling, and burning sensations), loss of tendon reflexes, and muscle weakness. Diabetic polyneuropathy, perhaps the most common neuropathy seen in general medicine, prototypically presents with distally symmetric sensory involvement in the "stocking and glove" distribution. Nocturnal pain can also be a common feature. Diabetic polyneuropathy may progress insidiously for years in an asymptomatic patient, but physical examination including monofilament testing and vibratory testing helps to identify patients who are at risk for ulcers.

DIAGNOSIS

A careful review of history and physical examination serves as a guide to ordering appropriate diagnostic studies. Extensive testing is not necessary in a patient with mild symptoms and a known underlying reason for the neuropathy (e.g., diabetes). A complete blood count can be helpful for the diagnosis of malignancy or lead poisoning; serum protein electrophoresis, for dysproteinemias; liver function tests, for malignancy; thyroid function tests, for thyroid disorder; serum creatinine, for renal failure; glucose and glycosylated hemoglobin, for diabetes mellitus; vitamin B_{12} level; antinuclear antibody, for autoimmune disorders; urine testing, for toxin poisoning and hereditary porphyrias; and serologic immunoassays, for human immunodeficiency virus. Electrodiagnostic studies can help to distinguish between demyelinating neuropathy (e.g., Guillain-Barré syndrome) and axonal neuropathy (e.g., diabetes). The latter are characterized by low-amplitude evoked action potentials and normal nerve conduction velocities, whereas the former exhibit slowed nerve conduction velocities, prolonged distal latencies, and evidence of demyelinating blocks. Finally, cutaneous nerve biopsy (usually of the sural nerve) is a more invasive but infrequently ordered diagnostic procedure.

MANAGEMENT

Management depends on the underlying disease process. Compression neuropathies are treated conservatively with localized treatment, antiinflammatory agents, and, in severe cases, surgery. Other systematic diseases are treated as indicated with the hope of stopping the progression of neuropathy. Some data suggest that angiotensin-converting enzyme inhibitors may be useful for diabetic neuropathy. Symptomatic dysesthesias can be ameliorated, although not cured, with tricyclics, gabapentin, or capsaicin.

Chapter 83

MULTIPLE SCLEROSIS

Christopher S. Alia

OVERVIEW

Multiple sclerosis (MS) is the most common of the demyelinating disorders and affects roughly one in 1,000 persons in the United States and Europe, the regions of highest prevalence. Often, the presenting symptoms are subtle or unusual, such as an isolated patch of numbness, and may be hard for the patient to describe, making diagnosis difficult. The clinical course of MS varies widely, as does the response to immunomodulating therapy, but it usually involves progressive neurologic dysfunction distributed over time and space.

PATHOPHYSIOLOGY

MS is a chronic demyelinating disease characterized by chronic inflammation and gliosis (scarring) of the lipid-rich myelin sheaths of the central nervous system (CNS). Current theory implicates an initial environmental exposure as the inciting event in a person who is genetically susceptible to the development of MS. An inflammatory reaction against the patient's myelin components results in the T-cell–mediated release of inflammatory cytokines, including interleukin-1, interferon, and tumor necrosis factor, and the eventual destruction of oligodendroglial cells (both B- and T-cell mediated). This process results in the development of plaques in the CNS white matter that can range in size from 1 to several millimeters. Eventually, these plaques become areas of complete demyelinization and loss of myelin-producing oligodendrocytes. These demyelinated areas can cause profound symptoms or imperceptible effects, depending on localization of the plaque.

MS is twice as common in women as men, with peak incidence occurring at the age of 30 years in women and slightly later in men. Genetically, there is an increased risk for developing MS in related individuals, including first-degree relatives, siblings, and twins, but simple genetic models do not explain this risk. The inheritance is therefore multifactorial and probably polygenic. Ethnic variability is well documented, having higher incidence in white populations than in African-American or Asian populations. Also, there is geographic variability, with temperate climates having a higher incidence of disease. Incidence increases proportionally with distance from the equator.

CLINICAL PRESENTATION

The clinical manifestations of MS are diverse and may include weakness, autonomic instability, and vision loss. The lesions are classically disseminated in time and space (two or more clinically distinct episodes of CNS dysfunction with at least partial resolution). The most common presenting symptoms are focal weakness of a limb; sensory disturbances, such as paresthesias or hypoesthesias; ataxia; and optic neuritis. Autonomic dysfunction often can be seen and can be manifested as urinary or fecal incontinence, hesitancy, and urgency. Cerebellar signs may include ataxia, vertigo, and changes in speech coordination. Generalized complaints include fatigue and cognitive dysfunction.

Eye findings are common in MS. Optic neuritis is a condition in which inflammation of the optic nerve leads to variable degrees of blindness. The result is usually a monocular visual field defect, but it can sometimes be binocular. The inflammation may be heralded by antecedent pain in an orbital or periorbital distribution. The pupillary response may be altered, and funduscopic examination may reveal optic disc swelling and perivascular cuffing. Internuclear ophthalmoplegia is a sixth cranial nerve palsy that results from a lesion in the medial longitudinal fasciculus, which is common in MS. The medial longitudinal fasciculus nerve tract connects the third and sixth cranial nerve nuclei and coordinates horizontal gaze, so that the affected patient is able to converge normally but delays adduction or is entirely unable to adduct and has nystagmus in the abducting eye. The patient may complain of visual blurring and diplopia as a result.

Trigeminal neuralgia, although far from exclusive to MS, may raise concern for MS when it presents at a young age and is bilateral and associated with other cranial nerve involvement. The patient experiences omnipresent sharp, shocklike facial pain, which often is constant. Lhermitte's sign is a brief sensation of electrical shock when the neck is flexed, which can migrate down the spine and to the legs. Although classically described in association with MS, Lhermitte's symptom is not pathognomonic of MS.

DIAGNOSIS

The diagnosis of MS is predominantly a clinical one. Examination findings of CNS lesions must be demonstrated. The differential diagnosis is extremely broad and can include a wide range of systemic and neurologic diseases, depending on the presenting symptoms.

The laboratory diagnosis of MS relies on spinal fluid analysis, magnetic resonance imaging (MRI), and occasionally evoked potentials. Spinal fluid analysis often reveals cell counts with monocyte predominance, elevation of cerebrospinal fluid total protein, immunoglobulin G, and oligoclonal immunoglobulins ("oligoclonal bands"). Eighty-five percent to 95% of MS patients exhibit oligoclonal bands in the cerebrospinal fluid during the course of the disease (but there may be up to 8% false-positives).

MS lesions can be well visualized, and diagnosis can be facilitated by the use of MRI. MRI testing is extremely sensitive; however, specificity is low, and false-positive tests are common. White matter lesions may be seen in as many as 10% of healthy 30- to 40-year-olds. Classic MS lesions appear as focal white matter densities (hypointense) in T1-weighted MRIs and appear as enhanced, bright-white foci on proton density and T2-weighted images. Lesions can be visualized in periventricular, cerebellar, and brainstem regions as well. With the administration of gadolinium contrast, T1-weighted images may show enhancement surrounding MS lesions suggestive of an impaired blood–brain barrier. Using criteria of three or more plaques, lesions abutting the lateral ventricles, and size larger than 5 mm optimizes accuracy with sensitivity of 81% and specificity of 96%. Serial MRI is helpful in localizing new lesions or expansion of previously defined lesions.

Evoked potentials are clinical tests that detect abnormality in conduction when the patient is subjected to certain stimuli. These stimuli may be sensory, visual, or auditory. Evoked potential abnormality is seen in 80% to 90% of MS patients but is of limited clinical usefulness. Testing is most helpful in detecting new lesions or abnormality in a patient already diagnosed with MS.

MANAGEMENT

The disease may follow a progressive course or a relapsing and remitting course. Management of MS therefore is aimed at disease modification and symptomatic treatment. In an acute flare or relapse, a course of intravenous methylprednisolone, 1 g daily for 3 to 7 days, is indicated. Disease-modifying agents that target prevention of new flares include immunomodulatory cytokines, such as interferon beta-1b (Betaseron) and interferon beta-1a (Avonex), as well as glatiramer acetate/copolymer-1 (Copaxone). Use does not improve the deficits already acquired but reduces exacerbations by 30%. Systemic immunosuppressants, such as azathioprine, cyclophosphamide, and methotrexate, and, recently, intravenous immune globulin, have also been used with limited success.

Therapies aimed at symptomatic relief include agents such as tricyclic antidepressants for neuralgia, neuromuscular relaxants for spasticity, autonomically active medications for bladder dysfunction, and treatment for coexistent depression and fatigue.

Chapter 84

BACK PAIN

Beth Anne Biggee

OVERVIEW

Back pain affects approximately 80% of the U.S. population at some time in their lifespan and 10% to 20% of the U.S. population each year. It is the second most common cause of lost time from work in the United States, and the fifth most common chief complaint in the physician's office.

The back contains the axial skeleton, spinal cord, nerve roots, muscles, tendons, ligaments, and important vessels and viscera. "Back" pain often originates from the spine. The spine is made up of vertebral bodies, intervertebral discs, longitudinal ligaments, and vertebral arches. Back pain can originate in the thoracic or lumbosacral spine. Spinal pain can be due to a systemic illness, such as infection, tumor, and rheumatologic conditions, or due to mechanical processes. As many as 90% of patients with back pain have lumbosacral involvement, mechanical in origin. Lumbosacral spinal pain due to a mechanical disorder includes back strain, herniated nucleus pulposus, spinal stenosis, spondylosis, and spondylolisthesis. It is important when evaluating a patient with lumbosacral spinal pain to include a differential diagnosis. The differential diagnosis can vary from compression fractures to dissecting abdominal aortic aneurysms and metastatic tumors.

PATHOPHYSIOLOGY

The lumbosacral spine consists of five lumbar vertebrae and five fused sacral vertebrae. The spine can be further divided into an anterior and a posterior portion. The anterior portion consists of vertebral bodies with intervertebral discs interposed. Intervertebral discs contain a center gelatinous nucleus pulposus and a peripheral tough annulus fibrosis. The anterior and posterior longitudinal ligaments surround the discs and bodies. The anterior spine absorbs shock from body motion. The posterior portion of the spine consists of vertebral arches and transverse and spinous processes. The arch is made up of two pedicles on the anterior surface and two laminae on the posterior surface. The pedicle and laminae fuse laterally to form transverse processes. The laminae fuse posteriorly to form the spinous process. Arising from the arch are two superior and inferior articular facets, which join each vertebrae vertically. The posterior spine protects the spinal cord and nerves. It also stabilizes the spine by serving as a site for muscle attachment.

The pathophysiology of mechanical low back pain is degeneration and narrowing of the structures in the spine secondary to age, overuse, and trauma. Usually a traumatic event, such as lifting a heavy object, can cause back strain or even disc herniation. With repetitive motions, such as lifting heavy boxes, bending, and twisting, the muscles and structures of the spine can degenerate and become chronically inflamed. The degeneration and inflammation can lead to osteoarthritis, narrowing, and instability with slippage of the vertebral spine. Strain or sprain of the back often causes low back muscle spasm. Such spasms are usually the sequelae of minor injuries to muscles, tendons, and ligaments. Injuries such as lifting heavy objects; sudden jerky movements of acceleration and deceleration, as in car accidents; and a minor fall with a twist of the low back can cause or exacerbate strain. Age of onset is usually between 20 and 40 years in an active individual.

Lumbar disc herniation is the extrusion of the nucleus pulposus through the annulus fibrosis that then compresses nerve roots or, rarely, the spinal cord itself. Degeneration of the disc increases with age. Sometimes, minor trauma or even such movements as a cough can cause a degenerated nucleus pulposus to prolapse, which can push the annulus posteriorly and then impinge nerve roots. Herniation, however, is due to severe disc disease, in which the nucleus extrudes through the annulus. Usually it is due to trauma, such as heavy lifting or sudden jerky movements. The most common discs affected are L4-L5 and L-5 to S-1. Wear and tear on the axial skeleton produces facet osteoarthritis. In this process, facet joints hypertrophy, and osteophytes form. These osteophytes can compress or irritate nerve roots. Disc degeneration causes forces to shift in the spine and leads to arthritis of the facet joints. Arthritis can progress to narrowing of the spinal canal, called *spinal stenosis*. Degeneration of the ligamentum flavum and bulging of degenerating discs can contribute. Arthritis can progress to the slipping of vertebrae over other vertebrae, called *spondylolisthesis*. Degenerating discs and spine cause instability, and vertebral bodies shift their forces across joints, leading to anterior displacement of one vertebra on another. The intervertebral disc degenerates and the spine loses height. The descending spine then compresses nerve roots.

CLINICAL PRESENTATION

Back Strain and Sprain

The patient complains of acute low back pain radiating to the paraspinous muscle of the affected side. The pain rarely can radiate to the buttocks but usually does not affect the thighs. The physical examination reveals worsened pain with twisting or bending to the affected side, with limited range of motion secondary to pain. The pain increases with bending and standing upright but not with sitting. The paraspinal muscle on the affected side is in spasm and feels tight on palpation. The neurologic examination in this condition is completely normal.

Disc Herniation

Once the nucleus extrudes through the ruptured disc, the patient experiences back pain, limited range of motion, and radicular pain. Radicular pain or sciatica is from the disc's impinging on one or many nerve roots, causing pain or paresthesias, or both, in a specific dermatomal distribution (radiating from back down buttock into thigh and calf of affected side). The sensitivity and specificity of sciatica for herniated disc are 95% and 88%, respectively. This sciatica is exacerbated by sitting and bending. Patients usually present with back pain radiating to the buttock down into the leg. The pain is acute and worse with sitting and bending, but it can be relieved when standing upright. Physical examination reveals reproduction or increase in radicular pain on the affected side when the examiner raises a straightened leg. The neurologic examination can be abnormal. Sensory deficits, weakness, and diminished or absent reflexes are hallmarks. L-4 disc herniation presents with pain on the anterior thigh and medial leg, with sensory loss to the medial leg. The patellar reflex is lost, and the anterior tibialis is weak. L-5 disc herniation presents with lateral leg pain and sensory loss. Extensor hallucis longus muscle (i.e., extension of the great toe) is weak. S-1 herniation presents with lateral foot pain and sensory loss with diminished or absent Achilles tendon reflex. The peroneus longus is weak.

Facet Arthritis

Low back pain is usually in the center of the spine, which worsens with movement. The pain usually increases at the end of the day. Pain is increased in the upright position and relieved with sitting or bending. The physical examination reveals pain that is worse with extension of the back or with bending to the affected side. Pain can extend into the thigh, but no neurologic deficits are found unless nerve root or spinal stenosis occurs.

Spinal Stenosis (Neurologic Claudication)

The patient usually is well over 60 years of age and presents with pain on standing or walking in one or both legs. The pain is not necessarily relieved just by resting, but by flexing forward or sitting, which decompresses the spinal stenosis. The physical examination is usually normal when sitting or flexing forward, but with prolonged standing or walking, the sensory, motor, or reflex examination can be abnormal and usually in dermatomal distributions.

Spondylolisthesis

As mentioned, spondylolisthesis can result from osteoarthritis of the lumbosacral spine. Patients complain of low back pain that is worse on standing and relieved on rest. Some can have referred pain into the leg. The physical examination reveals lordosis with increased pain on standing and bending that is relieved with sitting. The neurologic examination is usually normal.

DIAGNOSIS

Beware: The potential causes of lumbar back pain are numerous and sometimes dangerous. The key to recognition lies in maintaining a high index of suspicion despite a low prevalence, and investigating atypical symptoms (e.g., fever), unremitting or progressive pain incompletely relieved by lying down or at night, and back pain in patients with a known history of cancer or injection drug use. Unilateral or bilateral leg weakness and bladder, bowel, or sexual dysfunction suggest cauda equina syndrome, and absence effectively rules it out. Other causes of low back pain syndrome include adult scoliosis, ankylosing spondylitis, vertebral compression fracture, osteomyelitis, epidural abscess, neoplasm, lumbar adhesive arachnoiditis, Paget's disease, Reiter's syndrome, psoriatic arthritis, rheumatoid arthritis, diffuse idiopathic skeletal hyperostosis, polymyalgia rheumatica, fibromyalgia, Behçet's syndrome, dissection of an abdominal aortic aneurysm, appendicitis, cholecystitis, chordoma, endometriosis, multiple myeloma, pancreatitis, perforated ulcer, pyelonephritis, renal calculi, and psychiatric causes.

Back Strain

Diagnosis is made clinically through history and physical examination, and largely by excluding other etiologies—namely, lumbar disc herniation.

Disc Herniation

History of characteristic radicular pain, especially when accompanied by confirmatory physical findings, provides an accurate diagnosis. Magnetic resonance imaging should be reserved for patients with atypical findings and those in whom surgery is contemplated.

Facet Arthritis

Diagnosis is made by history and physical examination. Radiographs with facet joint narrowing, osteophytes, or periarticular sclerosis can aid diagnosis. Magnetic resonance imaging is indicated if neurologic symptoms ensue.

Spinal Stenosis

Diagnosis is made clinically; however, radiographs may reveal degenerative disease of the spine. Computed tomography scanning is more specific for joint disease and spinal canal findings. Magnetic resonance imaging is useful for identifying nerve root or spinal cord compression.

Spondylolisthesis

Radiographs can reveal the vertebral slipping in the lateral view. Magnetic resonance imaging is only useful for nerve impingement symptoms.

MANAGEMENT
Back Strain

Treatment is nonsteroidal antiinflammatory drugs (NSAIDs), physical therapy, and muscle relaxants for muscle spasms if needed. The sprain is usually a self-limiting acute event, but repetitive overuse, lifting, or twisting can lead to repetitive injury. More than 50% of patients improve after 1 week. Lifestyle modifications with physical therapy should instruct the patient on appropriate lifting techniques.

Disc Herniation

Treatment is with physical therapy, NSAIDs, and time. With conservative treatment, 50% of patients usually improve in 1 week, and 90% improve after 8 weeks. Only 5% or fewer require surgical decompression. If the patient is not better after 12 weeks, if sensory or motor losses progress rapidly, if intractable pain persists, or if bowel or bladder incontinence ensues, neurosurgical evaluation is necessary.

Facet Arthritis

Treatment is usually supportive, with physical therapy and NSAIDs; however, the arthritis can and does progress to the point of needing surgical decompression.

Spinal Stenosis

Treatment is conservative, with physical therapy, NSAIDs, facet joint corticosteroid injections, or epidural corticosteroid injections. Surgical decompression is for those with intractable pain.

Spondylolisthesis

Treatment is conservative, with physical therapy, such as flexion strengthening; NSAIDs; and corsets. Fusion surgery is indicated for patients with high-grade slipping and for nerve root impingement.

Chapter 85

MYASTHENIA GRAVIS

Gaby Weissman

OVERVIEW

Myasthenia gravis (MG) was first described clinically by Thomas Willis more than 300 years ago. The discovery of the role for the antibody to the acetylcholine receptor at the neuromuscular junction in 1973 marked the beginning of a better understanding of, and more targeted therapies for, this disease. Although MG is not the most common of the autoimmune diseases, it is not rare, with a prevalence of 50 to 125 cases per million of population.

PATHOPHYSIOLOGY

MG is a disease of the neuromuscular junction. Normally, acetylcholine is released from vesicles at the nerve terminal. This neurotransmitter then binds to a receptor on the skeletal muscle, leading to an end-plate potential. These end-plate potentials initiate an action potential in muscle fibers by summation, leading to muscle contraction. The acetylcholine is then degraded by acetylcholinesterase, thereby terminating its effects. In the case of patients with MG, there are antibodies to the acetylcholine receptor present that act by accelerating the degradation of the acetylcholine receptors, blocking the binding sites for acetylcholine within its receptor, and damaging the postsynaptic end of the neuromuscular junction. This process leads to a reduced number of receptors, simplified synaptic folds, and a widened synaptic space, all in the setting of a normal nerve terminal. These phenomena in turn lead to a decreased chance of an action potential's being created at any given muscle fiber, which causes weakness at that muscle.

B cells play a major role in the pathogenesis of the disease, as they produce the causative antibodies. In addition, there is a significant amount of data that suggests T cells also play a critical role in MG. Thymic hyperplasia is seen in 60% to 70% of patients and thymoma in 12%. The precise trigger that leads to the onset of MG has not been identified. This disease has a bimodal distribution, with one peak at the second and third decades, which mostly affects women, and a second peak affecting mostly men in the sixth and seventh decades.

CLINICAL PRESENTATION

The classic clinical features of MG relate to weakness and fatigability of the skeletal muscles, with increasing weakness on repeated stimulation. Most patients have weakness of the extraocular and eyelid muscles, which leads to ptosis and diplopia. In up to 15% of patients, the weakness is limited to those muscles alone. The face and bulbar muscles often also are affected, leading to a flattened smile and nasal speech, along with a difficulty in chewing and swallowing. Eighty-five percent of patients have generalized weakness affecting the limb muscles, often in a proximal distribution, as well as the respiratory muscles. Physical examination reveals a weakness in the muscular system without any alteration in sensation, coordination, or reflexes.

Severity is usually graded as follows: grade I is defined as focal disease, usually restricted to the ocular muscles. Grade II is generalized disease that is further subdivided into mild or moderate (IIa and IIb). Grade III is severe generalized disease, with grade IV being a life-threatening impairment in respiration that is also known as a *myasthenic crisis.*

DIAGNOSIS

As treatment for myasthenia is usually lifelong and with significant side effects, a definitive diagnosis must be made. Several steps are involved in making the diagnosis. A Tensilon test is often undertaken first. Edrophonium, a short-acting acetylcholinesterase inhibitor, is given. In MG, there is an unequivocal increase in the strength of the affected muscle groups. The next step is performing a repetitive nerve stimulation test. The nerve is stimulated continuously at a rate of three impulses per second, and surface electrodes over the muscle are used to measure the resultant action potentials. A positive result consists of a rapid reduction of the action potential amplitude by at least 15%. The next step is testing for the antibodies against the acetylcholine receptor. This test is positive in 80% to 90% of patients with MG but is only positive in 50% of patients with ocular muscle weakness alone. The rest of the patients have antibodies to the acetylcholine receptor, but they are not picked up by the standard assays. Other tests that may be done are those that measure the accelerated degradation or blockade of the acetylcholine receptors, or single-fiber electromyography. The latter test is 90% sensitive but is not specific, as it is positive in other disorders of nerves, muscles, or the neuromuscular junction.

An important part of the diagnosis is the exclusion of other diseases that may cause a similar constellation of symptoms. The list of these includes congenital myasthenic syndromes, drug-induced myasthenia (penicillamine, procainamide, quinines, aminoglycosides, and curare), Lambert-Eaton syndrome, hyperthyroidism, botulism, progressive external ophthalmoplegia, and an intracranial mass that compresses the cranial nerves. It is important to get thyroid function studies in all patients with myasthenia, as well as to screen for other autoimmune disorders, as they may change the prognosis or complicate therapy. Any patient with symptoms limited to the cranial muscles should get an imaging study to rule out an intracranial mass lesion.

MANAGEMENT

Several treatments are available for MG. The first involves anticholinesterase-blocking agents (pyridostigmine), which increase acetylcholine levels by inhibiting its degradation. This medication should be dosed to the patient's symptoms, although doses of pyridostigmine greater than 120 mg q3h often produce greater weakness owing to excessive depolarization. Muscarinic side effects (especially abdominal cramping, fasciculations, and excess oral secretions) can be reduced by low-dose atropine.

Immunosuppressive agents are another class of medications used in the treatment of MG, including prednisone, azathioprine, and cyclosporine. Steroids produce remission in 30% of patients and marked improvement in another 45%, with the onset of benefit in 2 to 4 weeks. These treatments carry significant side effects, and patients should be carefully monitored. Transient worsening of symptoms could occur during the first 3 weeks of treatment. Azathioprine is well tolerated but may take 3 to 12 months to show effect. Short-term immunotherapy with plasmapheresis and intravenous immune globulin are used for temporary and rapid stabilization of patients in a myasthenic crisis. Plasmapheresis works by removing acetylcholine receptor antibodies from the circulation, so the response is often rapid; however, it is also temporary, usually lasting weeks.

Thymectomy is a potentially curative therapy. The thymus is normally detectable on imaging until mid-adulthood. Twelve percent of myasthenia patients have thymic tumors, and persistence of the thymus past age 40 years raises the possibility of thymoma. It is recommended that the thymus be removed in patients between the ages of puberty and 60 years. Although some advocate performing a thymectomy in the elderly, there is a question as to the persistence of thymic tissue beyond the age of 60 years. A thymectomy should not be undertaken in patients until their functional status has been maximized to reduce postoperative complications.

When treating patients with MG, it is important to screen for disorders that may complicate treatment, especially with immunosuppressives. These disorders include tuberculosis, diabetes, gastrointestinal bleeding, peptic ulcer disease, renal disease, asthma, hypertension, and osteoporosis. In addition, there are disorders that exacerbate MG, including infection or hyperthyroidism or hypothyroidism, or the use of some of the listed medications that may mimic myasthenia.

Chapter 86

DEMENTIA

Joseph V. Agostini

OVERVIEW

Dementia is a disorder characterized by a decline in cognition that affects memory and includes at least one other abnormality: aphasia (language disturbance), apraxia (impaired motor ability despite intact motor function), agnosia (failure to recognize objects despite intact sensory function), or executive deficits (planning, organizing, sequencing, abstracting). Impairment in these domains leads to significant deterioration in social or occupational function and ultimately loss of independence in performing activities of daily living. Associated features of sleep disturbance, mood or anxiety symptoms, delusions (persecutory), and hallucinations (often visual) are common. The prevalence of dementia rises greatly with age, from 6% at age 65 years, 20% after age 80 years, and up to 45% after age 95 years. Mean survival is 8 years. Family history is a significant risk factor in early onset Alzheimer's dementia (at age 65 or younger), but the only known risk factor for dementia overall is increased age.

CLINICAL PRESENTATION

Dementia may be progressive, static, or remitting. Specific presentation depends partly on the cause of dementia. Dementia due to degenerative causes is characterized by progressive decline in function. In contrast, infectious, malignant, or vascular etiologies may present in a more abrupt, episodic manner, although the course of illness can be used only as a rough guide. Corroborating history from a spouse or other close family member provides important data concerning time of onset, degree and rapidity of decline, and overall changes in behavior or function.

Although there is an extensive differential diagnosis, Alzheimer's dementia is the most common (more than 60% of diagnoses), followed by vascular dementia (10–20%) likely due to cerebrovascular infarcts, hemorrhage, or hypoperfusion. Treatable causes of dementia (10%) may be infectious (syphilis, human immunodeficiency virus, Creutzfeldt-Jakob disease), neoplastic (metastatic and primary central nervous system lesions), immune (lupus, sarcoidosis), traumatic, toxic (alcohol, heavy metal poisoning), metabolic (vitamin B_{12} or folate deficiency, thyroid disease), neurologic (Parkinson's disease, Huntington's disease, hydrocephalus, multiple sclerosis), or psychiatric (depression). Dementia due to depression (pseudodementia) represents 25% of reversible causes of dementia.

DIAGNOSTIC STUDIES

Formal mental status testing is essential, and patients presenting in latter stages or those with deficits in hearing, speech, vision, and conversational skills may present particular challenges. Cognitive tests include the Mini–Mental State Examination, a 30-item clinician-administered tool that assesses across the domains of cognitive function: memory, executive function, attention, language, praxis, and visuospatial ability. Used in conjunction with patient presentation, scores lower than 21 suggest a high probability of dementia, and scores higher than 25 suggest dementia is less likely. The test may be influenced by patient education, language ability, and socioeconomic status. Neuropsychological testing may be useful as well.

Physical examination includes a comprehensive neurologic examination, with attention to hearing, vision, and gait, and a careful search for cardiac disease, peripheral vascular disease (bruits), and hypertension. Laboratory examination for reversible causes of dementia includes complete blood count, electrolytes, blood urea nitrogen, creatinine, glucose, liver and thyroid function, serum vitamin B_{12}, folate, syphilis serology, and urinalysis. Further testing, such as human immunodeficiency virus, erythrocyte sedimentation rate, and antinuclear antibody may be warranted. Review of current medications is important, especially anticholinergics, which impair memory. Neuroimaging is based on clinical suspicion for neurologic etiology (vascular, trauma) but is not diagnostic for Alzheimer's dementia. Lumbar puncture for cerebrospinal fluid analysis and electroencephalography may be useful in selected patients.

MANAGEMENT

Pharmacologic treatment of dementia is limited. Donepezil (Aricept) is a reversible acetylcholinesterase inhibitor used in Alzheimer's dementia, based on the theory that cholinergic neurons, which originate in the basal forebrain and project into the cerebral cortex and hippocampus, play a prominent role in memory function. When administered early in the course of Alzheimer's dementia, donepezil is thought to improve cognition, although evidence for its altering the progression of disease is not clear. Side effects include nausea, diarrhea, and insomnia. Newer agents, such as the N-methyl-D-aspartase (NMDA) receptor antagonist Namenda, may also be tried. The primary treatment of vascular dementia and reversible types of dementia is to treat the underlying causes, if possible. Low-dose antipsychotic agents target the associated perceptual disturbances and delusions in dementia. Family and caregiver involvement early is critical for education and long-term planning. Physicians should incorporate a multidisciplinary approach to the evaluation of social supports, living situation, daily care of the patient, and needs of the caregiver, in addition to ongoing attention to underlying medical and psychiatric conditions. Nursing home placement may be necessary in the latter stage of the illness.

Chapter 87

ACUTE DELIRIUM

Catherine Chiles

OVERVIEW

Delirium, or acute confusional state, is a common complication in hospital-ized patients that doubles the risk of mortality. Recognition is often difficult, because the symptoms may fluctuate throughout the course of a day and because caregivers may mistake the problem for another disorder, such as dementia. Delirium is often multifactorial in etiology. Risk factors include older age, prior cognitive deficit, acute concurrent illness (often infectious), medications, and sensory impairments (e.g., hearing or visual disturbance). For this reason, diagnosis and management depend on a careful evaluation of multiple domains and the implementation of interventions to address poten-tial contributing factors.

PATHOPHYSIOLOGY

Cortical and subcortical (e.g., thalamus, basal ganglia, and pontine reticular formation) structures are involved in the pathogenesis. At a neurotransmitter level, acetylcholine appears to play a key role, because anticholinergic drugs cause delirium, and hypoxia, hypoglycemia, and thiamine deficiency decrease central nervous system acetylcholine synthesis.

CLINICAL PRESENTATION

Delirium is characterized by acute (<24 hours) or subacute (<1 week) onset and fluctuating course. Other cardinal features include inattention, disorga-nized speech and thought, a varying level of consciousness, disorientation, and behavioral disturbance. Perceptual disturbances with vague delusions of harm often occur. Both hypoactive and hyperactive presentations may occur, but the former is more commonly underdiagnosed and leads to poorer out-comes. Dementia differs from delirium in that its typical onset is slower, it fol-lows an unrelenting as opposed to remitting course, and it does not impair attention, except in advanced cases.

DIAGNOSIS

The most important aspects of diagnosis are recognition that delirium is present and determining the underlying medical conditions that have caused the syndrome. Delirium recognition may be aided by a baseline mental status examination at admission, but it is often not done or not adequately docu-mented. The Confusion Assessment Method is a validated tool widely used by nonpsychiatrists to aid diagnosis. The Confusion Assessment Method criteria require the presence of acute onset and fluctuating course, inattention, and either disorganized thinking or altered level of consciousness. It has a sensitiv-ity of 94% to 100% and specificity of 90% to 95%.

Workup involves a complete medication review with attention to those drugs that may precipitate delirium, such as sedative-hypnotics, benzodiazepines, and medications with anticholinergic effects. Laboratory workup is based on clinical judgment and patient presentation. Certain patients may warrant a complete blood count, chemistry panel, chest x-ray, arterial blood gas, brain imaging, or lumbar puncture, depending on the differential diagnosis and the need to rule out such etiologies as infection, metabolic abnormalities, hypoxia, and neurologic event. A toxicologic screen is useful for patients presenting with acute delirium for whom the diagnosis is not readily apparent. Care should be taken to consider early shock, which may present as delirium without fever in sepsis or with the patient unable to relate a history of chest pain in myocardial infarction.

MANAGEMENT

Management of delirium requires a multidisciplinary approach, identifying and reversing the underlying cause. Reorientation can be improved by providing consistent communication and staffing, devices such as easily readable clocks and calendars, and a suitable environment (with adequate lighting, low noise, and familiar objects). Family involvement and education are also important. Physical restraints and other orders that restrict a patient's mobility should be discouraged, as they often lead to further physical and mental decline.

Pharmacologic treatment of delirium carries with it the risk of exacerbating extant cognitive impairment and making future assessments more difficult. If the benefit of treatment outweighs the risk of potential adverse effects, the lowest dose of medication should be initiated and response frequently reassessed. Antipsychotic agents are most commonly used, especially haloperidol, which can be administered via several routes and titrated from an initial dose of 0.5 mg.

Research suggests that many hospitalized patients have long-term effects of delirium and that delirium symptoms may linger. Appropriate discharge planning and follow-up are thus important.

Chapter 88

MOOD DISORDERS AND SUICIDE

Louis C. Sanfilippo and Vladimir Coric

OVERVIEW

Mood disorders are prevalent (10–20%), account for significant psychosocial morbidity, and have a suicide rate estimated to be between 15% and 20%, yet they are commonly missed diagnoses. Mood disorders can be divided into two categories: (i) primary mood disorders, which may be comorbid with other medical illnesses, and (ii) mood disorders caused by a general medical condition or substance. Primary mood disorders include major depressive disorder (MDD) and bipolar disorder (BD), which is differentiated from MDD by abnormally and persistently elevated mood. Mood disorder due to general medical condition or substance (medication or drug of abuse) is diagnosed when an etiology for the mood alteration can be established. Diagnosis requires thorough medical evaluation and a search for etiologies that may warrant specific medical intervention and treatments.

PATHOPHYSIOLOGY

Mood disorders arise from a combination of genetic, neurobiological, and psychosocial factors. Monozygotic twin studies suggest a higher level of heritability for BD than for MDD, although no specific genetic markers or chromosomes are identified. Norepinephrine, serotonin, and dopamine neurotransmitter systems are involved in the neurobiology of MDD. Abnormalities involving increased cortisol secretion and decreased left frontal cortical activity also have been observed in depressed individuals. Specific neurotransmitter system involvement has not been conclusively demonstrated in BD, but norepinephrine and dopamine are thought to play a role. The kindling hypothesis for BD suggests that manic episodes, like seizures, stem from underlying neuronal depolarization that predisposes to future episodes. Psychosocial stressors are known as precipitants for episodes of both MDD and BD.

CLINICAL PRESENTATION

An episode of MDD consists of core symptoms for at least 2 weeks and must include depressed mood or diminished interest in pleasurable activities (anhedonia), or both. Neurovegetative symptoms include increased or decreased sleep, weight loss or gain, and fatigue. Although characteristically patients display psychomotor slowing, they may become agitated when anxiety or irritability is prominent. Preoccupation with thoughts of worthlessness, hopelessness, guilt, and suicide is present in most patients with MDD. Impaired memory or concentration may present early and be part of the depressive episode. Severe symptoms include psychotic features, such as hallucinations and delusions, often with mood-congruent themes of guilt, nihilism, or persecution. Somatic complaints commonly lead to frequent primary care visits. Observable signs include psychomotor slowing, diminished eye contact, restricted affect, and speech that is soft in tone, with minimal spontaneity.

Patients with BD display manic behavior, but they are often charismatic and engaging, causing delays in detection and treatment. Typically, they are highly energetic, irritable, and agitated. Speech is commonly loud, rapid, and pressured (difficult to interrupt), sometimes marked by puns and rhyming. They may need less sleep than usual and be engaged in a variety of projects. BD patients have racing thoughts and overvalued ideas; frequent themes involve grandiosity, heightened religiosity, and increased sexualized behavior. Approximately one-half of patients with BD demonstrate frank psychosis, with mood-congruent delusions of omnipotence, power, and self-worth. They frequently exhibit extremely poor judgment and reckless, impulsive behaviors, such as promiscuity, unprotected sexual activity, and spending sprees. No specific clinical features of depression differentiate primary mood disorders from mood disorders due to general medical condition or substance.

Approximately 20% of patients diagnosed with MDD or BD will commit suicide. Known risk factors include adolescence or older age, male gender, white or Native American ethnicity, widowed or divorced marital status, recent losses, substance use, prior suicide attempt, access to lethal weapons or means, and major stressors (e.g., work, financial, legal pressure). Evaluation of the suicidal patient must include assessment of current suicidal thoughts;

intent or plan, or both; as well as history. Substance abuse, especially alcohol, contributes to impulsive behavior and is associated with suicide attempts and one-half of all completed suicides. Medical illnesses and chronic pain are seen frequently in patients who attempt suicide, especially in the older patient with few supports.

DIAGNOSIS

Diagnosis of MDD and BD is made when reversible causes have been excluded. When a specific medical condition or substance use is temporally related to the mood change, a diagnosis of mood disorder due to general medical condition or substance is made. When psychotic symptoms are present, disorders such as schizophrenia and schizoaffective disorder must be considered, but the history often reveals more pervasive psychosis and less-prominent mood symptoms. Depressive symptoms after the death of a loved one are seen in bereavement, but if symptoms are severe or extend beyond 2 months, MDD is diagnosed. Cognitive impairments similar to dementia may also be present in depression (pseudodementia); faster onset, preoccupation with morbid themes, and suicidality likely indicate depression.

Mood disorders often coexist with medical illnesses, blurring the distinction between the two categories. Medical conditions strongly linked to depression include stroke, coronary artery disease, multiple sclerosis, nutritional deficiencies (e.g., vitamin B_{12}), hypothyroidism, and pancreatic cancer. Parkinson's disease, infectious diseases such as human immunodeficiency virus, malignancies, and endocrine abnormalities (e.g., Cushing's disease, Addison's disease) also have been associated with depression. Mania may be seen in connection with multiple sclerosis, frontal lobe syndromes, epilepsy, hyperthyroidism, and Cushing's disease. Diagnosing a medical etiology involves: a careful history; physical examination, including mental status examination; and laboratory workup, including complete blood count with differential, platelets, electrolytes, blood urea nitrogen, creatinine, glucose, liver function tests, thyroid function tests, vitamin B_{12} and folate, rapid plasma reagent, urinalysis, chest x-ray, and electrocardiogram, and when clinically indicated, brain imaging and electroencephalography.

Mood disorders induced by substances cannot be distinguished by clinical presentation. If symptoms resolve after withdrawal of the suspected agent, mood disorder due to substance is likely. Substances commonly associated with depression include alcohol and opiates, as well as medications, such as steroids, barbiturates, sedatives, antihistamines, and calcium channel or beta-blockers. Withdrawal from amphetamine, cocaine, or caffeine may present as depression. Mania may be caused by cocaine or amphetamine intoxication, so urine drug screen is indicated. Medications associated with mania include steroids, dopamine agonists, and antidepressants. Caffeine intoxication (more than two to three cups or 250 mg) may also present as mania.

MANAGEMENT

Ensuring the patient's safety is the first concern. Actively suicidal patients in the hospital require one-to-one observation or physical restraint, and outpatients need hospitalization. Treatment with an antidepressant can induce mania or psychosis and activate suicidal thoughts in some patients; careful history and ongoing monitoring are key. If underlying medical etiologies have been excluded, treatment of MDD responds best to a combination of pharmacotherapy and psychotherapy, although milder forms of depression may benefit from therapy alone. Selective serotonin reuptake inhibitors are first-line agents and include citalopram, fluoxetine, paroxetine, and sertraline. Common side effects include diarrhea, nausea, headache, and decreased libido. Additional antidepressant agents targeting several neurotransmitter systems include bupropion, mirtazapine, nefazodone, and venlafaxine. Benzodiazepines, such as lorazepam or clonazepam, may be used initially to treat anxiety in depressed or manic patients but should be discontinued owing to the risk of habituation and depression.

BD is treated with mood-stabilizing agents, such as lithium, valproate, or carbamazepine. Side effects of lithium include nephrogenic diabetes insipidus, hypothyroidism, arrhythmias, tremor, and cognitive blunting. Lithium levels, thyroid function tests, blood urea nitrogen, and creatinine should be checked at least every 6 months during maintenance. Valproate is also commonly used in the treatment of BD and is particularly effective for acute episodes and rapid cycling. Side effects include sedation, weight gain, tremor, alopecia, thrombocytopenia, and rarely hepatotoxicity or pancreatitis. Valproic acid levels, liver function tests, and complete blood counts with platelets are routinely checked. Carbamazepine is also effective but requires white blood cell counts and liver function tests every 2 weeks in the first 2 months, and every 3 months thereafter owing to the risk of blood dyscrasias and hepatitis. BD patients presenting in a depressed phase usually require a mood stabilizer first. Similarly, psychotic symptoms of MDD or BD are treated first with an antipsychotic, such as olanzapine or risperidone, which minimize the risk of tardive dyskinesia. Olanzapine has antimanic properties in the acute phase as well.

Patients with mood disorders benefit from establishing better support systems, identifying environmental stressors, and changing maladaptive coping mechanisms. Education for patients about the illness and importance of maintenance treatments is critical to prevent relapse.

Chapter 89

SUBSTANCE ABUSE, TOXICITY, AND WITHDRAWAL

Sandra A. Springer

OVERVIEW

Addiction disorders are common problems in hospitalized settings as well as outpatient practices. Alcoholism alone has been reported to claim more than 100,000 lives annually. In addition, approximately 20,000 deaths were caused by illicit drug use in 1990 alone. This chapter describes major signs and symptoms of toxicity and withdrawal, as well as management strategies, primarily focusing on alcohol but also including heroin, cocaine, amphetamines, and barbiturates.

PATHOPHYSIOLOGY

Alcohol acts on various receptors throughout the central nervous system including the receptor for gamma-aminobutyric acid (GABA), which is an inhibitory neurotransmitter, leading to depressed neurologic function. Alcohol acts on many tissues, however, including the nervous system, liver, and gastrointestinal tract. Ethanol is metabolized through the alcohol dehydrogenase pathway, producing acetyl aldehyde, which is then converted to acetate. This process is toxic in several different ways: (i) a metabolic co-factor nicotinamide adenine (NAD^+) is converted to its reduced form, nicotinamide adenine dinucleotide (NADH). With increased NADH, hyperlactacidemia occurs, contributing to acidosis. Increased NADH also tends to oppose gluconeogenesis and favor hypoglycemia, ultimately causing increased ketone production and further acidosis (i.e., alcohol ketoacidosis). (ii) Acetyl aldehyde itself has direct toxic effects on important enzymes and cells. Although these processes lead to injury of many vital organs, the major cause of death from acute alcohol toxicity is respiratory depression. Coma and death may occur at very high blood alcohol concentrations.

The mechanism of alcohol withdrawal is not entirely known; however, one view is described as the Kalant model: The body adapts to the neurologic depressant effect of alcohol and, during withdrawal, one experiences unopposed neuronal excitability. Withdrawal from alcohol used to be associated with up to 15% mortality rates, primarily due to comorbid medical problems, including pneumonia and arrhythmias; however, with better identification and management of withdrawal, the mortality rate has decreased to below 3%.

CLINICAL PRESENTATION

The acutely alcohol intoxicated patient is often lethargic or somnolent at times, with slurred speech and motor and intellectual impairments at very high doses. Chronic alcohol ingestion may present with signs and symptoms of cirrhosis, alcoholic hepatitis, gastritis, peptic ulcer disease, neuropathy, and memory deficits. Alcoholic ketoacidosis may occur and reflects poor nutrition or vomiting, in addition to a decrease in fatty acid oxidation.

Patients in withdrawal may present with tremor, anxiety, tachycardia, hypertension, fever, diaphoresis, nausea, vomiting, or diarrhea occurring from less than 8 hours to 36 hours after the last drink. Hallucinations may occur and are usually visual. Patients with alcoholic hallucinations have an intact sensorium, and the hallucinations are not a predictor of delirium tremens (DTs). They occur usually 24 to 72 hours after the last drink. Alcoholic seizures are usually tonic-clonic in a patient with an intact sensorium, and fewer than 3% proceed to status epilepticus. The risk of having seizures is increased by a history of prior seizures. The time frame is usually approximately 12 hours after last drink and peaks at approximately 24 hours. Symptoms of DTs must include altered sensorium and usually consist of tachycardia, low-grade fevers, hypertension, diaphoresis, and hallucinations. DTs affect approximately 4% of patients with a long history of chronic alcohol abuse. The time frame usually is within 48 hours after last drink until 7 to 14 days after last drink, and they confer the greatest mortality risk.

There are long-term sequelae of alcohol abuse, including Wernicke's syndrome, a triad of ataxia; cognitive impairment; and impairment of ocular dysfunction (ophthalmoplegia, nystagmus). The cause is presumed to be from thiamine deficiency. Wernicke's can be reversed if thiamine is given immediately in daily 100-mg parenteral doses, with the first dose being before glucose administration. Korsakoff's syndrome is a chronic state characterized by selective disturbances of short-term memory, apathy, and confabulation with an otherwise intact sensorium. It is an irreversible progression of Wernicke's syndrome secondary to thiamine deficiency.

Alcohol also can directly or indirectly cause thrombocytopenia; coagulopathies can develop from liver disease that increase bleeding risk; anemia may develop also from direct alcohol effects and in combination with folate deficiency, common in chronic alcohol dependence.

DIAGNOSIS AND MANAGEMENT

Alcohol

The goal of treatment is to prevent the aforementioned sequelae of alcohol toxicity, as well as alcohol withdrawal seizures and DTs.

A careful history and physical examination must be obtained, with particular emphasis on determining alcohol use and quantity, and history of previous withdrawal seizures or DTs, as well as evaluation for other causes that can mimic alcohol toxicity and withdrawal symptoms, such as trauma (e.g., subdural hematoma), acidosis, hypoxia, hypercarbia, meningitis, hypoglycemia, and other toxic ingestions. Diagnostic studies should include complete blood counts, electrolytes, liver function tests, creatine phosphokinase, coagulation studies, alcohol level and toxin screen, and arterial blood gas. An osmolar gap should be measured, and if present, methanol or ethylene glycol poisoning should be considered. Head computed tomography may be performed to search for subdural hematoma. Patients should be closely observed. Parenteral thiamine should be administered before giving dextrose (oral thiamine is not absorbed well). One can also give a multivitamin and folate; no literature suggests reasoning for this therapy, but the cost is minimal. Hydration of the patient helps prevent sequelae of rhabdomyolysis.

Benzodiazepines are the main pharmacologic treatment of alcohol withdrawl, exploiting their similar action on the GABA receptor. A recent meta-analysis of the pharmacologic treatment of alcohol withdrawal showed less morbidity and mortality with the use of benzodiazepines compared to other treatments. The following considerations need to be pursued before the initiation of a benzodiazepine, however: In liver disease or the medically ill inpatient, however, lorazepam (PO, IM, IV, SL) and oxazepam (PO only) are the agents of choice because they are glucuronidated by the liver, but not oxidated, and have no active metabolites. Longer-acting benzodiazepines, such as chlordiazepoxide and diazepam, show a smoother withdrawal period, especially in the ambulatory patient at risk for withdrawal seizures. A patient having withdrawal seizures would benefit from a rapid-onset agent (owing to smaller volume of distribution), such as diazepam (5–10 mg). A patient exhibiting early signs of withdrawal without a history of seizures may benefit from a longer-acting, slower-onset agent, such as chlordiazepoxide. Some studies have shown that symptom-triggered dosing schedules are superior to fixed dosing schedules. The symptom-triggered dosing schedule is based on the use of the Clinical Institute Withdrawal Assessment for Alcohol, Revised (CIWA-AR) scale. Studies found shorter hospital stays and decreased amount of benzodiazepine used in the symptom-triggered dosing schedule. Individualized patient care is important, however, so patients with a history of withdrawal seizures or DTs should start on fixed dosing no matter what stage of withdrawal they manifest. Beta-blockers are used as adjunctive treatment to benzodiazepines; they decrease adrenergic symptoms (tachycardia, hypertension) when compared to placebo but do not alter the progression to withdrawal. Clonidine minimizes adrenergic symptoms but causes no difference in development of tremor or restlessness.

In addition to the acute treatment of withdrawal or intoxication, self-help groups, such as Alcoholics Anonymous, or inpatient detoxification programs, in which drugs such as (disulfiram) Antabuse and naltrexone may be administered and can be helpful. Antabuse deters use by increasing the adverse effects of alcohol through blocked metabolism, whereas naltrexone, a long-acting oral opioid antagonist, has been shown to decrease the pleasurable effects of alcohol.

Opioids

Overdose

Acute overdose of opioids requires emergency treatment. Signs include hypotension, constricted pupils, and decreased respiration. Management includes supporting vital signs, administration of intravenous fluids, including 50% dextrose solution in case of concurrent hypoglycemia, and naloxone (Narcan), a short-acting opioid antagonist. Effects of naloxone are seen within a few seconds to minutes; if there is no response, the airway should be protected by intubation and mechanical ventilation. If the patient does awaken, Narcan can wear off in 30 minutes, mandating hospital observation for at least 48 hours. As with alcohol intoxication, there should be a low threshold for evaluating other etiologies for the signs and symptoms seen in opioid intoxication, including trauma, infection, metabolic abnormalities, and other toxin ingestions.

Withdrawal

Opioid withdrawal is *not* life threatening, in contrast to alcohol and barbiturate withdrawal. Symptoms are divided into acute versus late symptoms. Acute withdrawal occurs within 12 to 36 hours after last use of opioids and includes symptoms of yawning, sweating, gooseflesh, insomnia, dilated pupils, anorexia, muscle cramps, and tremulousness. Late withdrawal symptoms occur approximately 48 to 72 hours after the last use of drug and include abdominal cramps, diarrhea, vomiting, hypertension, tachycardia, and tachypnea.

Clonidine may be given to decrease the discomforting symptoms. Long-term treatment includes methadone, a long-acting opioid agonist, which acts to decrease euphoria and must be started in a treatment program. Naltrexone can be used in combination with clonidine to hasten detoxification, and as a single agent for maintaining abstinence for up to 2 months. Buprenorphine, a mixed agonist/antagonist opioid, has been shown to be effective alone or in combination with naloxone as a maintenance therapy in the treatment of opioid dependence and is approved for use in physicians' offices. Support groups include Narcotics Anonymous.

Cocaine

Intoxication

Cocaine stimulates the dopaminergic receptors in the central nervous system, causing symptoms of euphoria, hyperalertness, and increased self-esteem, as well as transient delusional psychosis resembling paranoid schizophrenia or mania. Overdose can lead to tachycardia, respiratory acidosis, grand mal seizures, and respiratory and cardiac arrest. Management is supportive, as there are no direct antagonists for cocaine overdose.

Withdrawal

Cocaine withdrawal, like heroin withdrawal, is *not* life threatening. Symptoms include depression, anxiety, insomnia, irritability, and intense cocaine craving.

Treatment is supportive, including antiadrenergics, such as clonidine; self-help groups (Narcotics Anonymous); and inpatient detoxification groups.

Amphetamines

Symptoms of acute intoxication of amphetamines include psychosis due to their action on the dopamine system in the central nervous system; other symptoms are tachycardia, diaphoresis, and hypertension. Treatment is primarily aimed at stabilizing psychosis with antipsychotics. Withdrawal is also *not* life threatening.

Barbiturates

Signs and symptoms of barbiturate intoxication are similar to those of alcohol intoxication. Withdrawal from barbiturates *is* life threatening. The primary treatment is with tapered barbiturate or benzodiazepine.

Rheumatology and Allergy

Chapter 90

RAYNAUD'S PHENOMENON

Lisa Gale Suter

OVERVIEW

Raynaud's phenomenon (RP) of episodic, cold-induced digital ischemia was first described in 1862 by Maurice Raynaud. It has been estimated that 4% to 15% of the general population experiences RP. It is frequently familial, occurring in several generations, and is far more common in women. Patients who develop RP after the age of 20 years are more likely to have more severe attacks and digital ulceration, and to demonstrate nailbed capillary abnormalities on examination. These patients are at a significantly higher risk of developing systemic sclerosis or limited sclerosis and the CREST syndrome of *c*alcinosis, *R*P, *e*sophageal *s*trictures, and *t*elangiectasias. In these patients, RP can be associated with severe tissue fibrosis and ulceration.

PATHOPHYSIOLOGY

Although the pathophysiology of RP is not yet well understood, it is believed to result from vasospasm due to increased activity of alpha$_2$-adrenergic receptors. RP in the general population and in the population with systemic sclerosis may well represent two separate diseases, each with a different pathophysiology. A triad of factors is thought to impact on the normal regulation of microvascular tone and potentially go awry in RP: the vascular endothelium and its products, platelets and platelet activation, and the peripheral nervous system and its neuromediators. Imbalance or dysregulation of substances, such as endothelin, prostacyclin, and serotonin, may produce a more vasospastic environment in RP patients. In addition, vasodilation and vasopermeability may be affected by local damage or dysfunction of the peripheral sensory, sympathetic, or parasympathetic (or both sympathetic and parasympathetic) nervous systems, also contributing to an abnormal response to cold or other stimuli.

CLINICAL PRESENTATION

Patients note attacks of segmental digital pallor, usually on exposure to cold or stress. During these episodes, the digits can be painful or numb, occurring on the hands or feet, and may be followed by mottling or hyperemia during reperfusion. The attacks usually last 10 to 15 minutes after rewarming occurs.

DIAGNOSIS

The diagnosis of RP is clinical. It is important to evaluate the patient for evidence of systemic sclerosis or the CREST syndrome and for other underlying diseases with a thorough history and physical examination. Nailbed capillaroscopy, looking for capillary loop dilation or dropout, may help distinguish patients at risk of developing systemic sclerosis or other connective tissue disorders. RP is also frequently seen in other rheumatologic diseases, such as rheumatoid arthritis, systemic lupus erythematosus, Sjögren's syndrome, polymyositis, and dermatomyositis, and in the hand-arm vibration syndrome, cold agglutinin disease, and the paraproteinemias, and other arterial disease, such as Buerger's disease and atheroemboli; it also can be due to drugs, such as clonidine or amphetamines.

MANAGEMENT

Mild to moderate RP usually can be controlled by behavioral modification and prevention, including avoiding exposure to the cold; avoiding vaso-damaging or -constricting substances, such as tobacco or caffeine; and maintaining a normal body temperature. For more severe RP, vasodilators, such as slow-release calcium channel blockers, are the first line of treatment. Nifedipine, the best-studied drug, has been shown to reduce the frequency and severity of attacks in a double-blind study. Amlodipine, prazosin, angiotensin-converting enzyme inhibitors, and topical nitrates have also been used with varying rates of success as second-line agents. Severe RP can be treated with intravenous prostacyclin or sympathectomy. It is also important to provide proper skin care, as many systemic sclerosis patients have digital ulcers. Soaking the affected digit in half-strength hydrogen peroxide, allowing it to air dry, and then applying an antibiotic ointment and a loose dressing is one commonly used strategy for superficial ulcer care. More severe ulcers may require oral antibiotic therapy, débridement, or surgical intervention.

Chapter 91

RHEUMATOID ARTHRITIS

Bridget Ann Martell

OVERVIEW

Rheumatoid arthritis (RA) is a disease characterized by a chronic, symmetric, and erosive synovitis of peripheral joints. The disease affects approximately 1% of the general population and 4% to 10% of those older than age 65 years. Considered a systemic autoimmune disease, RA is known to affect most organ systems, including the heart, lung, eye, skin, and nerves. RA is usually a progressive disease, with 16% of patients being completely disabled after 12 years of disease. Predictors of disease severity are human leukocyte antigen haplotype (DR1 and DR4), initial degree of synovial inflammation, presence of serum rheumatoid factor, and rheumatoid nodules. The life expectancy of patients with RA is 10 to 15 years less than for the general population, thereby highlighting the need for early detection and intervention.

PATHOPHYSIOLOGY

Although the etiology of RA has remained elusive, some factors that predict the risk of disease development include age older than 65 years; female gender, with women affected 2.5 times more than men; and the presence of human leukocyte antigen haplotypes DR1 and DR4. Bacterial or viral infections may also play a role. *Escherichia coli* and Epstein-Barr virus genes share homology with sequences of HLA-DRDW4 that are involved in signaling T-cell clonal expansion or deletion. These infections, therefore, may trigger T-cell activation. Additionally, viruses, especially Epstein-Barr virus, have been shown to affect the activation of cellular-mediated immunity by blunting T-cell responses.

The activation of CD4 T lymphocytes stimulates release of specific cytokines, such as tumor necrosis factor-alpha, initiating injury of the synovial endothelial cells. Ultimately, as tissue invasion continues, the synovial membrane is transformed into a highly vascularized tissue known as a *pannus*. Chronically, as this process continues unabated, the joint synovium becomes hypertrophic and edematous, and eventually granulation and fibrosis develop. This development leads to decreased vascularity of the synovium, and permanent joint damage and immobility ensue.

CLINICAL PRESENTATION

The diagnosis of RA, for the most part, is a clinical one. It is usually an insidious disease, with the development of symptoms such as malaise, fever, weakness, joint swelling, and stiffness lasting for weeks to months. Rarely, a patient may present as a palindromic arthritis, characterized by episodic monoarticular arthritis with episodes lasting 3 to 5 days. Eventually, the patient evolves into a pattern of classic RA.

Not all joints are involved in RA, and of them, distinct features can be noted. *Cervical spine* RA is common, whereas involvement of the thoracic and lumbar spine is quite rare. Tenosynovitis of the transverse ligament of C-1 and disease progression of the apophyseal joints may result in atlantoaxial subluxation, with ultimate C1-C2 instability. *Shoulders* are involved rarely and often present with frozen shoulder syndrome, as patients limit shoulder motion owing to pain. *Elbow* involvement is easy to detect, as active synovitis or synovial thickening can be palpated laterally between the epicondyle and the olecranon. Compressive neuropathies are common, as the ulnar nerve passes through this space. *Hands* are involved in almost all patients with RA, specifically at the wrist, metacarpophalangeal, and proximal interphalangeal joints, with sparing of the distal interphalangeal joint. Swan neck and boutonniere deformities of the digits are common. Carpal tunnel syndrome may result from peripheral nerve entrapment from active synovitis of the wrist. *Hips* are commonly involved joints in RA, but early disease may go unnoticed because the joints are hard to palpate. Pain characteristically radiates to the groin or thigh. *Knee* involvement is easily detected as active synovitis and joint effusion. A complication of the disease can be the rupture of a Baker's cyst, which mimics thrombophlebitis. *Foot and ankle* joints affected are, typically, the metatarsophalangeal, talonavicular, and ankle joints. Tarsal tunnel syndrome, similar to carpal tunnel, may occur at the ankle joint.

Extraarticular manifestations are present in most patients with RA and become more likely with increasing severity of disease. *Skin* involvement manifests as subcutaneous nodules (rheumatoid nodules), which may be seen in 25% to 50% of patients and are commonly found over pressure points of the olecranon, extensor surfaces of the forearm, Achilles tendon, and, occasionally, the ischial area. Vasculitic changes, such as purpura, splinter hemorrhages, and distal tissue necrosis, also may be seen. The *eye* may be affected by episcleritis, which is common and self-limited. Scleritis is rare but an ophthalmologic emergency, because left untreated it may cause ulceration and erosion through the sclera into the choroid. *Respiratory* involvement includes inflammation of the cricoarytenoid joint, presenting as dysphonia and dysphagia. RA pulmonary disease may manifest as basilar interstitial fibrosis, bronchiolitis obliterans (with or without organizing pneumonia), solitary or multiple pulmonary nodules, or pleurisy and pleural effusion. *Cardiac* disease in RA most commonly presents as pericarditis and pericardial effusions, present in up to 50% of patients but rarely symptomatic. It occasionally can progress to a chronic constrictive pericarditis. Rheumatoid nodules may involve the myocardium or valvular structures. *Renal* disease is rare and presents with involvement of the glomeruli. Proteinuria or increased creatinine should cause investigation into a possible drug reaction or amyloidosis. *Neurologic* problems include cervical myopathy, entrapment neuropathies (most commonly carpal tunnel syndrome), and vasculitis neuropathies, such as mononeuritis multiplex. *Hematologic* involvement is almost universal in RA patients as anemia of chronic disease. Felty's syndrome is the constellation of RA, splenomegaly, leukopenia, and leg ulcers and is most commonly seen in association with severe, nodule-forming RA with high titers of rheumatoid factor.

DIAGNOSIS

Diagnosis is made on the basis of the American Rheumatism Association's 1987 revised criteria for classification of RA, as listed in Table 91–1. Early disease is

TABLE 91–1 The American Rheumatism Association 1987 Revised Criteria for Classification of Rheumatoid Arthritis

Feature	Criteria
1. Morning stiffness	Lasting ≥1 hr before maximal improvement.
2. Arthritis of ≥3 joints	≥3 areas of soft tissue swelling or fluid. 14 possible areas are right or left PIP, MCP, wrist, elbow, knee, ankle, and MTP joints.
3. Arthritis of hand joints	≥1 swollen area in a wrist, MCP, or PIP joint.
4. Symmetric arthritis	Simultaneous involvement of the same joint areas on both sides of the body. Bilateral involvement of PIPs, MCPs, or MTPs is acceptable without absolute symmetry.
5. Rheumatoid nodules	Subcutaneous nodules over bony prominences or extensor surfaces, or in a juxtaarticular region.
6. Serum rheumatoid factor	Demonstration of abnormal amounts of serum rheumatoid factor by any method for which the result has been positive in <5% normal control subjects.
7. Radiographic changes	Changes seen on posteroanterior hand and wrist, which includes erosions, or bony decalcification localized in or most marked adjacent to involved joint. (Osteoarthritic changes alone do not qualify.)

MCP, metacarpophalangeal joint; MTP, metatarsophalangeal joint; PIP, proximal interphalangeal joint.
Note: For classification of RA, a patient should clinically fulfill four of the seven criteria with criteria 1 through 4 being present for at least 6 weeks.

often confined to the hand and wrist, and plain radiographs can be most useful. Newer techniques, including magnetic resonance imaging and high-frequency ultrasonography, are now being used to detect erosions earlier.

MANAGEMENT

Drugs used in the treatment of RA work to offer patients symptomatic relief or modify disease progression, or both. Of those that provide relief of pain and inflammation, nonsteroidal antiinflammatory drugs are the most commonly used, despite the risk of gastrointestinal bleeding. Glucocorticoids have also been standard therapy to decrease symptomatic pain and swelling. Disease-modifying antirheumatic drugs have been shown to decrease rate of progression, decrease erosions, and decrease disability. Combination therapy with multiple drugs is known to be superior to single drug treatment, as assessed by multiple randomized control trials. These drugs include methotrexate, azathioprine, cyclophosphamide, hydroxychloroquine, sulfasalazine, and the anticytokine drug etanercept, to name a few. The benefits of dynamic exercise also cannot be overemphasized. Three-times-weekly aerobic and isometric exercise improves aerobic capacity and muscle strength, and causes marked improvement in daily functioning, although its effect on disease progression is unknown. Finally, treatment of comorbid conditions in RA patients is extremely important, as they are more likely to die of coronary artery disease than age-matched peers.

Chapter 92

SYSTEMIC LUPUS ERYTHEMATOSUS

Bridget Ann Martell

OVERVIEW

Systemic lupus erythematosus (SLE) is a multisystem autoimmune disease characterized by immune dysregulation that results in autoantibody production, complement activation, and ultimately immune complex deposition. SLE occurs more often in women than in men, with a ratio of 9:1, and more commonly in blacks and Asians. Although it can occur at almost any age, most people affected are between 15 and 45 years old. A genetic predisposition exists, with human leukocyte antigen–DR2 and DR3 haplotypes being at increased risk of disease. Inherited complement deficiencies also increase disease susceptibility. Conceptually, it is believed that a deficiency in complement components may delay the clearance of foreign antigen, thus setting off an aggravated immunologic assault. Triggering events are thought to influence disease development within susceptible groups and severity of disease, because concordance between monozygotic twins is not complete.

PATHOPHYSIOLOGY

SLE likely results from the local deposition of immune complexes onto vascular endothelium that then triggers an inflammatory response, cytokine release, and activation of the complement cascade. Histologically, fibrinoid necrosis of small vessels and deposition of immunoglobulins and complement factors are seen. It is likely that the antibodies themselves are not directly cytotoxic, but rather the ensuing inflammatory cascade that damages cells. The pathophysiology of neurologic lupus may differ slightly, in that the immune complex deposition may cause direct vascular occlusion, and the activation of antiphospholipid may directly damage the vascular endothelium as well as cause clotting.

CLINICAL PRESENTATION

More than 90% of lupus patients initially present with a constellation of constitutional symptoms, which include malaise, fever, arthralgia, myalgia, headache, lymphadenopathy, fever, and loss of appetite and weight. Almost all organ systems can be involved and show specific manifestations. The musculoskeletal system is a common site of presentation, with 40% to 60% of patients having arthralgias or, less often, arthritis. Any joint may be involved, but wrists, hands, and knees are most common. The syndrome of arthritis in lupus has been coined "rupus" and is symmetric and nonerosive, and may be migratory or chronic, or both. The arthritis is deforming and can cause subluxation, ulnar deviation, and contractures. The pattern of nonerosive, deforming arthritis known as *Jaccoud's arthropathy* is correctable if caught early and is very rare. Skin is often the organ system that heralds disease, and over the course of the illness, 70% to 80% of patients will have some dermatologic or vascular manifestation. The most common cutaneous signs are malar rash, alopecia, bullous lesions, urticaria, photosensitivity, and panniculitis. Discoid lupus is manifest by raised erythematous patches on the skin and may not have systemic involvement. Vasculitic findings include digital ulcers, purpura, livedo reticularis and thrombophlebitis. Raynaud's phenomenon may be seen and is due to vasoconstriction. Finally, painless oral and nasopharyngeal ulcers may be seen. Eye involvement in lupus may be severe, ranging from conjunctivitis, scleritis, and arterial or venous occlusions to neuro-ophthalmic involvement. Scleritis and retinal vasculitis are often indicative of increasing disease activity. Lung findings in SLE are inflammatory and include most often pleurisy, pleural effusion, and pneumonitis. Pulmonary hemorrhage portends a poor prognosis. Patients also may develop pulmonary hypertension. Heart involvement is also related to inflammation and may include pericarditis, pericardial effusion, myocarditis, Libman-Sachs endocarditis, and premature coronary artery disease. Gastrointestinal involvement is difficult to diagnose, as patients typically complain of diffuse abdominal pain; however, serious complications can occur, such as peritonitis, intestinal obstruction and perforation, bowel vasculitis, pancreatitis, and inflammatory bowel disease. Hepatosplenomegaly is also common. A prominent aspect of disease is renal involvement, with more than 50% of patients having clinical nephritis as defined by persistent proteinuria. The classification of renal disease is outlined in Table 92–1.

Neurologic involvement occurs in 20% to 80% of patients with active disease. Central nervous system manifestations range from mild cognitive dysfunc-

TABLE 92-1   Classification of Renal Disease

I. Normal glomeruli
II. Pure mesangiopathy
IIIA. Focal segmental glomerulonephritis
IIIB. Focal segmental glomerulonephritis
IV. Diffuse glomerulonephritis
V. Diffuse membranous glomerulonephropathy
VI. Advanced sclerosing glomerulonephritis

tion, mood disorders, and headaches to cranial neuropathies, organic brain syndrome, stroke, seizures, movement disorders, spinal cord lesions, and dementia. Peripheral nerves are affected by neuropathies, polyneuropathies, autonomic dysfunction, and, rarely, mononeuritis multiplex. Hematologic manifestations include anemia, leukopenia, lymphopenia, thrombocytopenia, and clotting abnormalities as a result of the lupus anticoagulant. This clotting disorder is demonstrated by an abnormal partial thromboplastin time that is not corrected in a mixing study, the presence of anticardiolipin antibody, a falsely positive VDRL test, or some combination of these.

DIAGNOSIS

The American College of Rheumatology criteria for the diagnosis of SLE is provided in Table 92-2. A patient is said to have SLE if four of the 11 criteria are present serially or simultaneously, but these criteria are more useful for research purposes. For example, a patient who presents with lupus nephritis can be diagnosed with lupus even if he or she does not meet four of the criteria.

Clinical manifestations of the disease, as noted by physical findings, remain the most sensitive method of diagnosis and may predate laboratory findings by months. Autoantibody detection in serum is an important diagnostic modality, however. Many autoantibodies may be seen in SLE; however, the following are most clinically useful. Antinuclear antibody (ANA) is very sensitive and is present in virtually all SLE patients. Although a positive ANA does not rule in the diagnosis (as it is often positive in other inflammatory disorders and in a certain percentage of the normal population), a negative ANA almost always rules out SLE. Anti–double-stranded DNA is more specific and, when positive, therefore may help establish the diagnosis. Similarly, anti-sm is also specific for the diagnosis of SLE. Anti-Ro and -La are important to obtain in SLE patients considering pregnancy, because they predict an increased risk of neonatal lupus.

Laboratory markers are also important in following disease activity. Ones that are commonly followed are Anti dsDNA, C3, C4, urinalysis, and complete blood counts. Of note, ANA titers do not parallel disease activity.

Neuroimaging with magnetic resonance imaging or positron emission tomography scanning is expensive and does not add to the information gathered by physical examination and laboratory analysis.

MANAGEMENT

Treatment depends on disease severity. Hydroxychloroquine (Plaquenil) is useful in treating skin and joint problems as well as fatigue. Plaquenil has been shown to prevent flares of lupus, so, unless there is a contraindication, all patients should be on Plaquenil. Nonsteroidal antiinflammatory drugs are

TABLE 92–2 The American College of Rheumatology Criteria for the Diagnosis of Systemic Lupus Erythematosus

Criteria	Characteristics
1. Malar rash	Fixed erythema, flat or raised, over the malar eminences, tending to spare the nasolabial folds
2. Discoid rash	Erythematous raised patches with adherent keratotic scaling and follicular plugging: may have atrophic scarring in older lesions
3. Photosensitivity	Skin rash as an unusual reaction to the sun
4. Oral ulcers	Painless oral or nasopharyngeal ulceration
5. Arthritis	Nonerosive arthritis involving ≥2 peripheral joints, characterized by tenderness, swelling, or effusion
6. Serositis	Pleuritis or pericarditis
7. Renal disorder	Persistent proteinuria (>0.5 g/day) or cellular casts in urinalysis
8. Neurologic disorder	Seizures or psychosis in the absence of offending medications or other metabolic causes
9. Hematologic disorder	Hemolytic anemia with reticulocytosis, or Leukopenia of <4,000 mm^3, or Lymphocytopenia of <1,500 mm^3, or Thrombocytopenia of <100,000 mm^3
10. Immunologic disorder	Positive LE prep, or Anti-DNA antibody, or Anti-Sm antibody, or False-positive serologic test for syphilis with known negative fluorescent treponemal antibody test
11. Antinuclear antibody	An abnormal titer in the absence of drugs known to incite "lupuslike syndrome"

LE, lupus erythematosus.
Note: The classification is based on 11 criteria; a patient is said to have systemic lupus erythematosus if four of the 11 criteria are present serially or simultaneously.

most helpful for treating arthralgias and mild pleuritis or pericarditis. Prednisone is commonly used to treat the inflammatory manifestations of SLE. The dosage depends on the severity of the disease and specific organ involved. Life-threatening disease is generally treated with high-dose steroids and cytotoxic agents.

Chapter 93

SCLERODERMA

Nha-Ai Nguyen-Duc

OVERVIEW

Scleroderma is a chronic disorder that involves fibrosis of the skin and internal organs. This disease usually presents in the third to fifth decades of life, affecting women two to three times more often than men. Two forms of the disease are recognized: Limited disease is seen in approximately 80% of patients, diffuse disease in 20%. Clinical course and prognosis differ depending on the form of the disease. Patients with limited disease usually have skin tightening limited to the face, neck, and extremities up to the level of the elbows and knees. They also often present with the CREST syndrome, which includes *c*alcinosis, *R*aynaud's phenomenon, *e*sophageal dysmotility, *s*clerodactyly, and *t*elangiectasias. In contrast, patients with diffuse disease develop skin thickening of the proximal extremities and trunk with involvement and progression of disease of the internal organs, leading to death within a few years. Patients with limited disease have a better prognosis overall.

PATHOPHYSIOLOGY

Although the etiology remains unclear, postulated mechanisms include interactions among the immune system, fibroblast abnormalities, small vessel damage, and environmental factors, ultimately causing excess production and deposition of collagen in the skin and internal organs. Antigens exposed by the disease activate the immune system, most importantly the T-cells, which then regulate the function of other immune cells, such as mast cells, neutrophils, and eosinophils and basophils. Cytokines, such as tumor necrosis factor-α and interleukin-1, stimulate fibroblasts, likely resulting in fibrosis. Endothelial cell damage may also result from activation of the cellular immune system and cytokine production.

CLINICAL PRESENTATION

Patients usually present with nonspecific symptoms, such as fatigue and musculoskeletal complaints. More than 90% of patients experience Raynaud's phenomenon but, in contrast to primary Raynaud's, often have enlarged capillary loops and loss of normal capillaries in the nail fold of their digits. Skin thickening is often the first specific clinical sign and symptom. Musculoskeletal complaints include myalgias and arthralgias. Occasionally, a friction rub is present over tendon sheaths, due to inflammation and fibrosis, and is an important poor prognostic sign. Late manifestations include muscle atrophy and weakness. Shortness of breath often signifies pulmonary involvement. Patients with limited disease are at higher risk of developing pulmonary hypertension in the next 10 years, as compared to those with diffuse disease. Pulmonary function tests reveal a decreased diffusing capacity, with low lung volumes and decreased lung compliance. These patients have an increased mortality. The gastrointestinal manifestations are seen equally in limited and diffuse disease and include

253

dysphagia and heartburn due to esophageal dysfunction, asymptomatic large mouth diverticula in the small bowel due to muscular atrophy, and abdominal pain and distension from pseudo-obstruction. Intestinal fibrosis is the major cause of mortality in diffuse disease. Cardiac manifestations of scleroderma occur late and almost exclusively in diffuse disease and include pericarditis, heart block, and right heart failure from pulmonary hypertension. Renal crisis often presents as accelerated hypertension, with normal or high creatinine and proteinuria. The majority of patients with this feature present have diffuse disease. Disease is due to obstruction of smaller renal blood vessels and portends a grave prognosis, although use of angiotensin-converting enzyme inhibitors has decreased mortality.

DIAGNOSIS

Diagnosis of scleroderma is based mainly on clinical findings. Anemia and an elevated erythrocyte sedimentation rate are nonspecific findings. Antinuclear antibody is almost always positive, and usually in high titers. One-third of patients with diffuse disease have anti-Scl-70 present, which suggests serious internal organ involvement and thus is a poor prognosis. Anti-centromere antibody can be detected in approximately one-half of patients with CREST syndrome and is highly specific for limited disease. Although these autoimmune antibodies are fairly specific, they are not sensitive, and their absence does not rule out scleroderma.

MANAGEMENT

Management and treatment of scleroderma are largely symptomatic and supportive. It is important to identify those patients who have diffuse disease, because therapy for these patients should be aggressive. Management of skin changes is largely conservative, which includes avoiding excess bathing and moisturizing the skin with creams containing lanolin. Calcinosis can neither be prevented nor dissolved. Arthralgias and myalgias can be controlled with nonsteroidal antiinflammatory drugs and then low-dose corticosteroids if nonsteroidal antiinflammatory drugs are inadequate. High-dose steroids should be avoided, as they have been shown to increase the risk of renal crisis. Physical therapy may benefit those with tenosynovitis.

All patients with esophageal disease should be treated with H_2 blockers and antacids. Proton pump inhibitors should be used in those with refractory esophagitis. Modified behavior, such as avoiding late-night meals and elevating the head of the bed, should be recommended. Prokinetic drugs seem to benefit a few patients with delayed gastric emptying. Advising patients to modify their behavior by eating small, frequent meals and remaining upright for 1 to 2 hours after eating should be emphasized. Management of pulmonary disease depends on the disease process. Inflammatory alveolitis has been treated using corticosteroids; cyclophosphamide may also be effective. Pulmonary interstitial disease in the fibrotic phase usually requires no therapy. Patients with pulmonary hypertension carry the worst prognosis but may be treated with supplemental oxygen and anticoagulation, and by controlling right heart failure and using prostacyclin. Cardiac complications of scleroderma are treated similarly to those of primary cardiac disease. Renal hypertensive crises must be treated aggressively in the hospital with angiotensin-converting enzyme inhibitors. Other antihypertensives also may be added to control blood pressure.

Chapter 94

DERMATOMYOSITIS AND POLYMYOSITIS

Beth Anne Biggee

OVERVIEW

The inflammatory myopathies (polymyositis and dermatomyositis) are autoimmune disorders that are characterized by chronic inflammation of skeletal muscle, as in polymyositis, and the skin, as in dermatomyositis. Disease is most commonly classified according to whether it occurs in childhood or adult life and whether it is associated with a connective tissue disease or malignancy. Gender plays a role, with women overall being at 2.5 times higher risk than men; however, if associated with a connective tissue disease, the incidence becomes ten times higher for women. Blacks also are at increased risk, with a ratio of 3:1 compared to whites.

PATHOPHYSIOLOGY

Polymyositis and dermatomyositis are idiopathic; however, genetic predisposition may play a role in disease activity. The diseases are manifested by inflammation and necrosis of affected skeletal muscle. Autoimmune factors and cellular immunity are likely the underlying mechanism of disease; however, a specific antigen or etiologic factor has not been identified. Autoantibodies found in polymyositis are abundant and can be associated with clinical presentation, prognosis, response to therapy, and genetic human leukocyte antigen haplotypes.

CLINICAL PRESENTATION

Inflammatory myopathies cause weakness in the neck, shoulders, and hips that is symmetric and diffuse. The muscles may be tender as well. The onset may be gradual or may have a rapidly progressive course. Patients first describe weakness in the lower limb proximal muscles, with difficulty in climbing stairs or rising from a chair. Eventually, weakness in the upper proximal muscles presents as difficulty in brushing teeth or combing hair. Neck weakness can present as difficulty in holding their heads from a pillow, and they may complain of difficulty chewing and swallowing. Respiratory problems may result from weakness of the respiratory muscles, alveolitis, or interstitial lung disease, and cardiac involvement may include myocarditis and inflammation of the conduction system of the heart. Patients may also present with constitutional symptoms, polyarthritis, and vasculitis, such as Raynaud's phenomenon.

Dermatomyositis also presents with cutaneous findings that include the classic heliotrope rash, a purple discoloration of the upper eyelids. Sun-exposed areas may show a reddish discoloration, especially over the face, neck (V sign), and shoulder (shawl sign). The nailbed may also be red from periungual erythema or cuticular telangiectasias, and "mechanic's hands," with rough scaling skin that cracks over the fingertips, may be seen. Gottron's sign is scaly or smooth erythematous patches of thick skin over dorsal proximal interphalangeal, metacarpophalangeal, knee, or elbow joints or over the medial malleoli. The only pathognomonic skin finding in adults is Gottron's papules, which are violaceous and flat-topped papules found over the dorsum of the interphalangeal joints of the hands only. Skin manifestations may occur at any time of the disease course.

DIAGNOSIS

Diagnosis is made by differentiating polymyositis from the other myopathies, such as drug-induced, noninflammatory, inclusion body, and infectious. Careful history and physical examination can help distinguish among these entities, but serology, electromyography, and muscle biopsy are usually needed to confirm the diagnosis. Signs of inflammation and chronic disease, such as a nonspecific high sedimentation rate and anemia of chronic disease, are present. High creatine kinase, aldolase lactic dehydrogenase, and transaminases suggest inflammation of muscle. Autoantibodies are usually present. Antinuclear antibody is positive in more than 75% of cases. Rheumatoid factor is evident in less than 50% of cases. Anti-Jo-1 is seen in 20% to 30% of patients with articular, lung, and Raynaud's involvement. Anti-Mi-2 is seen 5% to 10% of the time and is associated with dermatomyositis. Muscle biopsy usually shows inflammation with necrosis around blood vessels. Electromyography can also be useful in distinguishing polymyositis from other myopathies based on characteristic patterns.

MANAGEMENT

The inflammatory myopathies are most commonly treated with high-dose steroids, and most patients require a lower dose as maintenance therapy thereafter. For refractory cases, methotrexate, azathioprine, cyclophosphamide, or intravenous immune globulin have been used with success. A search for malignancy is indicated and is found at a relative risk of 1.8 for men and 1.7 for women with polymyositis, and 2.4 for men and 3.4 for women with dermatomyositis.

Chapter 95

TEMPORAL ARTERITIS

Joseph V. Agostini

OVERVIEW

Temporal, or giant cell, arteritis is an inflammatory disease characterized by injury to medium and large-sized arteries. The temporal branch of the carotid artery is commonly involved and lends its name to the disease, but the disease may occur systemically. It is closely linked to polymyalgia rheumatica, a syndrome notable for aching, stiffness, and pain of the neck, shoulders, and pelvic girdle.

PATHOPHYSIOLOGY

Histologic examination reveals vasculitis with an inflammatory infiltrate characterized by mononuclear cells and, often, multinucleated giant cells. Serial sections of vessel biopsies need to be examined owing to the discontinuous nature of the disease, and specimens of several centimeters are recommended to improve diagnostic sensitivity.

CLINICAL PRESENTATION

The mean age at diagnosis is approximately 70 years, and the diagnosis is unlikely before the age of 50 years. Patients can present with headache, scalp pain over the temporal area (which may be noted by the patient while combing hair or putting on glasses), and jaw claudication. The most feared presenting symptoms involve ocular complaints, ranging from diplopia to blindness as a result of ischemic optic neuritis. Constitutional symptoms, such as weight loss, fever, malaise, and night sweats, also occur. Polymyalgia rheumatica symptoms can be present at the time of diagnosis or independently.

DIAGNOSIS

Laboratory studies can be helpful but not necessarily diagnostic. Findings include anemia, elevated erythrocyte sedimentation rate (ESR), anemia of chronic disease, and elevated transaminases. Antineutrophil cytoplasmic antibodies and antinuclear antibodies are not positive. In 1990, clinical criteria were identified for the diagnosis of temporal arteritis. Having three or more of the criteria has a sensitivity and specificity of more than 90% for having temporal arteritis. They are as follows: age older than 50 years, new localized headache, temporal artery tenderness or diminished temporal artery pulse, ESR over 50, and temporal artery biopsy positive for necrotizing arteritis.

MANAGEMENT

Corticosteroids are the mainstay of treatment, but there is no complete consensus on exact dosage or course of treatment. Rapid response to 40 to 60 mg prednisone per day is common. Dosage tapering and the optimal length of treatment should be guided by the patient's clinical response and monitoring of the ESR. Pharmacotherapy should not be withheld to await a biopsy, as irreversible blindness may occur, particularly in the presence of ocular symptoms. Patients with polymyalgia rheumatica typically respond to lower doses of prednisone, 15 to 20 mg per day, for initial treatment. Prognosis for temporal arteritis and polymyalgia rheumatica is quite good. Most patients can expect complete remission; however, relapse is common.

Chapter 96

SERONEGATIVE SPONDYLOARTHROPATHIES

Christopher B. Ruser

OVERVIEW

The seronegative spondyloarthropathies are a heterogeneous group of inflammatory disorders characterized by a spectrum of articular and extraarticular manifestations, including involvement with the eye, gastrointestinal (GI) tract, genitourinary (GU) tract, and skin. This group of disorders includes ankylosing spondylitis (AS), Reiter's syndrome, enteropathic arthropathy, and psoriatic arthritis. Most of the spondyloarthropathies are human leukocyte antigen (HLA)-B27 associated but have variable prevalences of HLA-B27. It has been variously proposed that HLA-B27 serves as a specific receptor for an infective agent, or that the presence of this gene induces tolerance to organisms with which it cross-reacts. These are rare disorders; for example, the prevalence of AS in North America is believed to be 0.1% to 0.2%. If untreated, however, they may result in significant morbidity and debilitation.

PATHOPHYSIOLOGY

Ankylosing Spondylitis

AS involves the axial skeleton and large proximal joints and is associated with HLA-B27 in more than 95% of patients. The etiology of AS remains unknown, but it is at least twice as common in men than in women and usually presents from age 15 to 40 years. At the cellular level, the disease begins with inflammation of fibrocartilage, progressing to involve bone and bony-ligamentous junctions (also known as *enthesopathy*). Inflammation can be followed by fibrosis with secondary ossification and ankylosis. This process is most dramatically demonstrated in the spine, where vertebral bodies may ultimately become fused (known as *syndesmophytes*), resulting in the characteristic radiographic appearance of "bamboo spine."

Reiter's Syndrome

Reiter's syndrome, the classic triad of arthritis, conjunctivitis, and urethritis often, but not invariably, occurs after a GI or GU infection with *Yersinia, Salmonella, Shigella, Campylobacter,* or *Chlamydia.* It is more strongly HLA-B27 associated than AS and also has a poorly understood pathophysiology.

Enteropathic Arthritis

Enteropathic arthritis describes the joint manifestations associated with inflammatory bowel disease (Crohn's or ulcerative colitis) and is also poorly understood. A peripheral arthritis may occur in up to 20% of patients with Crohn's and 12% of patients with ulcerative colitis. Axial arthritis is less common and hard to distinguish from AS. It occurs in approximately 6% of patients with inflammatory bowel disease.

Psoriatic Arthritis

An asymmetric oligoarticular arthritis occurs in at least 5% to 7% of patients with psoriasis, with psoriasis preceding the joint disease in 75% of the cases.

CLINICAL PRESENTATION

Ankylosing Spondylitis

Patients typically present with low back pain that is worse in the morning and is relieved by physical activity. The pain may involve the buttocks, thigh, peripheral large joints, or ligamentous insertions. On physical examination, pain and tenderness may be elicited at the sacroiliac joints with associated paraspinal spasm. As the disease progresses, loss of spinal motion can be demonstrated, and patients are at increasing risk of vertebral fractures, discitis, and spinal stenosis. Extraaxial joints may also show loss of range of motion. Extraarticular manifestations include uveitis, restrictive lung disease, and aortic insufficiency.

Reiter's Syndrome

Patients may present with a history of an antecedent GI or GU illness, complain of arthritis (usually oligoarticular, involving low extremities more than upper), and have continued urethritis or visual problems (conjunctivitis or, more rarely, uveitis). The syndrome may also have mucocutaneous findings, including circinate balanitis, keratoderma blennorrhagicum (rash on the palms and soles), and mucosal ulcers.

Enteropathic Arthritis

Patients typically present with abrupt onset of oligoarticular arthritis in a migratory pattern; knees and ankles are most commonly affected. The peripheral arthritis usually correlates with flares of the bowel disease, but in the case of spondylitis, may antedate bowel problems by months to years.

Psoriatic Arthritis

Psoriatic arthritis commonly presents with a large joint oligoarthritis, arthritis of distal interphalangeal joints, and dactylitis (sausage digit, caused by flexor tenosynovitis). There are five patterns of arthritis: spondylitis, symmetric small joint arthritis (which resembles rheumatoid arthritis), asymmetric large joint oligoarthritis, classic arthritis confined to distal interphalangeal joints, and the rare arthritis mutilans with sacroiliitis.

DIAGNOSIS

Ankylosing Spondylitis

AS remains a clinical diagnosis, but radiographic findings often can aid in the diagnosis. These include erosions and pseudowidening of the sacroiliac joints, as well as the bony bridging seen in the spine. Peripheral joints usually show concentric narrowing of the joint space, particularly at the hips and shoulders. The erythrocyte sedimentation rate (ESR) is often elevated as well.

Reiter's Syndrome

Laboratory findings are relatively nonspecific and may include an elevated ESR, normocytic anemia, or relative thrombocytosis. Pyuria and a neutrophil-rich urethral discharge may occur. Joint fluids reveal a predominantly neutrophilic inflammation with a cell count as high as 5,000 to 50,000 per mm^3. On occasion, infective organisms may be recovered from urethral discharge or joint aspiration. To rule out other infections, such as disseminated gonococcus, all recovered fluids should be sent for Gram stain and culture.

Enteropathic Arthritis

Laboratory findings are again nonspecific. Patients may have an elevated ESR, an elevated white blood cell count, and a normocytic anemia. Joint fluids reveal a sterile inflammatory pattern with 5,000 to 50,000 white blood cells, predominantly neutrophils.

Psoriatic Arthritis

Diagnosis is usually made in the context of psoriatic skin changes and can be distinguished from rheumatoid arthritis on the basis of distal interphalangeal involvement, asymmetry, lack of nodules, and negative rheumatoid factor.

MANAGEMENT

Ankylosing Spondylitis

Nonsteroidal antiinflammatory drugs (NSAIDs) are considered primary in control of inflammation and resulting pain. Indomethacin, up to 200 mg daily in divided doses, can be used as first-line treatment. In general, comparable relief can be achieved with all modern NSAIDs. Disease-modifying agents, such as sulfasalazine and methotrexate, have moderate success in terms of symptomatic relief and have been shown to be of benefit in patients with peripheral arthritis. Intraarticular corticosteroids may provide relief in the setting of an acutely inflamed joint. Pharmacotherapy should be coupled with patient education and aggressive physical therapy. Patients with AS may ultimately require surgical intervention, most commonly for hip replacement, but occasionally for knee replacement or lumbar spine corrections. Extraarticular diseases often need to be treated jointly with subspecialists—for example, ocular steroids for uveitis.

Reiter's Syndrome

As with AS, most patients respond well to initial antiinflammatory therapy with NSAIDs. Approximately 30% of patients develop a chronic form of the disease, with occasional flares. Second-line treatments include sulfasalazine, methotrexate, and azathioprine with variable results. Some evidence supports the use of a 3-month course of tetracycline to decrease the rate of relapse in patients who have positive cultures for *Chlamydia*.

Enteropathic Arthritis

Treatment should be aimed at control of the underlying bowel disease. A conservative approach to arthritis management should be pursued, given the potential dangers of NSAIDs with underlying bowel disease, but second-line agents, such as sulfasalazine and methotrexate, may be used. Symptomatic relief may be obtained by intraarticular injections of corticosteroids. Improvement of underlying bowel disease or surgical resection usually results in significant improvement of peripheral arthritis but has little effect on axial arthritis.

Psoriatic Arthritis

Treatment is best focused on the skin disease; however, NSAIDs should be considered as first-line treatment for the joint manifestations. Severe or unresponsive disease may respond to disease-modifying drugs.

Chapter 97

VASCULITIS

Gaby Weissman

OVERVIEW

The vasculitides make up a heterogeneous group of disorders characterized by vascular and perivascular inflammation. These disorders can be difficult to diagnose, as patients often present with multisystem involvement or nonspecific symptoms, or both. Kussmaul and Maier first described a necrotizing vasculitis, which they named *periarteritis nodosa,* in 1866. Since then, many more vasculidities have been described. Although all have vascular inflammation as their *sine qua non,* the particular organ systems affected and the course of the disease vary. Primary vasculitidies are classified based on the size of the vessels affected, as outlined in the following:

- Large vessels predominantly affected:
  - Takayasu's arteritis
  - Giant cell arteritis
  - Isolated angiitis of the central nervous system
- Medium vessels predominantly affected:
  - Polyarteritis nodosa
  - Churg-Strauss syndrome
  - Wegener's granulomatosis
  - Isolated central nervous system vasculitis
- Small vessels predominantly affected:
  - Microscopic angiitis
  - Schönlein-Henoch syndrome
  - Cutaneous leukoclastic angiitis

Secondary vasculidities may result from infection, connective tissue disease, drug hypersensitivity, malignancy, essential mixed cryoglobulinemia, hypocomplementemic urticaria, post–organ transplant, or endocarditis. Pseudovasculitis mimics vasculitis and is associated with antiphospholipids, endocarditis, cholesterol emboli, or atrial myxoma.

PATHOPHYSIOLOGY

The pathophysiology of these disorders has not been fully elucidated, and it is evident that the different diseases within this syndrome may have differing pathogenic mechanisms. However, several mechanisms have been identified that, alone or in combination, may lead to the vascular inflammation seen.

Immune complex formation and deposition appear to be major factors in developing these disorders and have been described after pneumococcal pneumonia, serum sickness, and hepatitis B infection. The response to the immune complexes includes activation of the complement cascade and inflammation. Another mechanism is the production of antiendothelial antibodies, which has been proposed in the etiology of Wegener's granulomatosis, Kawasaki's disease, and polyarteritis nodosa (PAN). These antibodies promote endothelial damage via complement-mediated lysis, antibody-dependent cellular cytotoxicity, or enhancement of thrombosis and myointimal proliferation. T-cell–dependent endothelial cell injury may also occur and contribute to vasculitis. Another mechanism implicated involves antineutrophil cytoplasmic antibodies (ANCAs). c-ANCA, directed against proteinase 3, is fairly specific to Wegener's granulomatosis. ANCAs with a perinuclear staining pattern (p-ANCA) are directed at myeloperoxidase. There is some evidence that ANCAs play a direct role in disease formation. Last, there often is an increase in the coagulation activity seen in the affected vascular beds, leading to thrombosis and necrosis.

CLINICAL MANIFESTATIONS

Some clinical features are common throughout all causes of vasculitis. Constitutional symptoms including fever, muscle aches, fatigue, and a decreased appetite are common. Patients may also report a significant weight loss. In addition, specific organ systems may be affected. The most commonly involved organ is the skin, and patients may present with palpable purpura, ulcers, livedo vasculitis, or even distal infarctions. Lungs may be affected and can present as hemoptysis or dyspnea. Kidney involvement may manifest as proteinuria or hematuria. Gastrointestinal tract symptoms can include gastrointestinal bleeding, abdominal pain, and liver enzyme abnormalities. Nervous system symptoms include headache, mononeuritis, stroke, altered mental status, and peripheral neuropathy. The specific organ system affected depends on the particular vasculitis in question and the extent of its activity.

The differential diagnosis should include illnesses that may mimic a vasculitis, such as emboli (calcium, cholesterol, or infectious), sepsis, malignancy, lymphoma, and intravenous drug abuse. The secondary causes of vasculitis, as listed previously, also should be ruled out.

DIAGNOSIS

Because the vasculitidies often present with nonspecific clinical complaints, laboratory examinations can be very useful in making the diagnosis. An accurate diagnosis is essential, given that the treatments are likely to be prolonged and have potential or significant side effects. Inflammatory markers are often elevated, such as white blood cell count, erythrocyte sedimentation rate, C-reactive protein, or liver enzymes. In addition, tests for suspected secondary etiologies should also be done, such as cultures for infections, drug levels, cryoglobulin levels, and antiphospholipid antibodies, and appropriate workup for any suspected malignancy. Some vasculitidies have tests that aid in the diagnosis, such as c-ANCA for Wegener's granulomatosis and p-ANCA for PAN. In general, however, a biopsy of the affected tissue that is most easily accessible should be obtained. There is the possibility of missing affected tissue on biopsy, and the diagnostic accuracy of this test is highly dependent on the type of tissue biopsied and the degree of disease activity. Another useful test that may be obtained is angiography. It is often considered in patients who have a suspected systemic vasculitis but have no obvious choice for biopsy site. Angiography of the involved vessel bed may show long segments of smooth arterial stenosis alternating with areas of normal artery or aneurysms (in the case of PAN). Smooth, tapered occlusions and thrombosis may be seen as well. Arterial plaques, irregularities, and ulcerations are usually absent.

MANAGEMENT

Treatment depends on the type of vasculitis, the extent of involvement, and the pace of the disease process. It is beyond the scope of this discussion to present in detail the different vasculidities and their treatments. Instead, a general guideline is provided.

As a general rule, glucocorticoids are often used and in many cases may be sufficient for the management of the disease process. Initially, high-dose daily corticosteroids are used. The patient's clinical condition should be closely monitored for improvement, and laboratory markers, such as the erythrocyte sedimentation rate, often return to normal. Once the patient has returned to baseline, the dose of the steroids should be tapered to the lowest possible dose that will control the disease process. Sometimes, cytotoxic immunosuppressants are needed. General indications for their use include rapidly progressive disease with significant visceral involvement, disease that does not respond to corticosteroids, or the inability to wean down the corticosteroids. Once started, cytotoxic drugs are often continued for 1 year once remission is achieved, and thereafter the dose is slowly tapered. In addition, treatment of any secondary etiologies, such as malignancy, is the primary therapy in those cases. If the vasculitis is associated with hepatitis B or C, interferon therapy is often indicated. Intravenous immunoglobulin has been tried in some conditions.

The prognosis is dependent on the specific vasculitis. Most respond to treatment, but many have reactivations and require long-term treatment.

Chapter 98

GOUT

Beth Anne Biggee

OVERVIEW

Gout is one of the crystal deposition arthritides. It is a metabolic disease caused by deposition of monosodium urate crystals in joints and other soft tissues. This crystal deposition can result in acute attacks of gouty arthritis, which over time can lead to a chronic form of tophaceous gout. It is more common in men than in women, and the peak incidence is between ages 50 and 60 years. Gout is the most common cause of inflammatory arthritis in men older than 30 years of age.

PATHOPHYSIOLOGY

Acute gouty arthritis is caused by deposition of urate crystals in the joints. Cells such as macrophages engulf the crystals, releasing inflammatory mediators. Foreign-body reaction can ensue, typically 10 years after gouty attacks and resulting in tophi. Tophi are foreign-body granulomas surrounding urate crystals. They form in articular and periarticular soft tissues, causing chronic tophaceous gout. The urate crystals that cause acute gouty arthritis and chronic tophaceous gout are due to overproduction (10%) or underexcretion (90%) of urate. Uric acid is the end product in purine metabolism. Inherited disorders of urate metabolism, such as enzyme deficiencies, most commonly the enzyme uricase, can result in gout. Excessive purine or alcohol in the diet can lead to overproduction of urate. Excessive cell destruction and turnover, as in cancers, lymphoproliferative disorders, hemolytic anemias, and cytotoxic drugs, can lead to high uric acid levels and cause gout. Decreased renal function, especially in the setting of diuretics or dehydration, can lead to underexcretion of urate. Drugs, such as cyclosporine, ethambutol, low-dose aspirin, and Glucotrol, can lead to underexcretion of uric acid. Stress, such as surgery, trauma, or infection, can also precipitate acute attacks.

CLINICAL PRESENTATION

Acute gouty arthritis is sudden and usually monoarticular, and affects the great toe (podagra), feet, ankles, and knees most frequently. The joint is swollen, warm, tender, and red. Patients can have an associated fever as well. The symptoms usually subside slowly over 3 to 10 days.

Gouty arthritis also can be chronic and can lead to joint deformities. The intercritical period or time between attacks shortens over time and, if left untreated, can lead to chronic tophaceous gout. Tophi can form under skin (in pulp of fingers, toes, and ear lobes), and within joints, tendons, or bones. Usually, they appear as white-yellow raised collections just underneath the skin. They are not associated with inflammatory skin changes and are usually not tender, unless they ulcerate, but they can be disfiguring.

DIAGNOSIS

The diagnosis of acute gouty arthritis is made by arthrocentesis (aspiration of joint fluid). History and physical examination are not sufficient to diagnose gout. Other crystal deposition diseases, such as calcium pyrophosphate dihydrate crystals, can present similarly. In addition, an infected joint may present like gout or can coincidentally be present in a gouty joint. Joint aspiration fluid should always be examined under a polarized microscope. Negatively birefringent, needle-shaped crystals are seen. White blood cell counts can vary from 20,000 to 100,000 per mm^3, with more than 50% being neutrophils. Gram stain and culture should be sent to rule out infection. Uric acid levels can be checked and are often elevated; however, diagnosis should not be made on uric acid levels alone. Uric acid levels may be normal in an acute attack and rise later, after symptoms resolve. In addition, uric acid may be elevated in some individuals in the absence of symptoms. X-rays are often done but do not diagnose gout, although some patients have characteristic findings. Most often, x-rays show nonspecific findings, such as soft tissue swelling, bony erosions, and calcification.

MANAGEMENT

Acute gouty arthritis can be treated with nonsteroidal antiinflammatory drugs, such as ibuprofen, naproxen, or indomethacin, for 3 to 4 days and tapered over 1 to 2 weeks. These antiinflammatory drugs help reduce swelling and erythema and offer pain relief. Colchicine also is used to treat acute gout. It prevents inflammatory cells from migrating to affected joints and phagocytosing the urate crystals by inhibiting polymerization of microtubules. Side effects, such as nausea, vomiting, and diarrhea with cramps, occur. At high doses, renal failure and bone marrow suppression have been known to occur.

Corticosteroids, such as prednisone, can also be used to reduce inflammation, particularly in severe attacks. Intraarticular corticosteroid injections can also reduce inflammation locally.

Prophylaxis for gout is typically considered in patients who experience two or more attacks a year. Colchicine may be used to prevent attacks despite the uric acid level. Correction of hyperuricemia also prevents attacks and can be accomplished by use of allopurinol, a xanthine oxidase inhibitor. Allopurinol should not be started during an acute attack, as it may exacerbate the attack. In addition, colchicine is often used concomitantly when starting allopurinol to prevent an acute attack. Probenecid, an agent that increases excretion of uric acid, also can be given to prevent recurrences but is less commonly used. All patients with gout should be told to avoid foods high in purines, such as meats, spinach, beans, and anchovies, and to avoid alcohol, especially beer. They should also avoid dehydration and diuretics.

Tophaceous gout treatment requires the use of long-term urate-lowering drugs, as they may help with resorption of the urate within the tophus. Therefore, allopurinol is probably more useful in tophaceous gout than is colchicine. Surgery, in addition to antibiotics, is occasionally indicated for tophi that are infected or if they are impinging on important structures.

Chapter 99

FIBROMYALGIA

Lisa Gale Suter

OVERVIEW

Fibromyalgia is a clinical syndrome characterized by chronic widespread pain and fatigue, poor sleep pattern, and discrete tender points on examination. It affects 3 to 4 million Americans, most of whom are women, and results in profound societal costs in the form of lost work time and decreased productivity. It coexists with multiple other common diseases that are equally hard to define, including chronic fatigue syndrome, depression, irritable bowel syndrome, and migraine headaches, thus further complicating diagnosis and treatment.

PATHOPHYSIOLOGY

Multiple hypotheses have been proposed in an attempt to explain fibromyalgia, including altered nociception; slow-wave-sleep abnormalities and decreased sleep efficiency; neuroendocrine or neurotransmitter imbalances, or both; abnormal muscle metabolism; various viral or infectious etiologies; and changes in cerebral blood flow. None of these theories has led to the identification of a definitive causal agent, but research continues. Nonrestorative sleep patterns are present in more than 75% of fibromyalgia patients, most frequently seen as faster alpha wave intrusion in non–rapid eye movement sleep. It is unclear whether these findings are causative or rather are a consequence of fibromyalgia, as studies have also demonstrated the development of fibromyalgialike symptoms in nonaffected persons subjected to disturbances in non–rapid eye movement sleep. In addition, studies suggest that increased nociception may play a role, as substance P levels are increased in the cerebrospinal fluid of fibromyalgia patients, and these patients have decreased regional blood flow to the thalamus and caudate nucleus, where noxious stimuli are signaled. Alterations in the hypothalamic-pituitary-adrenal axis and in insulinlike growth factor-1 and serotonin levels have also been implicated, but the data are inconclusive and may be related to abnormalities in stage 4 sleep in fibromyalgia, rather than the primary pathophysiology of the disease.

CLINICAL PRESENTATION

Most patients present with chronic widespread pain, fatigue, and sleep disturbances, but other features include headaches, paresthesias, irritable bowel syndrome, dysmenorrhea, facial pain, functional disability, depressive symptoms, and Raynaud's phenomenon–like symptoms. This syndrome can coexist or be confused with depression, somatization, or other psychiatric diagnoses, systemic lupus erythematosus, Lyme disease, rheumatoid and osteoarthritis, nerve entrapment, or other orthopedic or rheumatologic diseases.

DIAGNOSIS

In 1990, the American College of Rheumatology developed classification criteria for fibromyalgia, consisting of widespread pain (in areas above and below the waist and on both sides of the body) for at least 3 months, tenderness on digital palpation at a minimum of 11 out of 18 tender points, and axial skeletal pain. In the original American College of Rheumatology study, the combination of the first two criteria demonstrated a sensitivity of 88% and a specificity of 81% in differentiating fibromyalgia from other types of prolonged musculoskeletal pain. Diagnosis requires eliminating other possible diseases with a thorough history and physical examination, and a minimal battery of tests, such as an erythrocyte sedimentation rate and thyroid function tests. The physical examination is unremarkable beyond the aforementioned tender points, and significant joint, muscular, or neurologic findings should signal the need for an investigation of alternative causes of the patient's symptoms.

MANAGEMENT

Amitriptyline, cyclobenzaprine, and alprazolam taken at bedtime all have been shown to decrease symptoms in fibromyalgia patients in short-term, randomized, blinded, controlled studies. The efficacy of these medications has been shown to wane over time, however, and treatment should be targeted toward optimizing sleep patterns and maintaining daily activities. Nortriptyline may well prove more effective as a long-term treatment, as patients report fewer side effects compared with amitriptyline. There are no data to support the use of sedative hypnotic medications or opioids, with the exception of occasional benzodiazepines or zolpidem use in the management of patients who have difficulty falling asleep. Tramadol has shown promise for short-term pain relief in fibromyalgia patients, but long-term data are unavailable. Nonsteroidal antiinflammatory drugs and corticosteroids generally have not been shown to be effective in the treatment of fibromyalgia, but nonsteroidal antiinflammatory drugs are commonly used in an effort to control pain. Multiple other nonmedical interventions have been studied and may be useful in the long-term management of fibromyalgia, including biofeedback, aerobic exercise, hypnotherapy, acupuncture, meditation, massage, and local injections of steroids or anesthetics at tender points. Any concomitant medical or psychiatric diagnoses should also be treated to optimize therapeutic success. Most patients receive some level of relief with medical intervention, but many will relapse and require alternative treatment. Some patients may even note the persistence of symptoms at a lower and often more tolerable level for years.

Chapter 100

ANAPHYLAXIS, ANGIOEDEMA, AND URTICARIA

Michael A. Nelson

OVERVIEW

Anaphylaxis is an immunoglobulin E (IgE)–mediated systemic allergic reaction that is thought to be responsible for 500 deaths in the United States each year. Anaphylactoid reactions are virtually identical but occur through non-IgE-mediated pathways. Atopic individuals have no higher incidence of anaphylaxis but are more likely to die if it occurs. Patients with a history of anaphylaxis are at higher risk of occurrence and may have more severe reactions with subsequent exposures.

Angioedema and *urticaria* are conditions in which inflammation causes extravasation of fluid into interstitial spaces. Angioedema involves the deeper dermis and subcutaneous tissues and is not pruritic. It can be distinguished from edema in that it can be asymmetric and occur in nondependent areas. Urticaria occurs in the superficial dermis and is manifested as pruritic, well-circumscribed erythematous wheals with blanched centers. Urticaria and angioedema are classified into acute (<6 weeks) or chronic, with acute episodes affecting 10% to 20% of the population during its lifetime.

PATHOPHYSIOLOGY

Anaphylaxis results when the allergen to which a person has been exposed cross-links specific IgE antibodies to receptors on tissue mast cells and blood basophils. This cross-linking triggers a cascade that culminates in the extracellular release of histamine, tryptase, inflammatory cytokines, and platelet-activating factor. Histamine is the major secretory product and causes venular and arterial vasodilation, increased vascular permeability, and diastolic hypotension. Anaphylactoid reactions are due to various mechanisms that result in the same degranulation process as anaphylaxis.

Anaphylaxis and anaphylactoid reactions have numerous causes, including beta-lactams (penicillin may account for 75% of anaphylaxis deaths in the United States), nonsteroidal antiinflammatory drugs, and aspirin (through non-IgE mechanisms involving arachidonic acid metabolites), radiocontrast dye, and blood products.

The causes of angioedema and urticaria can be divided into immunologic causes, which involve complement or IgE, or nonimmunologic causes. IgE, complement, or kinin each can trigger mast cell degranulation, although complement can increase vascular permeability independent of mast cell activation. The mast cell degranulation leads to pruritus and urticaria in 90% of people. C1-inhibitor deficiency results in angioedema and urticaria via lack of regulation of complement activation that can be hereditary or acquired. Acquired forms are often secondary to lymphoproliferative diseases, malignancies, systemic lupus erythematosus, or autoantibodies, whereas hereditary forms are autosomal dominant and present in late adolescence.

Drugs are a common etiology; specifically, aspirin and penicillin are responsible for 50% of cases. Angiotensin-converting enzyme inhibitors cause angioedema in 0.1% to 0.7% of patients taking them by decreasing the vasoconstrictor angiotensin II and increasing the vasodilator bradykinin. Autoantibodies, by interacting with various antigens, can induce urticarial reactions. Additionally, physical causes of urticaria are well described, including mechanical trauma, temperature changes, light exposure, exercise, and water.

CLINICAL PRESENTATION

Anaphylactic and anaphylactoid reactions result in myriad symptoms involving the skin, lungs, gastrointestinal tract, heart, and nervous system. Most deaths result from bronchospasm, suffocation from upper airway edema, or intravascular collapse. The most common symptom is urticaria, and patients also may complain of pruritus, diaphoresis, flushing, or angioedema. Fifty percent of reactions involve the respiratory tract, and symptoms include hoarseness, stridor, a choking sensation, or a "lump" in the throat. Laryngeal edema can lead to mechanical obstruction of breathing and death. Lower airway manifestations include dyspnea, tachypnea, wheezing, and cyanosis. Cardiac manifestations include arrhythmias, perhaps induced by hypoxia, hypotension, and cardiac arrest. Shock occurs in 30% of anaphylactic reactions. Gastrointestinal manifestations include nausea, vomiting, cramping, and diarrhea. Neurologically, patients may experience weakness, syncope, or seizures.

The hallmark of urticaria is the wheal, which develops classically in crops over a 24-hour to 72-hour duration. The lesions blanch with pressure. Angioedema is nonpitting and occurs in nondependent areas, such as the face. Noncutaneous manifestations include bowel swelling with nausea, vomiting, and coliclike pain, and laryngeal edema, which can result in asphyxiation and death.

DIAGNOSIS

Anaphylaxis is straightforward to diagnose in patients who have the full-blown syndrome, particularly in the setting of a known exposure. In less pronounced cases, however, the diagnosis is more difficult, and a detailed medical history looking for potential triggers is critical. Plasma histamine levels become elevated within 5 to 10 minutes after mast cell activation but normalize within 30 to 60 minutes. Urine N-methyl-histamine, a metabolite of histamine, remains elevated for several hours, and a 24-hour urine sample may help with the diagnosis. Serum tryptase levels peak 1 hour after onset of symptoms and remain elevated for 6 hours.

Cutaneous manifestations of angioedema and urticaria are often diagnostic. A detailed history of potential exposures is important but identifies an underlying trigger in less than one-half of the cases. To differentiate angioedema from other diseases with similar appearance, it is important to note that IgE-mediated angioedema occurs without fever, leukocytosis, or an elevated erythrocyte sedimentation rate and usually lasts 24 to 48 hours. Vasculitis urticaria lasts longer than 72 hours, typically. Important laboratory studies to obtain include a workup for vasculitis-associated urticaria, such as erythrocyte sedimentation rate, and hepatitis serologies. If C1 esterase deficiency is suspected, C4 levels are obtained initially, which then, if low, may be followed up with C1 esterase inhibitor levels. The markers for mast cell degranulation, such as serum B-tryptase levels, also can be obtained. In chronic urticaria, autoimmune disease should be investigated with serum protein electrophoresis and thyroid function tests.

MANAGEMENT

Management of anaphylaxis begins with the assessment of airway, breathing, and circulation. Early assessment of possible airway compromise is critical, as emergent intubation or tracheotomy may be required. Epinephrine is the first-line treatment of anaphylaxis and should be given intravenously in patients with severe respiratory or circulatory involvement in doses of 0.5 to 1.0 mL of 1:10,000 concentration every 5 to 10 minutes as needed. Subcutaneous epinephrine may be used in less severe cases in doses of 0.3 to 0.5 mg and may be repeated in 15 to 20 minutes as needed. Patients on beta-blockers may not respond well to the epinephrine and should be given 1 to 5 mg of IV glucagon, followed by 5 to 15 mg per minute of continuous infusion. Hypotension requires placement of large-bore intravenous access to replete fluids aggressively and may require the use of vasopressors. Bronchospasm may be treated with inhaled beta agonists or intravenous aminophylline. H_1 and H_2 blockers should be given until symptoms of anaphylaxis have completely resolved. Corticosteroids, although not useful acutely, are often given concomitantly to help curtail recurrences or protracted reactions. All patients need to be observed for an extended period of time for signs of rebound anaphylaxis and should be aggressively counseled about trigger avoidance and the use of self-injectable "epinephrine pens." They should also be referred to an allergist.

H_1 antihistamines are the mainstay of treatment of angioedema and urticaria. Cycloheptadine and hydroxyzine are effective when H_1 blockers are insufficient and, rarely, some patients may respond to a combination of H_2 and H_1 blockers when H_1 blockers are inadequate. Systemic glucocorticoids should be limited to treatment of persistent vasculitis angioedema and urticaria, given their side effects, and should be avoided in idiopathic, allergen-induced, or physical urticarias. There have been reports of benefit with short courses of oral cyclosporine for chronic angioedema and urticaria.

For those with inherited or acquired C1-inhibitor deficiency, antihistamines, epinephrine, and steroids are often ineffective. Danazol and stanozolol work by effectively increasing levels of C1 inhibitor and C4 by enhanced hepatic synthesis. Fresh-frozen plasma has been used to increase levels of C1 inhibitor but may cause worsening edema through increased levels of mediator substrates, and it is therefore not recommended.

Chapter 101

ERYTHEMA MULTIFORME, STEVENS-JOHNSON SYNDROME, AND TOXIC EPIDERMAL NECROLYSIS

Karen S. Taraszka

OVERVIEW

Erythema multiforme (EM), Stevens-Johnson syndrome (SJS), and toxic epidermal necrolysis (TEN) encompass an overlapping spectrum of acute, self-limited exanthems. EM is a relatively common, mild form frequently related to herpes simplex virus (HSV) infection. SJS and TEN are less common, life-threatening forms with mucocutaneous involvement usually due to a drug reaction.

PATHOPHYSIOLOGY

The etiology and pathophysiology of these diseases are unclear. EM is frequently linked to HSV infection. In approximately 80% of patients with recurrent EM, clinical HSV lesions precede the exanthem. Although HSV has not been cultured from keratinocytes in EM lesions, HSV antigens, DNA, and RNA can be identified. *Mycoplasma pneumoniae* infection is also associated with the spectrum of SJS-TEN.

In contrast, drugs appear to be the leading causative agents in SJS and TEN. Based on case reports and a case-controlled study, the drugs most commonly associated with SJS and TEN include sulfonamides, such as trimethoprim-sulfamethoxazole and sulfasalazine; aminopenicillins; fluoroquinolones; cephalosporins; macrolides; tetracyclines; imidazole antifungals; phenytoin; valproic acid; carbamazepine; phenobarbital; and allopurinol. EM can also be due to drug hypersensitivity. These diseases are thought to result from cell-mediated immune destruction of keratinocytes' expressing foreign antigens, such as HSV antigens or drug-related haptens.

CLINICAL PRESENTATION

The skin lesions of EM appear abruptly and are distributed symmetrically in an acral distribution on the extensor surfaces of the extremities but can also be present on the palms and soles, thighs, buttocks, and trunk. EM presents with erythematous, edematous papules or plaques that are in fixed positions for 1 week or longer. The center becomes dusky or blisters and gives rise to the classic lesion of EM, the target lesion. The lesions can be pruritic and burning. Typically, much less than 10% of the total body surface area is affected. Mucosal lesions are seen in 70% of patients and most commonly involve the oral mucosa. This benign disease typically lasts 1 to 4 weeks and is without complications.

SJS and TEN often are preceded by a nonspecific viral-like prodrome. An erythematous macular or maculopapular rash begins on the face, neck, and central trunk and then may spread to the extremities. Individual lesions are round to irregularly shaped macules or patches with a dusky center. Target lesions can appear at the periphery. Lesions increase in number and size and may coalesce. Large, flaccid blisters form and rupture, leading to denudation and erosions. Frequently, there is involvement of two or more mucosal surfaces (oral, anal, conjunctival, or urogenital). Mucosal lesions also can occur throughout the pulmonary and gastrointestinal tract. Sequelae from mucosal scarring, such as blindness and esophageal stricture, can occur. SJS and TEN are part of an overlapping spectrum. Generally, the term SJS is used to refer to disease limited to less than 10% of the body surface area, and TEN to disease involving more than 30% of the skin.

DIAGNOSIS

On skin biopsy, EM shows occasional keratinocyte necrosis, dermal edema, lymphohistiocytic infiltrate in the dermis, and vacuolar degeneration of basal epidermal cells that can lead to subepidermal blistering. HSV may be detected by polymerase chain reaction of the biopsy. In SJS and TEN, keratinocyte necrosis predominates and may affect the entire epidermis, and there is less dermal infiltrate.

MANAGEMENT

When evaluating a patient with EM, SJS, or TEN, attempt to identify the etiologic agent (infection vs. drug). Discontinue suspected drugs and treat infections when appropriate. Dermatology should be consulted to assist in diagnosis and treatment.

Symptomatic treatment of EM can include topical steroids, analgesics, antihistamines, liquid antacids, liquid anesthetics, and oral hygiene. Patients with recurrent EM due to recurrent HSV outbreaks benefit from antiviral treatment with oral acyclovir or valacyclovir early in the HSV episode.

In SJS and TEN, with more extensive skin and mucous membrane involvement, morbidity and mortality are increased. The mortality rate in TEN is between 5% and 50% with septicemia. Particular attention should be paid to early detection of infection, with a low threshold for initiating antibiotic therapy. Management includes careful mucous membrane hygiene and wound care. Depending on the severity of erosions or ulcerations, consider a petrolatum gauze dressing or an absorptive dressing. Corticosteroids have been shown to increase the mortality of SJS-TEN when given after extensive skin involvement and blistering have developed. Some authors have found administration of a short course of high-dose steroids (80–120 mg methylprednisolone PO q.d. and tapering over 1 week or sooner if tolerated) useful early on in drug-induced SJS-TEN to prevent progression of skin involvement and blistering. Some studies suggest a benefit of treatment with intravenous immune globulin. When there is widespread mucocutaneous involvement, the patient should be managed in a burn unit, with particular attention to fluid loss and thermoregulation. With gastrointestinal involvement, aggressive nutritional support is required. The patient should be followed closely for conjunctival involvement and, if present, ophthalmology should be consulted.

Endocrinology

Chapter 102

DIABETIC KETOACIDOSIS AND HYPERGLYCEMIC HYPEROSMOLAR NONKETOTIC STATE

Amy M. Nuernberg

OVERVIEW

Diabetic ketoacidosis (DKA) is the initial presentation in 25% to 30% of type 1 diabetics. The mortality rate is approximately 5%, but the morbidity is much higher. It is important to recognize this condition early, because the associated shock and acidosis can be life threatening.

Hyperglycemic hyperosmolar nonketotic state (HHNK) accounts for many fewer hospitalizations than does DKA, but the mortality rate for HHNK can be 20% to 60%, much higher than for DKA. Also, HHNK is a common first presentation of type 2 diabetes.

PATHOPHYSIOLOGY

Diabetic Ketoacidosis

DKA results from insulin deficiency, with glucagon levels concurrently increased and glucose utilization impaired. The low insulin, high glucagon state results in lipolysis, creating serum fatty acids that are converted into ketoacids. An anion gap acidosis develops. Serum hyperglycemia leads to glucosuria, which causes osmotic diuresis leading to hypovolemia. Decreased tissue perfusion worsens acidosis, and patients can develop frank shock.

Hyperglycemic Hyperosmolar Nonketotic State

Decreased insulin sensitivity or increased catecholamines, or both; glucagon; or growth hormone results in significant hyperglycemia. This in turn causes a profound osmotic diuresis and dehydration. This hypovolemia leads to decreased renal perfusion and a hyperaldosterone state. Worsening renal function causes decreased glucose excretion and thus worsens hyperglycemia. Hyperaldosteronism is responsible for worsening urinary losses of potassium, sodium, calcium, magnesium, and phosphate. Hyperosmolarity and decreased cerebral perfusion pressure result in changes in mental status, often impairing response to thirst mechanisms. Hemoconcentration thus continues to progress, but the presence of insulin prevents ketoacidosis.

CLINICAL PRESENTATION

Diabetic Ketoacidosis

DKA generally develops in type 1 diabetics who have a pure insulin deficiency. Type 2 diabetics with severe insulin resistance may also present in DKA or with a combined DKA-HHNK picture. The initial evaluation of type 1 and type 2 diabetics who are acutely ill is therefore nearly identical.

Symptoms resulting from hyperglycemia include polydipsia, polyuria, and polyphagia. Symptoms resulting from acidosis include nausea, vomiting, and abdominal pain. Patients also may have symptoms related to a precipitating event, such as infection or myocardial infarction (MI). Signs elicited on physical examination may include fruity acetone breath, tachypnea and hyperpnea (Kussmaul breathing), hypothermia, hypotension, and signs of hypovolemia.

Hyperglycemic Hyperosmolar Nonketotic State

HHNK symptoms are generally limited to those resulting from hyperglycemia and hypovolemia, as well as symptoms of any precipitating stress. Polyuria and polydipsia are most common, along with the confusion, lethargy, weakness, and obtundation that accompany hyperosmolarity. Many patients present comatose, thus the term *hyperosmolar coma*. Signs include those of profound dehydration, such as hypotension, as well as central nervous system manifestations, such as changes in mental status or coma.

DIAGNOSIS

Diabetic Ketoacidosis

Measurement of glucose and ketones in both serum and urine is the first step in diagnosis. A basic metabolic panel in DKA shows an anion gap. Of course, the differential diagnosis of anion gap acidosis includes ingestions such as methanol, salicylic acid, paraldehyde, and ethylene glycol, and states such as lactic acidosis or uremia. The differential diagnosis of ketosis includes prolonged starvation or complications related to alcohol abuse. Classic laboratory findings in DKA include the following:

- Anion gap acidosis (usually anion gap >20)
- Arterial blood pH lower than 7.3 (and PCO_2 <35 mm Hg)
- Serum bicarbonate less than 15 mEq per L
- Serum ketones (as well as ketonuria)
- Glucose higher than 250 mg per dL (and glucosuria)

The major diagnostic dilemma once DKA is recognized is to elucidate a precipitant. The most common triggers include insulin noncompliance and infection. Most patients have leukocytosis with or without infection. Other precipitants include myocardial ischemia and infarction, surgery, trauma, and even emotional stresses. Cardiac enzymes should be checked in the majority of cases of DKA. Although MI may not be the initial precipitant, the dehydration and tachycardia that result, and the presence of premature atherosclerosis in diabetics, makes the risk of secondary cardiac ischemia significant.

Hyperglycemic Hyperosmolar Nonketotic State

Classic laboratory findings in HHNK include the following:

- Serum osmolarity higher than 310 mOsm per L (generally >350 mOsm/L)
- Glucose higher than 600 mg per dL (generally >800–1,000 mg/dL)
- Absent ketonemia and ketonuria

- Arterial pH higher than 7.35 with HCO_3^- higher than 15
- Elevated blood urea nitrogen and creatinine

The usual precipitants are similar to those of DKA, including infections, most commonly urinary tract infections or pneumonia, especially in gram-negative bacteremia. Undiagnosed secondary diabetes can quickly develop into HHNK. The differential diagnosis of secondary diabetes includes Cushing's syndrome, acromegaly, steroid use, thiazides, phenytoin, pancreatitis, or total parenteral nutrition administration. As with DKA, cardiac enzymes should be part of the standard workup, because of both MI as a possible precipitant and as a possible result of profound hypovolemia in patients with preexisting coronary disease.

MANAGEMENT

Diabetic Ketoacidosis

The key to management is to correct the major abnormalities, which include dehydration, hyperglycemia with ketone formation, acidosis, and electrolyte derangements.

Intravenous Fluids

In DKA, osmotic diuresis from glucosuria causes profound volume loss. Gastrointestinal losses from vomiting or diarrhea are also common in acidotic patients. The average fluid deficit in DKA patients is 3 to 6 L. Fluid repletion with normal saline (NS) should be initiated early. If the patient is hypotensive, immediate crystalloid resuscitation obviously is indicated. If the patient has stable vital signs, the fluid deficit should be calculated—one-half of the deficit should be replaced over the first 12 hours, and the second half over the following 24 hours.

Insulin Therapy

An initial bolus of 10 U or 0.1 U per kg of regular insulin is followed by an intravenous drip starting at 10 U per hour or 0.1 U per kg per hour. The goal is to decrease serum glucose by approximately 75 mg per dL per hour (to prevent cerebral edema) until serum glucose reaches 250 mg per dL. Once achieved, the insulin drip is "clamped": The insulin drip is continued so that ketoacids continue to be metabolized, correcting the acidosis, but the serum glucose should be maintained around 250 mg per dL by initiating a concurrent 5% dextrose in water (D_5W) or $D_5W/0.5$ NS drip. The goal of the clamp is to improve the acidosis, and it should be continued until the anion gap has closed. Once the acidosis, ketosis, and hyperglycemia are corrected, the transition can be made to subcutaneous insulin. A dose of regular insulin should be given subcutaneously 0.5 to 1.0 hour before discontinuation of the insulin drip. Generally, patients should be kept on nothing by mouth until this transition is made, to avoid worsening hyperglycemia and ketosis.

Electrolytes

Hyponatremia is commonly seen, because hyperglycemia causes movement of water into the blood vessels, diluting the sodium; however, because of the urinary loss of water in excess of natriuresis, some DKA patients will have hypernatremia. Serum sodium should be corrected to estimate its value in the setting of normal serum glucose by adding 1.6 mEq per L to the measured serum sodium for every 100 mg per dL above 100 mg per dL the serum glucose is. The fluid deficit should be calculated with this corrected value. The anion gap, however, should be calculated with the measured serum sodium, not the corrected value. Whole-body potassium depletion occurs in DKA patients with normal renal function.

Lack of insulin and acidosis, however, causes shift of potassium out of cells, so measured serum potassium may be deceptively normal or high on presentation. Administration of insulin can cause a dramatic fall in potassium levels, and thus aggressive potassium repletion is often necessary. If the serum potassium is low on presentation, then 20 to 60 mEq potassium chloride (KCl) should be administered before giving insulin. If measured potassium is normal or high, KCl can be added to 0.45% NS once serum sodium is less than 4.5 mEq per L, with additional intravenous repletion as needed. Adding KCl to 0.9% NS results in a hypertonic solution that slows correction of osmolality. If renal function is impaired, potassium repletion should be more cautious, based on frequent (every 1 to 2 hour) electrolyte measurements. Hypophosphatemia is common with DKA, again because of urinary losses. Aggressive replacement is generally not indicated, however. Once volume is replaced and the patient is eating normally, phosphate levels generally normalize without sequelae.

Bicarbonate

Bicarbonate therapy should not be a routine part of DKA management. In general, insulin therapy results in metabolism of the ketoacids, which regenerates HCO_3^-. Thus, exogenous alkali is not indicated. Bicarbonate also has never had a proven mortality benefit in DKA. The exception is when arterial pH is dangerously low—for instance, lower than 7.00. In this case, bicarbonate may help to counteract the dangerous results of acidemia. For instance, the cardiotoxic effects of acidosis include impaired contractility, lowered threshold for ventricular fibrillation, and reduced cardiac output. Additionally, severe hyperkalemia can be treated initially with bicarbonate. A bicarbonate drip is initiated as 3 ampules in 1 L D_5W, or 2 ampules in 1 L 0.25 NS.

Hyperglycemic Hyperosmolar Nonketotic State

Intravenous Fluids

In HHNK, fluid resuscitation is the essential treatment and should precede any other therapeutic interventions. Fluid resuscitation can begin with NS, because it still is hypotonic relative to the patient. Rapid infusion of 1 to 2 L is usually appropriate. The free water deficit in HHNK can easily exceed 10 L and should be calculated to guide management. Hypotonic fluid, such as 0.45% NS, is appropriate for the cautious repletion of one-half the total deficit in the first 12 to 24 hours.

Insulin

Insulin therapy does not need to be used emergently. In fact, use of insulin before adequate rehydration may result in total vascular collapse and shock because of the removal of osmotically active glucose from the intravascular space. If the patient presents with a mixed picture of DKA and HHNK, insulin can be used earlier with caution. Often, subcutaneous insulin can be used to manage HHNK, but an insulin drip similar to that with DKA is preferred.

Electrolytes

The profound electrolyte derangements are similar to those in DKA, but they depend on the degree of renal dysfunction, both preexisting and that induced by dehydration. Hyponatremia is common, but the sodium value corrected for hyperglycemia often is elevated, reflecting hypovolemia. Potassium levels are variable, again based on the degree of renal dysfunction. The use of insulin causes potassium to shift intracellularly, so as in DKA, repletion should be guided by frequent serum measurements.

Chapter 103

HYPERCALCEMIA

Douglas W. Bowerman

OVERVIEW

Hypercalcemia may be an ominous finding, because the most common cause in the hospitalized patient is cancer. Therefore, the recognition and evaluation of this condition are very important. Hypercalcemia is defined as mild (calcium level, 10.6–11.5 mg/dL), moderate (calcium level, 11.6–14.0 mg/dL), and severe (calcium level, >14 mg/dL). Calcium varies with albumin and should be corrected by adding 0.8 mg per dL to the measured calcium for every 1 mg per dL that the albumin is below 4 mg per dL.

PATHOPHYSIOLOGY

Hypercalcemia is usually due to overproduction of parathyroid hormone (PTH) or malignancy, but several other mechanisms can result in hypercalcemia. A useful mnemonic for the differential diagnosis of hypercalcemia is PAM F. SCHMIDT. P stands for pheochromocytoma, A for Addison's disease, M for multiple myeloma, F for familial hypocalciuric hypercalcemia (FHH), S for sarcoid, C for cancer, H for hyperparathyroidism, M for milk alkali syndrome, I for immobility, D for vitamin D and drugs (thiazides and tamoxifen), and T for thyrotoxicosis. Neoplasm can cause hypercalcemia in several ways, including ectopic PTH production, direct lytic bone metastases, humoral hypercalcemia, osteoclast-activating factors, and production of active vitamin D metabolites.

CLINICAL PRESENTATION

Signs and symptoms are usually due to the effects of the high calcium concentration on cellular membrane, resulting in decreased excitability, or to the deposition of calcium in tissues. Central nervous system signs include depression, confusion, fatigue, somnolence, and, eventually, coma. Neuromuscular effects are manifested as weakness and hyporeflexia. Cardiac signs can range from bradycardia to a shortened QT interval. There is also increased digoxin sensitivity. Gastrointestinal symptoms are common and result from slowing of peristalsis; they include nausea, vomiting, anorexia, constipation, and dyspepsia. Polyuria, renal colic, nephrocalcinosis, and renal failure can occur as well.

DIAGNOSIS

The first step in diagnosis is to measure the ionized calcium level to verify the hypercalcemia. The phosphate level may help narrow the differential diagnosis. Phosphate is low in primary hyperparathyroidism and in humoral hypercalcemia of malignancy. Phosphate is high in granulomatous disease, immobility, thyrotoxicosis, milk alkali syndrome, and metastatic bone disease, and with high vitamin D levels. Elevated PTH levels should stimulate a nuclear medicine study of the parathyroid glands. If uptake is high in one gland, then primary hyperparathyroidism due to an adenoma or carcinoma is

277

likely. If uptake is high in all glands, then primary hyperparathyroidism due to hyperplasia or tertiary hyperparathyroidism should be considered. If the PTH level is low, the other diagnoses listed should be investigated. A 24-hour urine calcium may be measured, and if the urine calcium is low, the diagnoses of FHH, thiazide use, and milk alkali syndrome should be considered.

MANAGEMENT

Management should be directed at the underlying cause of the hypercalcemia. Initially, though, the hypercalcemia should be managed so as to prevent cardiac and central nervous system effects. Rehydration with normal saline at 200 to 250 mL per hour is the first step. Rehydration works by inducing a diuresis, which results in an obligate loss of calcium. A loop diuretic may be added to help with diuresis or if the patient is in danger of volume overload. Bisphosphonates (pamidronate, 30–90 mg IV over 6 to 12 hours, is preferred, but etidronate, zoledronate, and alendronate are also available) are used for the severe hypercalcemia seen with malignancy and work by inhibiting osteoclast activity. The effect can be profound enough to cause hypocalcemia but is temporary. Keep in mind that infusion of pamidronate can be associated with fever, malaise, and an increased white blood cell count. Calcitonin, 4 to 8 U per kg IV or IM, is rarely used, as tachyphylaxis develops within 24 hours of administration. Its effects are temporary, as with the bisphosphonates. Glucocorticoids may be useful if the causes of the hypercalcemia are vitamin D–mediated mechanisms. Most often, only rehydration is needed to effectively treat hypercalcemia. Unless the hypercalcemia is severe, or if the patient has symptoms, rehydration should be attempted and the calcium rechecked. If progress is not satisfactory, then the other options can be attempted.

Chapter 104

THYROTOXICOSIS AND THYROID STORM

Seonaid F. Hay

OVERVIEW

Thyrotoxicosis is the condition of having excess thyroid hormone, usually occurring because of an excess production by the thyroid gland (hyperthyroidism) but in some cases due to exogenous sources of thyroid hormone. The most common cause of thyrotoxicosis in the United States is Graves' disease, but other important causes include toxic multinodular goiter, toxic adenomas, subacute thyroiditis (postviral, postpartum, and Hashimoto's), high intake of iodine, excess or surreptitious intake of levothyroxine, and ectopic thyroid tissue (struma ovarii). Thyroid storm is the manifestation of extreme thyrotoxicosis. Thyroid storm is rare, but the presenting symptoms and signs are very common and, if missed, can be fatal.

CLINICAL PRESENTATION

Thyroid hormone affects nearly every organ system, and most of the symptoms can be traced to an increased metabolic state. Patients may present with anxiety, tremor, hyperdefecation, weight loss in the setting of increased appetite, increased energy or fatigue, heat intolerance, and palpitations. On examination, a stare (sclera visible above the iris) or lid lag may be noted, both from increased sympathetic tone. Exophthalmos occurs if the thyrotoxicosis is from Graves' disease and is caused by infiltration of the extraocular muscles by immune complexes. Sinus tachycardia or atrial fibrillation may occur, and patients typically have a rise in their systolic blood pressure. High-output heart failure may occur in extreme cases. A goiter may be palpated in Graves' disease. Other causes, such as a multinodular goiter or adenoma, may be palpated within the thyroid. In postviral thyroiditis, the thyroid is tender and warm to the touch. The skin usually feels warm, soft, and moist, and in Graves' disease, there may be a classic dermopathy, pretibial myxedema, from infiltration of the skin of the shin by immune complexes. Deep tendon reflexes are increased symmetrically, and a proximal muscle myopathy may be present. Long-standing thyrotoxicosis can lead to osteoporosis due to increased bone resorption.

DIAGNOSIS

Thyroid function tests should be checked in all patients with suspected thyrotoxicosis. Elevation of the free (or unbound) thyroxine index with suppression of thyroid-stimulating hormone (TSH) is the most common pattern. Elevations can be seen in T_3, the active thyroid hormone, and occasionally is solely elevated in the absence of thyroxine elevation. TSH also can be elevated if the pituitary or hypothalamus is the site of the primary defect. Subclinical hyperthyroidism is characterized by a low TSH and a normal free thyroxine index and is associated with few symptoms but a threefold increase in the risk of atrial fibrillation. A 24-hour radioiodine scan can be helpful in determining the cause of the thyrotoxicosis. Graves' disease shows diffusely increased uptake of iodine; toxic nodules or an adenoma show "hot" nodules; thyroiditis or exogenous sources of thyroxine show decreased uptake. Antibodies against the TSH receptor (also known as *thyroid-stimulating immunoglobulins*) can be measured in patients with Graves' disease.

MANAGEMENT

Beta-blockers treat thyrotoxicosis by blocking the action of thyroid hormone on tissues and can be started on all thyrotoxic patients without contraindications. Methimazole and propylthiouracil (PTU) act by blocking the synthesis of thyroid hormone. Methimazole has the advantage of once-a-day dosing; however, PTU should be used in pregnancy. Both drugs have the significant side effect of agranulocytosis, and patients should be monitored for signs and symptoms of bacterial infections. Glucocorticoids block conversion of T_4 to T_3 and are immunosuppressive in Graves' disease; however, their efficacy has not been proven. Radioablation of the thyroid or surgical removal is offered to most Graves' patients in the United States, with most physicians recommending radioablation.

Management of thyroid storm focuses on controlling the clinical phenomena while treating the underlying problem. Hypotension is usually a manifestation of high-output failure and should be managed with intravenous fluids, preferably normal saline. Dextrose 5% injection may be added to the intravenous fluids because of the high metabolic state and need for glucose. Fever should be treated, especially if dangerously high (>104°F), with antipyretics and cooling blankets. Atrial fibrillation should be rate controlled with digoxin, beta-blockers, or calcium channel blockers and should resolve with decreasing thyroid hormone levels. Steroids should be given, both to treat the underlying problem and to prevent precipitation of adrenal crisis. Because of the high metabolic state, more steroids are needed than can be endogenously produced. Iodine and PTU can also be used to decrease hormone release. Beta-blockers may be used, but with caution.

Chapter 105

HYPOTHYROIDISM AND MYXEDEMA COMA

Lisa Sanders

OVERVIEW

Hypothyroidism is a relatively common disorder. In regions of adequate iodine supply, such as the United States, incidence runs around 0.8% to 1.0%; however, in iodine-poor regions, up to 20% of a population can be thyroid deficient. Myxedema coma is an uncommon (<0.1% of cases of hypothyroidism result in myxedema coma) but deadly complication of hypothyroidism, with a mortality of 30% to 60% in most series. The name *myxedema coma* is misleading, as few patients with this complication have significant myxedema and even fewer coma, although a change in mental status is necessary for the diagnosis. Early recognition and therapy are essential in myxedema coma, and treatment should be begun on the basis of clinical suspicion.

PATHOPHYSIOLOGY

Hypothyroidism can be primary, secondary, or tertiary. In the vast majority of cases, it is caused by thyroid disease (primary). Much less frequently, it is caused by decreased secretion of thyrotropin [thyroid-stimulating hormone (TSH)] from the anterior pituitary (secondary) and rarely by decreased secretion of thyrotropin-releasing hormone from the hypothalamus (tertiary). The most common cause of primary hypothyroidism is chronic autoimmune thyroiditis (Hashimoto's), which is caused by T-cell and antibody-mediated destruction of thyroid tissue. Incidence runs around 5% in the adult population and approximately 15% in the elderly population; most of these patients have a goiter. The second most common cause is iatrogenic: Thyroidectomy, radioablation, and external radiation are well-known causes of hypothyroidism. Drugs may also cause hypothyroidism: Lithium and amiodarone are the most common of these drugs, but interferon alpha and interleukin-2 may cause it as well. Drugs containing iodine may cause hypothyroidism by inhibiting iodide organification in the thyroid gland. Patients with normal thyroids are not affected, but those with abnormal glands may become hypothyroid after only a few days' exposure. Commonly used drugs that contain iodine include some cough medicines, theophylline, amiodarone, topical antiseptics, such as povidone-iodine (Betadine), and many intravenous contrast agents.

Myxedema coma can occur as the culmination of severe, long-standing hypothyroidism or can be triggered in a patient by an acute event, such as infection, myocardial infarction, cold exposure, or the administration of sedating drugs, primarily narcotics. It is almost exclusively a disease of older women and winter: The vast majority of patients are older than 60 years, 80% of cases occur in women, and more than 90% occur during winter.

CLINICAL PRESENTATION

Thyroid hormone works in almost every tissue in the body, so response to a deficit of the hormone affects multiple organ systems. The classic symptoms of hypothyroidism include fatigue, constipation, weight gain, cold intolerance, a deep voice, coarse hair, and dry, pale, cool skin. Carpel tunnel syndrome is common. Elderly patients may present with atypical symptoms, including depression or decreased mobility. Some elderly patients are asymptomatic.

On examination, skin may feel rough, nails may be brittle, and hair may be sparse (Queen Anne's eyebrow, in which the lateral one-third of the eyebrow is missing, is a classic sign.) Macroglossia is common, and the relaxation phase of reflex movements is delayed. Diastolic hypertension is common. Nonpitting edema, from deposition of glycosaminoglycans with associated water retention, is also found in long-standing disease. Pericardial effusion also may be seen. Common associated laboratory abnormalities include normocytic anemia, hypercholesterolemia, hyperhomocysteinemia, and elevated creatine phosphokinase.

The hallmarks of myxedema coma include hypothermia, hyponatremia, and decreased mental status. Changes in mental status can vary from confusion to psychosis and, rarely, to coma. Myxedema coma should be in the differential diagnosis of any patient admitted with hyponatremia associated with mental status changes. Hypotension, bradycardia, hypoglycemia, and hypoventilation with respiratory acidosis also are common.

DIAGNOSIS

Anyone suspected of being hypothyroid will need measurement of TSH, as well as free T_4 and T_3. If myxedema coma is suspected, then cortisol should be measured as well, as adrenal insufficiency can accompany myxedema coma. Adrenal insufficiency is most commonly seen in primary hypothyroidism caused by autoimmune thyroid disease, because the adrenal glands are another common target of autoantibodies. In addition, secondary hypothyroidism may be associated with multiple pituitary deficits, including adrenocorticotropic hormone.

Elevated TSH is the *sine qua non* of primary hyperthyroidism. In overt hypothyroidism, free T_4 levels are low; however, in subclinical hypothyroidism, free T_4 and T_3 may be normal. In secondary and tertiary hypothyroidism, TSH may be normal or low, but free T_4 and T_3 levels are low as well. When pituitary or hypothalamic deficits are suspected, magnetic resonance imaging is necessary to determine which organ is involved.

MANAGEMENT

Myxedema coma is a medical emergency and, if suspected, should be treated before confirming laboratory results are available. Treatment consists of thyroid hormone and supportive measures for the effects of hypothyroidism, as well as treatment of any suspected precipitating factor, such as infection. Until adrenal insufficiency can be ruled out, the patient should be given stress-dose steroids (hydrocortisone, 100 mg IV every 8 hours.) There is some controversy about how thyroid hormone should be given, and because myxedema coma is rare, no studies have been done to compare treatments. Historically, T_4 has been given intravenously because of impaired intestinal absorption. The first dose is usually large: 0.2 to 0.4 mg. The dose should be reduced in older and smaller patients, or if the patient has a history of coronary artery disease or arrhythmias. Daily doses of 0.05 to 0.20 mg are given thereafter. Some experts support the use of T_3 in addition to T_4, as T_3 is the more biologically active form of the hormone, and systemic conversion of T_4 to T_3 is depressed in hypothyroidism or acute illness, or in the presence of steroids. Proper dosing is important; high serum T_3 levels have been associated with higher rates of mortality. The recommended dose is 5 to 20 mg followed by 2.5 to 10.0 mg every 8 hours thereafter. When T_3 is used, the initial dose of T_4 should be decreased from 0.2–0.4 mg to 0.2–0.3 mg and then 0.05 mg daily thereafter.

Supportive therapy is extremely important in the treatment of myxedema. Hypothermia should be treated with passive rewarming with blankets. More active rewarming can worsen hypotension by causing peripheral vasodilation. Hypotension that is refractory to fluids can be treated with vasopressor drugs until the T_4 has had time to act. Empiric antibiotics should be considered if clinically indicated until cultures are proved negative.

Less severe hypothyroidism is usually treated on an outpatient basis. Synthetic thyroxine is the drug of choice for these patients, with the usual replacement dose in adults being 1.6 mg per kg per day. T_4 has a half-life of 7 days, so TSH should be checked after steady state is reached, 6 weeks after initiation of therapy.

Elderly patients or patients with known coronary artery disease should be treated more conservatively. A starting dose of 25 to 50 mg per day is usually required, with a 25-mg increase in dose every 3 to 6 weeks until replacement is adequate.

Successful treatment of hypothyroidism reverses all symptoms associated with the hypothyroid state, although some symptoms—especially the neuromuscular and psychological symptoms—may take several months to resolve.

Chapter 106

THYROID NODULE

Michelle Lee

OVERVIEW

The thyroid nodule is a common problem in clinical practice. Its prevalence in the United States ranges anywhere from 4% to 7%, and depending on the population can even approach up to 50%. Although the risk of malignancy among patients with thyroid nodules is relatively low (5–10%), the need to rule out thyroid carcinoma must be addressed.

PATHOPHYSIOLOGY

The most common type of thyroid malignancy (70–80% of thyroid carcinomas) is papillary cancer, which often presents as a single nodule. It is usually the least aggressive of the thyroid cancers. The second most common type of thyroid carcinoma is follicular, followed by medullary, then anaplastic (the most aggressive of the thyroid carcinomas), and thyroid lymphoma. Finally, metastatic cancer (particularly breast and renal cell primaries) can also result in a thyroid nodule, although it is rare. Benign causes of thyroid nodules include multinodular goiter, Hashimoto's thyroiditis, cysts (colloid, simple, or hemorrhagic), follicular adenomas, and Hürthle cell adenomas.

CLINICAL PRESENTATION

Frequently, thyroid nodules are discovered in asymptomatic patients on routine neck palpation by the clinician or incidentally by the patient. At other times, they are found incidentally on imaging studies, such as carotid ultrasound or neck computed tomography or magnetic resonance imaging done for other reasons. Most patients with thyroid nodules are euthyroid, both clinically and biochemically; however, approximately 20% of patients who have an autonomously hyperfunctioning solitary thyroid nodule may have symptoms of thyrotoxicosis, including nervousness, emotional lability, insomnia, tremors, frequent bowel movements, heat intolerance, weight loss, and palpitations. Usually, these are patients who older than 40 years of age or have a nodule larger than 3 cm in diameter.

DIAGNOSIS

A thorough history and physical examination is the first step in diagnosing thyroid nodules. The prevalence of thyroid nodules increases with age, exposure to ionizing radiation, and iodine deficiency. They are more common in women than in men but have a higher likelihood of being cancerous in men. The risk of malignancy also increases in nodules that are larger than 2 cm and in patients younger than 20 years of age and older than 60 years of age. Other risk factors for cancer include a family history of thyroid carcinoma, particularly medullary cancer; rapid growth; and complaints of hoarseness, although benign goiters can also lead to vocal cord paralysis with a subsequent hoarse voice. A history of radiation to the head and neck areas can predispose to papillary carcinoma, which may not present until 10 to 20 years after exposure. Attention should be paid to nodule size, texture, fixation, and the presence of cervical adenopathy, which is often associated with papillary cancer. A hard nodule, as well as fixation to adjacent tissues, suggests a cancerous etiology as well.

Few laboratory tests are necessary in the evaluation of thyroid nodules. Checking the serum thyroid-stimulating hormone (TSH) is generally sufficient, although thyroid function tests are often routinely done and are usually normal. Low TSH can suggest an autonomously functioning adenoma that is benign (this accounts for less than 5% of all thyroid nodules.) High TSH may be indicative of Hashimoto's thyroiditis but does not exclude cancerous etiologies. An elevated serum calcitonin is often seen in medullary thyroid cancer, but it generally should only be checked in patients who have a family history of either multiple endocrine neoplasia type II or of medullary carcinoma. Serum thyroglobulin is a useful marker for following recurrence of papillary and follicular tumors. The most useful and preferred first-line test for evaluating thyroid nodules is fine-needle aspiration (FNA) biopsy. It is an outpatient office procedure with few complications and is considered the most accurate and cost-effective approach in diagnosing thyroid nodules. The specificity of FNA ranges from 72% to 100%, with a sensitivity between 65% and 98%. False-negative rates range from 0% to 5%, with false-positive rates that are less than 5%. Suspicious or indeterminate results refer mostly to follicular lesions in which follicular carcinoma cannot be distinguished from benign follicular adenoma.

Additional diagnostic modalities that are used in the evaluation of thyroid nodules include ultrasound and thyroid scanning. They are best used as adjunctive tests to FNA. Ultrasonography provides information regarding whether the nodule is cystic, solid, or mixed, with purely cystic nodules almost always being benign. Thyroid scanning or scintigraphy reveals whether a nodule is cold (approximately 85%), hot, or indeterminate and is useful in assessing patients with a palpable nodule and a low TSH. It is also useful as an adjunct in assessing FNA results that fall into the suspicious or indeterminate category. Risk of carcinoma in a cold nodule ranges from 5% to 10%. Five percent of all nodules are hot and are usually not cancerous. Indeterminate or warm results may be further evaluated with suppression scanning. In this test, thyroid hormone is administered in doses that suppress TSH secretion, and a second scan is performed. Radioiodine uptake is low in the nonautonomous nodule and high in autonomous tissue.

MANAGEMENT

Management is directed by the cytologic results of the FNA biopsy. Five percent are malignant and are managed by surgical excision. Seventy-five percent of nodules are found to be benign and are managed medically. Benign nodules may be followed clinically with serial examinations and possibly repeat FNA in 6 to 12 months, especially if the nodule grows or is clinically suspicious. They also may be treated with levothyroxine suppression, in which levothyroxine is given in doses that suppress TSH secretion, shrinking the thyroid nodule. This treatment is controversial, because complications include inducing subclinical hyperthyroidism, which may carry the risk of exacerbating osteoporosis or inducing atrial fibrillation, and it is unclear whether suppressive therapy is even effective. Suspicious or indeterminate cytology results may be followed up with TSH level and thyroid scan. If these reveal a normal TSH and a cold nodule, surgical excision is usually recommended. In the patient with a single hot thyroid nodule and symptoms of hyperthyroidism, treatment options include radioiodine ablation, alcohol ablation (percutaneous ethanol injection), or surgery. Likewise, toxic multinodular goiter can be managed either by surgery or by medical means with radioactive iodine ablation. Five percent of multinodular goiters may carry a malignant nodule and consequently merit surgical management if local compressive symptoms occur or if biopsy of a dominant nodule reveals malignancy.

Chapter 107

ADRENAL INSUFFICIENCY

Christopher S. Alia

OVERVIEW

The adrenal cortex, under feedback regulation from the hypothalamus and pituitary, is responsible for the production of cortisol. Cortisol is one of the major regulatory hormones involved in fat, protein, and carbohydrate metabolism; the response to stress and inflammation; and immune system regulation. The production of epinephrine by the adrenal medulla is also dependent on cortisol secretion. Therefore, interference with adrenal cortical functions can be serious and potentially fatal if untreated.

PATHOPHYSIOLOGY

Primary adrenal insufficiency is most commonly precipitated by autoimmune destruction of the adrenal glands. This condition is known as *Addison's disease* and accounts for approximately 65% of cases. Previously, tuberculosis was the most common cause of glandular destruction resulting in insufficiency, and it remains a predominant cause in developing countries. Other precipitants include infectious etiologies, metastatic invasion, adrenal hemorrhage and infarction, iatrogenic causes, and infiltrative disorders. Infectious causes include tuberculosis, histoplasmosis, coccidioidomycosis, cryptococcosis, *Mycobacterium avium-intracellulare*, and cytomegalovirus. The predominance of these fungal and viral pathogens makes adrenal insufficiency an important diagnosis in immunocompromised hosts, including those with human immunodeficiency virus and acquired immunodeficiency syndrome. Iatrogenic causes include medication-induced causes, such as phenytoin, ketoconazole, mitotane, and rifampin, and also surgical removal of the adrenals. Infiltrative causes include amyloidosis and sarcoidosis.

Secondary adrenal insufficiency results from pituitary or hypothalamic dysfunction or as a result of exogenous administration of corticosteroids, resulting in suppression of the hypothalamic-pituitary-adrenal axis. Tumors, such as pituitary adenomas or craniopharyngiomas; postpartum hemorrhage (Sheehan's syndrome); and head trauma can all result in impaired pituitary or hypothalamic function and resultant adrenal insufficiency.

CLINICAL PRESENTATION

Patients presenting with primary adrenal insufficiency have weakness, fatigue, myalgias, nausea, vomiting, anorexia, and weight loss. They produce excess adrenocorticotropic hormone (ACTH) owing to lack of feedback inhibition, which can lead to hyperpigmentation. In addition, patients may experience hypotension, often manifesting with postural changes or presyncope due to concomitant mineralocorticoid deficiency and interference with aldosterone production. Hyponatremia and hyperkalemia also are commonly seen.

Secondary adrenal insufficiency manifests similarly to primary, with the exception that hyperpigmentation is usually absent because ACTH levels are suppressed or inappropriately normal. In addition, the hypotension and electrolyte abnormalities are seen less often, because mineralocorticoid is not deficient. Mineralocorticoid levels are normal, because ACTH affects the adrenal cortex and not the rest of the gland.

DIAGNOSIS

The diagnosis is made based on clinical setting, the constellation of symptoms, and useful laboratory tests and diagnostic maneuvers. Useful markers in primary adrenal insufficiency include hyponatremia, hyperkalemia, acidosis, hypoglycemia, elevated blood urea nitrogen, and slight increase in plasma creatinine. In addition, hematologic studies may show mild normocytic anemia and lymphocytosis. In secondary adrenal insufficiency, the same markers can be seen, with the exception of the hyperkalemia, acidosis, and creatinine changes, because rather than aldosterone deficiency and salt wasting, there is cortisol deficiency, vasopressin increase, and water retention.

Confirmatory testing includes measurement of plasma cortisol between 8 a.m. and 9 a.m. If the value is equal to or less than 3 mg per dL, adrenal insufficiency is diagnosed. If the value is greater than 19 mg per dL, adrenal insufficiency is ruled out. If the value is between 3 and 19 mg per dL, then it is necessary to proceed to the corticotropin stimulation test.

After a basal plasma cortisol level is drawn, 250 mg of cosyntropin is injected intravenously or intramuscularly before 10 a.m. Thirty to 60 minutes after the injection, a plasma cortisol measurement is taken. If the absolute value of the cortisol level after injection is greater than 18 to 20 mg per dL, adrenal insufficiency is ruled out. This test is confirmatory in primary adrenal insufficiency, because endogenous corticotropin production is maximal, and additional exogenous corticotropin does not induce further adrenal activity. In severe secondary adrenal insufficiency, this test is diagnostic because the adrenal cortex has undergone significant atrophy and cannot produce an adequate response to exogenous corticotropin. The test may be normal in patients with mild or recent-onset secondary adrenal insufficiency. If still suspected, three other tests may be confirmatory. Measurement of cortisol levels after insulin-induced hypoglycemia, metyrapone administration, and corticotropin-releasing hormone administration are alternative means of determining secondary adrenal insufficiency. Further testing as to the etiology of the adrenal insufficiency should be pursued after the diagnosis of insufficiency has been made.

MANAGEMENT

Patients who are symptomatic should have replacement of cortisol in the form of hydrocortisone. Hydrocortisone is administered as 25 mg daily divided in doses of 15 mg in the early morning and an additional 10 mg in the early afternoon. If inadequate to relieve symptoms, or if the patient has comorbid conditions, higher doses may be required. Doses may also require adjustment during acute illness. If primary adrenal insufficiency is present, the patient will also require mineralocorticoid replacement in the form of fludrocortisone. The dose is 50 to 200 mg once daily to replace deficient aldosterone. Dose adequacy is evaluated based on blood pressure, serum chemistries, and plasma renin activity.

Adrenal crisis (acute adrenal insufficiency) requires fluid resuscitation to correct hypovolemia and hyponatremia, and high-dose hydrocortisone replacement (100 mg IV every 8 hours). Hydrocortisone replacement doses are then tapered as the clinical course improves.

Chapter 108

HYPERADRENAL STATES

Amy M. Nuernberg

OVERVIEW

The adrenal gland is anatomically composed of the cortex and the medulla. The medulla secretes catecholamines, such as epinephrine and norepinephrine. The cortex has three distinct regions, each responsible for production and secretion of a different steroid hormone. The outer region is the *zona glomerulosa*, which produces aldosterone; the middle region, or *zona fasciculata*, produces cortisol; and the inner region, or *zona reticularis*, secretes androgens.

Because these adrenal products have very different physiologic functions, hyperadrenal states encompass several distinct diseases. Among these are hypercortisolism, or Cushing's syndrome, hyperaldosteronism, adrenal hyperandrogenism, and pheochromocytoma. Although we make brief mention of the latter two diseases, we focus on the first two entities, as they are most common.

CUSHING'S SYNDROME

Pathophysiology

Cortisol secretion is normally controlled through the hypothalamic-pituitary-adrenal axis. Corticotropin-releasing hormone is secreted from the hypothalamus, which stimulates adrenocorticotropic hormone (ACTH) secretion by the anterior pituitary. ACTH in turn triggers cortisol secretion by the adrenal cortex. Cushing's syndrome can thus originate in the pituitary by an *ACTH-dependent* mechanism, or in the adrenal cortex by an *ACTH-independent* mechanism. Alternatively, ACTH can be secreted by an ectopic focus. The most common causes of Cushing's syndrome are (i) an ACTH-secreting pituitary adenoma ("Cushing's disease," approximately 70% of cases); (ii) a cortisol-secreting adrenal tumor, or micronodular adrenal disease (approximately

15%); and (iii) an ectopic source of ACTH, most commonly a nonpituitary tumor (e.g., small-cell lung, pancreatic, or thyroid malignancies) or an intrathoracic carcinoid (approximately 15%).

Pseudo–Cushing's syndrome occurs when patients have chronic physiologic elevation of cortisol which occurs most commonly in alcoholism and depression.

Clinical Presentation

Cushing's syndrome has many classic signs and symptoms as a result of glucocorticoid excess. Visible findings include central obesity with a dorsocervical fat pad ("buffalo hump") and supraclavicular fat pads; rounded, plethoric "moon facies"; purple striae; hirsutism; acne; and thin, fragile skin. Other signs are hypertension and proximal muscle wasting. Patients may complain of polyuria, which is usually caused by both increased free water clearance (a direct action of cortisol) and glucosuria (from secondary diabetes). Patients are osteoporotic and may present with vertebral compression fractures or avascular necrosis, especially of the femoral heads. Women may have oligo- or amenorrhea and infertility. Laboratory abnormalities include hyperglycemia, hyperlipidemia, hypothyroidism, granulocytosis, thrombocytosis, and increased alkaline phosphatase.

Diagnostic Studies

The first steps in establishing a diagnosis of Cushing's syndrome are confirming increased serum or urinary cortisol and lack of diurnal variation or normal suppression to dexamethasone. Thus, a good first test is determination of 24-hour urinary free cortisol. A result higher than 50 mg per day is consistent with Cushing's syndrome; a level higher than 200 mg per day is more diagnostic. Patients with pseudo–Cushing's syndrome states, for instance, can have results between 50 and 200 mg per day. Alternatively, an overnight low-dose dexamethasone suppression test can be used in screening. The patient takes 1 mg PO dexamethasone at 11 p.m., when endogenous cortisol should be at its trough, and plasma cortisol is measured the following morning at 8 a.m. Lack of suppression (a.m. cortisol of >5 mg/dL) suggests Cushing's syndrome. This test may be easier to perform in the outpatient setting, but pituitary adenomas may demonstrate suppression to dexamethasone. Pseudo–Cushing's syndrome states, such as obesity, also may give false-positives. High levels of estrogens (e.g., pregnancy or oral contraceptive pills) can also cause lack of suppressibility. Phenobarbital and phenytoin increase dexamethasone metabolism, causing false-positives. Second, once hypercortisolism is confirmed, ACTH is measured to determine whether the hypercortisolism is ACTH dependent or independent. Third, the clinician must identify the source of cortisol or ACTH hypersecretion. If ACTH is suppressed, a computed tomography scan of the adrenals is warranted. If ACTH is elevated, magnetic resonance imaging of the brain can be used to look for pituitary tumors. Bilateral inferior petrosal sinus sampling to measure local venous ACTH can confirm pituitary pathology. Thoracic and abdominal computed tomography scan can identify tumors that could be ectopic sources of ACTH. Overnight or 2-day high-dose dexamethasone suppression or a peripheral corticotropin-releasing hormone test can also help differentiate pituitary disease from ectopic ACTH or adrenal sources of cortisol.

Management

The treatment of Cushing's syndrome is primarily surgical. In the case of pituitary adenomas, transsphenoidal resection is the standard of care. Pituitary radiation may be used adjunctively in some cases. Surgical resection is also generally used for adrenal adenomas and carcinomas.

The treatment of bilateral adrenal hyperplasia is more complex. Bilateral adrenalectomy is sometimes performed, but the hyperplasia may result from hypersecretion of ACTH, and thus the treatment often aims to find and resect this source. In cases in which no clear source of ACTH overproduction is found, adrenalectomy, pituitary resection, and medical therapy have all been used.

If the patient is not a surgical candidate, palliative medical therapy can include ketoconazole, which inhibits steroidogenesis; metyrapone or amino-glutethimide, both of which block steroid synthesis; or mifepristone (RU486), which competitively inhibits glucocorticoid binding. Mitotane therapy is generally used as chemotherapy for postoperative treatment of adrenal carcinoma.

PRIMARY HYPERALDOSTERONISM

Pathophysiology

Aldosterone is a mineralocorticoid that acts on the renal tubules to reabsorb sodium, secrete potassium, and expand extracellular fluid volume. Mineralocorticoid excess thus results in renal potassium wasting and sodium retention. Secretion of aldosterone is controlled primarily by the renin-angiotensin system, which responds to hypovolemia or decreased renal perfusion pressure. Angiotensin II is the primary regulator of aldosterone, but aldosterone secretion can also be triggered by hyperkalemia or in response to ACTH.

Primary hyperaldosteronism is caused by aldosterone oversecretion, most commonly from a unilateral adrenal adenoma, or Conn's syndrome (60–75%). Bilateral adrenal hyperplasia is responsible in approximately 20% to 40% of cases, and adrenal carcinoma is a rare cause, occurring in approximately 1% of cases. Renin activity in primary hyperaldosteronism is suppressed.

Secondary hyperaldosteronism is due to overactivity of the renin-angiotensin system—for instance, in congestive heart failure, cirrhosis with ascites, renal artery stenosis, or renin-secreting tumors. Aldosterone and renin are elevated.

Clinical Presentation

Classically, patients present with hypertension and hypokalemia, both of which should be present to make the diagnosis. Symptoms can be very non-specific, including fatigue, muscle weakness, and headache. In more severe cases, signs and symptoms include paresthesias, tetany, and periodic paralysis.

Polydipsia and polyuria also occur as a result of a hypokalemia-induced renal concentrating defect. Glucose intolerance can result from hypokalemia's inhibiting insulin secretion. Patients do not usually have peripheral edema because of an "escape" from sodium retention with chronic mineralocorticoid excess, and serum sodium is normal.

Primary hyperaldosteronism is a cause of secondary hypertension in less than 1% of patients with hypertension. It is more common in women, often presenting in the third and fourth decades.

Diagnostic Studies

The first step in making the diagnosis is documenting hypokalemia with concurrent hypertension. The patient must have adequate salt intake (>120 mEq KCl/day) for at least 4 days before electrolyte determination. Similarly, the patient must be off diuretic therapy for 2 to 4 weeks to eliminate confounding volume depletion and urinary potassium losses.

One common screening test is measurement of the ratio between plasma aldosterone and plasma renin activity. Aldosterone is determined in the morning, after the patient has been upright for 2 to 4 hours. Plasma renin activity is determined virtually simultaneously. A ratio of more than 25 is suggestive of primary hyperaldosteronism, and a ratio of more than 50 is diagnostic. The test can be confounded by antihypertensives, especially angiotensin-converting enzyme inhibitors, beta-blockers, and spironolactone.

Diagnosis can be confirmed with determination of aldosterone excretion via 24-hour urine collection. Again, it should be done after KCl repletion. A urine aldosterone value of more than 10 to 14 mg per day with urine sodium higher than 250 mmol per day is diagnostic. Alternatively, baseline serum aldosterone can be measured, followed by repeat measurement after oral salt-loading with 10 g per day NaCl; lack of aldosterone suppression after salt-load is highly suggestive of primary aldosteronism.

Management

The treatment of unilateral adrenal adenomas is generally surgical resection. Preoperative therapy with spironolactone, a mineralocorticoid antagonist, should be used to normalize blood pressure and potassium.

In patients with bilateral adrenal cortical hyperplasia, or in nonsurgical candidates, spironolactone is the treatment of choice. Amiloride also can be used, with or without spironolactone. Bilateral adrenalectomy is generally *not* indicated; it results in normalization of serum potassium, but it may not correct the hypertension.

Spironolactone is also used to suppress the renin-angiotensin-adrenal axis in some forms of secondary aldosteronism, such as cirrhosis and congestive heart failure.

ADRENAL HYPERANDROGENISM

The adrenal cortex produces dehydroepiandrosterone (DHEA) and DHEA sulfate, both weak androgens. These are converted to more potent androgens, namely androstenedione and testosterone, in the adrenal glands and peripheral tissues, such as adipose. ACTH is the major determinant of adrenal androgen production.

One major cause of adrenal hyperandrogenism is congenital adrenal hyperplasia (e.g., 21-hydroxylase or 11-beta-hydroxylase deficiencies), which is not discussed in detail here. Additionally, adrenal tumors can secrete androgens. Adrenal adenomas are rarely androgen secreting, but carcinomas more commonly secrete androgens along with cortisol. ACTH-dependent Cushing's syndrome also results in androgen hypersecretion with mixed manifestations of androgen and glucocorticoid excess. An often overlooked source of adrenal androgen syndromes is exogenous intake of DHEA as a performance-enhancing drug.

In men, adrenal androgen excess can present with acne, virilization, or infertility, or some combination of these. In women, the manifestations include oligo- or amenorrhea and hirsutism. The differential diagnosis of hirsutism in women is broad, but adrenal androgen excess is among the causes.

Diagnostic testing depends on the suspected cause of virilization or other symptoms, but serum DHEA/DHEA sulfate levels can be checked in hirsute women in whom the cause is unclear. Treatment obviously is also etiology dependent. Androgen-secreting tumors (or pituitary adenomas) may be resected. Palliative therapies include ketoconazole, mitotane, metyrapone, aminoglutethimide, and mifepristone (RU486). See Management under Cushing's Syndrome for description of these medications.

PHEOCHROMOCYTOMA

This rare but potentially catastrophic entity is characterized by paroxysms of hypertension, palpitations, profuse sweating, anxiety, and headache. Patients experience tremor and weight loss. These symptoms and signs are caused by release of epinephrine and its metabolites from a catecholamine-secreting adrenal medullary tumor. Pheochromocytoma classically follows the "rule of tens": 10% are bilateral, 10% malignant, 10% metastatic, 10% familial, and 10% extraadrenal.

Differential diagnosis includes hyperthyroidism (which must be ruled out), acute intermittent porphyria, tyramine crisis, and amphetamine or cocaine intoxication. Diagnosis is made by demonstrating increased urinary catecholamines and their metabolites, namely 24-hour urine collection for unconjugated catecholamines, vanillylmandelic acid, and the metanephrines. Plasma catecholamine measurements have been proposed by some.

Treatment always begins with alpha-blockade, generally with phenoxybenzamine. Only after adequate alpha-blockade is achieved can beta-blockade be added or surgical intervention attempted. Ultimately, resection of the tumor is desired, with continuing adjunctive medical therapy.

Chapter 109

PITUITARY DISORDERS

Gaby Weissman

OVERVIEW

The pituitary gland and hypothalamus form a neurohormonal axis that is critical in regulating many of the metabolic and reproductive functions of the body. It forms a complex mechanism that can be disrupted at many levels. The disease may be primarily in the pituitary itself, often in the form of microadenomas or macroadenomas, and may lead to significant illness.

PATHOPHYSIOLOGY

To understand the diseases of the pituitary gland, one needs to review the anatomy and function of the normal neuroendocrine axis. The hypothalamus sits at the base of the brain, below the third ventricle and above the optic chiasm. The pituitary gland lies below the hypothalamus in the *sella turcica*, a bony cavity. The pituitary gland is positioned outside the dura and below the optic chiasm. It is connected to the hypothalamus via the pituitary stalk. The pituitary is divided into two main parts, the anterior (adenohypophysis) and posterior (neurohypophysis) portions. Each is distinct in function and embryology, as well as in possessing a separate blood supply. The posterior pituitary can be considered an enlargement of the pituitary stalk and hence gets direct stimulation via neural signaling from the hypothalamus. The anterior pituitary receives only hormonal signals via the blood stream from the hypothalamus and is not directly connected to it via neurons, as the posterior portion is.

The two portions of the pituitary also have very different functions. The adenohypophysis produces six hormones. The first is corticotropin (ACTH), which is regulated by corticotropin-releasing factor produced in the hypothalamus, as well as by serum levels of cortisol. It acts in the adrenal gland to increase the production of cortisol. At pathologically high levels, ACTH may have extracortical effects as well. The next hormone produced is growth hormone (GH). This hormone is regulated by the hypothalamic peptide GH-releasing hormone, which exerts a positive influence, and somatostatin, which plays an inhibitory role. GH serves to stimulate growth. It also has other actions, including antiinsulin effects and maintenance of normal body composition. Another product of the anterior pituitary is prolactin (PRL). PRL is suppressed by dopamine and stimulated by thyrotropin-releasing hormone. PRL serves to initiate and maintain lactation. At high levels, it can suppress the hypothalamic production of gonadotropin-releasing hormone and lead to hypogonadism. The anterior pituitary also produces thyroid-stimulating hormone (TSH). This glycoprotein is regulated by thyrotropin-releasing hormone levels and circulating thyroid hormone levels. TSH serves to stimulate the production of T_3 and T_4. Finally, the anterior pituitary produces gonadotropins, follicular stimulating hormone (FSH), and luteinizing hormone (LH). These hormones are primarily regulated by gonadotropin-releasing hormone. FSH acts to stimulate gametogenesis in both genders, acting on the Sertoli cells in men and on the granulosa cells of the ovary to promote follicular development. LH stimulates testosterone secretion in men and is important in follicular rupture and luteinization in women.

The posterior pituitary is involved in completely different pathways. It produces oxytocin and vasopressin, also known as *antidiuretic hormone* (ADH). ADH is used in the regulation of plasma osmolarity. Its release is stimulated by an increase in the osmolarity and acts to decrease it by effects on the kidneys and thirst. Oxytocin release is stimulated by mechanical distention of the reproductive tract and suckling of the nipples, and it is important in milk letdown parturition.

Several pathologic processes can affect this axis and hence cause disease. Developmental abnormalities of the hypothalamus and pituitary may be seen, often in association with defects of other midline structures, such as a cleft lip or palate. The empty sella syndrome is seen when a defect in the diaphragma sella is present and there is a free communication of cerebrospinal fluid, leading to increased pressure in the sella and compression of the pituitary with concomitant enlargement of the sella. Infectious agents can, on rare occasions, cause pituitary disease. If a viral encephalitis involves the hypothalamus, it may result in pituitary dysfunction. An abscess can also form in the sella after bacteremia. Noninfectious granulomas may also form in the pituitary, most commonly secondarily to sarcoid in adults. Hemochromatosis can also cause parenchymal pituitary damage. Autoimmune disorders are another mechanism by which pituitary dysfunction may occur and are most often seen in postpartum women. Ischemic damage to the pituitary is most common as a complication of severe postpartum hemorrhagic or infectious shock. This syndrome of panhypopituitarism is known as *Sheehan's syndrome*. Accidents, trauma, and radiation can all lead to pituitary dysfunction. Finally, pituitary adenomas can occur and can either be functional or nonfunctional tumors. Extrapituitary tumors, such as craniopharyngiomas that abut the gland, can also lead to pituitary dysfunction.

CLINICAL PRESENTATION

The clinical symptoms seen are dependent on the particular part of the pituitary that is affected, and many can be predicted based on understanding the particular actions of the hormone that are affected. Because the hormones released by the pituitary are constantly regulated by various feedback mechanisms, a primary excess or deficiency of these needs to be distinguished from a high or low level caused by an appropriate response to a derangement in a target hormone.

ACTH deficiency leading to a cortisol deficiency causes anorexia, weight loss, hypoglycemia, hyponatremia, and hypotension. A deficiency in ACTH rarely leads to significant potassium abnormalities or circulatory collapse, as aldosterone is influenced by other mechanisms more than ACTH. ACTH excess leads to Cushing's disease, which presents with central obesity, cutaneous atrophy, muscle wasting, diabetes, and hypertension. GH deficiency in children leads to dwarfism. In adults, GH deficiency leads to an increase in body fat, decreased muscle mass, and subtle neuropsychiatric effects. GH excess in children leads to gigantism, whereas in adults it leads to acromegaly. PRL deficiency leads to a failure of proper lactation in the postpartum period. PRL excess leads to amenorrhea due to the inhibition of LH-releasing hormone. Galactorrhea is seen in one-third of patients with a prolactin-secreting adenoma. Hypoestrogenemia also occurs owing to the lack of gonadotropins stimulating the ovaries. The hypoestrogenenemia, in turn, leads to vaginal mucosal atrophy and osteoporosis. A primary TSH deficiency in the pituitary leads to hypothyroidism and its attendant symptoms, whereas a high level of TSH secretion in the pituitary leads to hyperthyroidism, with its distinct symptomatology. Primary gonadotropin deficiency is usually due to hypothalamic dysfunction, except in near-total pituitary destruction, and leads to amenorrhea in women. In men, there is a decrease in serum testosterone leading to a decrease in libido and impotence. LH and FSH excess causes premature puberty in children. Pituitary disease can lead to abnormal ADH levels and hence an abnormal serum osmolarity. An abnormally low level of ADH leads to pituitary diabetes insipidus, in which one is not able to conserve water and hence has polyuria, polydipsia, and a predisposition to a high serum osmolarity.

In addition to the direct effects of the pituitary hormones, pituitary disease, especially tumors, can have nonhormonal clinical effects. Tumors in the pituitary gland or sella can invade the sphenoid sinus or the nasopharynx, sometimes leading to cerebrospinal fluid rhinorrhea. They may also invade the cavernous sinus or carotid sheath if they expand laterally. Because the optic chiasm lies superior to the pituitary, it is susceptible to mass effect from lesions in this area. A bitemporal hemianopsia is the classic visual defect associated with a pituitary lesion. A growth into the cavernous sinus here also can affect cranial nerves III, IV, V1, V2, and VI. Finally, pituitary hemorrhage can lead to a severe headache and an abrupt loss of vision.

DIAGNOSIS

The diagnosis of a pituitary abnormality in adults requires the observation of the clinical features, followed by the appropriate blood tests and imaging studies. Once the clinician is alerted to a possible pituitary disease, one can check the level of the appropriate hormone (this is true in discussing diseases of the anterior pituitary). As mentioned, it is always important to determine whether it is a primary disease of the pituitary or a dysfunction of the target organ with an appropriate compensatory response by the pituitary. Hence, measurements of the pituitary hormones are almost always done in conjunction with levels of the target hormones that they promote. Imaging of the pituitary is another important arm of diagnosis. Plain radiographs have for the most part been supplanted by computed tomography and magnetic resonance technology, the latter being preferred for its better resolution. These studies can identify tumors as well as help guide therapy.

MANAGEMENT

Treatment of pituitary disease depends on the hormone involved. From a medical standpoint, many of the hormonal deficiencies can be supplemented, as in thyroid disease or in supplementing adrenal steroids in the case of an ACTH deficiency. Multiple hormones are required in the case of panhypopituitarism.

Treatment of hypersecretion is often medical, although surgical and radiation therapy is used if the medical treatment fails to control the endocrine abnormalities or the mass effects of the tumor. Bromocriptine or cabergoline is often used in the treatment of prolactinomas. Acting as dopamine agonists, both inhibit prolactin production and cause tumor regression. The first-line treatment for acromegaly is surgery; however, radiation plus octreotide, a somatostatin analog, may be used if the patient has a subtotal resection or recurrence. Nonsecreting microadenomas may be just observed; however, if they become symptomatic or macroadenomas, they are treated with surgery.

With the increased use of computed tomography and magnetic resonance imaging, "incidentalomas" have become a more common finding. They should be evaluated for hormonal overproduction. In the case of asymptomatic lesions larger than 10 mm, treatment with radiation, surgery, or both is sometimes recommended. Those smaller than 10 mm often can be followed with serial images and treated only if changes in the tumor are seen, or if symptoms occur.

Chapter 110

OSTEOPOROSIS

Joseph V. Agostini

OVERVIEW

Osteoporosis, resulting in decreased bone mineral density, is a common problem in older adults that leads to increased morbidity and mortality owing to fractures. A minority of osteoporosis cases may be secondary to other disorders, such as hyperparathyroidism or hyperadrenocorticism. Osteomalacia, a related disorder, refers to a defect in mineralization (inadequate calcium and phosphorous deposition) during the organic phase of bone growth.

PATHOPHYSIOLOGY

Bone formation and resorption constitute a coupled process, carried out by the activity of osteoblasts and osteoclasts, respectively. The remodeling process usually results in the maintenance of bone mass, but age-related bone loss begins to occur in women at 40 years of age and in men at 50 years of age. It commonly affects the spine, hip, and radius bones. Women experience rapid bone loss during the perimenopausal period due to estrogen deficiency and increased osteoclast activity.

CLINICAL PRESENTATION

Physical examination findings of osteoporosis include dorsal kyphosis (the "dowager's hump"), scoliosis, and decreased height. Patients often present with fractures, which may be the result of minor trauma. Common presentations include hip, radius (Colles'), and vertebral compression fractures. Risk factors for osteoporotic fractures include age, tobacco use, low body-mass index, history of vertebral fracture, postmenopausal status without estrogen supplementation, steroid use, limited exercise, and white or Asian race.

DIAGNOSIS

Bone mineral densitometry is used as a diagnostic tool for osteoporosis. Dual-energy x-ray absorptiometry results are reported in T scores (standard deviations from the mean in young adults) and Z scores (standard deviations in age-matched controls). Osteopenia, or decreased bone mass, is defined as a score of 1.0 to 2.5 standard deviations below the mean, whereas 2.5 standard deviations or more below the mean defines osteoporosis. Whether to screen a patient should be guided by the presence of risk factors and the degree to which ordering the test influences recommendations for treatment. Plain radiographs are a less sensitive method of detecting low bone mineral density. Laboratory studies are usually normal.

MANAGEMENT

Clinical management of osteoporosis focuses on risk factor modification and pharmacotherapy. Patients should be counseled on the merits of tobacco cessation, physical activity, and adequate nutrition. Older patients should be questioned about risk factors for falling. The risks and benefits of estrogen replacement therapy, along with concurrent progesterone administration if indicated, should be addressed in all postmenopausal women with osteoporosis. Estrogen replacement may decrease fracture risk by up to 50%, but ongoing therapy is necessary for maximal benefit. Discontinuation of therapy leads to a resumption in bone loss. Calcium (1,000–1,500 mg/day for postmenopausal women) and vitamin D (400 IU daily) in combination are useful for prevention and treatment of osteoporosis. Bisphosphonates, such as alendronate and risedronate, inhibit osteoclast activity and thus decrease bone resorption. They are more costly to use, and patients (particularly older hospitalized patients who remain recumbent) should be given instructions to prevent esophagitis. Other therapies include raloxifene, a selective estrogen receptor modulator, and calcitonin, which may be beneficial for its analgesic effect in some patients.

Section 9

Renal and Electrolyte

Chapter 111

HYPERKALEMIA

Lynn E. Sullivan

OVERVIEW

Hyperkalemia is a laboratory diagnosis that is an indicator of potentially serious systemic disease. It can be caused by an array of different disease states and, if left untreated, leads to fatal cardiac arrhythmias.

PATHOPHYSIOLOGY

The most frequent causes of persistent hyperkalemia are diminished renal excretion. There are three primary causes of diminished renal excretion: renal failure, hypovolemia, and hypoaldosteronism. Systemic diseases in which there is a defect in tubular potassium secretion, such as sickle cell disease, lupus erythematosus, and amyloid or obstructive uropathy, can have associated hyperkalemia. Additional causes of hyperkalemia include adrenal insufficiency, Addison's disease, and hyporeninemic hypoaldosteronism. Certain drugs acting by a variety of different mechanisms can cause elevations in serum potassium concentration. Examples of these medications are beta-blockers, nonsteroidal antiinflammatory drugs, angiotensin-converting enzyme inhibitors, toxic levels of digoxin and the potassium-sparing diuretics, spironolactone, amiloride, and triamterene. The majority of potassium is intracellular; therefore, massive cellular breakdown, as seen in trauma, rhabdomyolysis, and hemolysis, can cause large elevations in serum potassium concentration. Acidosis shifts potassium out of the cell, causing hyperkalemia. This phenomenon is seen in diabetic ketoacidosis, in which patients present with acidosis, hyperkalemia, and the insulin-deficient state of diabetes. Pseudohyperkalemia can be seen in patients with a significantly high number of platelets or white blood cells, as these cells clot and liberate intracellular potassium, or in those who have had an improper venipuncture technique, which causes hemolysis and hyperkalemia.

CLINICAL PRESENTATION

Most episodes of hyperkalemia are characteristically without symptoms. Moderate hyperkalemia can cause ascending muscle weakness and decreased deep tendon reflexes, and paresthesias in the distal extremities are not uncommon. In addition, hyperkalemic periodic paralysis can occur, in which case the hyperkalemia is a secondary cause of the paralysis. The most serious sequelae of hyperkalemia are life-threatening cardiac arrhythmias, including bradycardia, complete heart block, ventricular fibrillation, and asystole.

DIAGNOSIS

If a laboratory test reveals a high serum potassium concentration, the first step is to check an electrocardiogram (ECG) and send a second vial of blood to recheck the level and rule out hemolysis as a cause. If the potassium level is truly elevated, evaluation of the ECG is crucial (see color plate). The initial finding is tall, peaked T waves, followed by a decrease in the height of the P waves and widening of the QRS complex. The P waves then disappear, and the final change is the merging of the QRS complex into the T waves, creating the sine wave pattern. Cardiac arrhythmias include bradycardia, complete heart block, ventricular fibrillation, and asystole.

MANAGEMENT

In the case of mild to moderate hyperkalemia, sodium polystyrene sulfonate (Kayexalate) can be given (15–60 g every 3 to 4 hours). Kayexalate is a cation exchange resin that binds potassium and should be given with an osmotic agent, such as sorbitol. Each gram of Kayexalate removes 1 mEq of potassium. The patient must have a bowel movement to eliminate the potassium. In the cases of severe hyperkalemia with ECG changes noted, calcium gluconate (10–30 mL of 10% solution infused over 1–5 minutes) should be given to temporarily antagonize the cardiac effects of hyperkalemia. To drive potassium intracellularly, 10 U of regular insulin in 500 mL of 10% glucose solution should be administered over 60 minutes, or 10 U of insulin can be given with 1 ampule of 50% glucose over 5 minutes. Nebulized albuterol or intravenous sodium bicarbonate also shifts potassium into the cell. If using nebulized albuterol, the dose should be a minimum of 5 mg, and up to 10 to 20 mg may be needed. This method can cause a rapid drop in serum potassium concentration by up to 1.5 mEq per L very rapidly, and its use is limited by tachycardia. When other methods have failed, or if the patient has minimal urine output, hemodialysis must be used. The patient should be kept on a cardiac monitor, and repeat ECGs should be obtained to confirm resolution of abnormalities.

Chapter 112

HYPOKALEMIA

Lynn E. Sullivan

OVERVIEW

Hypokalemia is a common problem that can result from a number of causes. In the case of severe hypokalemia, cardiac arrhythmia can occur; therefore, it is important to recognize hypokalemia, ascertain its cause, and treat it promptly.

PATHOPHYSIOLOGY

The primary causes of a low serum potassium concentration include the redistribution of potassium into cells, gastrointestinal losses, and increased renal losses:

- Cellular shift: The majority of potassium is within the intracellular compartment, and this concentration gradient is maintained by a membrane sodium-potassium pump. The following conditions cause a shift of potassium into the cells: an elevated pH (either metabolic or respiratory alkalosis); the use of insulin, which causes potassium to go into the cells; beta-adrenergic activity (seen with epinephrine, or albuterol in the treatment of asthmatics); significant increase in blood cell production when treating vitamin B_{12} or folate deficiency; hypokalemic periodic paralysis (a rare familial disorder); and hypothermia.
- Gastrointestinal losses: Seen in a patient with nasogastric tube suctioning, diarrhea, and laxative abuse. In the setting of vomiting, the primary loss of potassium is of renal origin. The potassium content of stomach secretions is low; therefore, little potassium is lost in gastric secretion. Vomiting causes volume depletion, however, and the resultant hyperaldosterone state causes loss of potassium in the urine. Potassium loss is greater in lower gastrointestinal losses.
- Increased renal losses: Urinary potassium loss can occur secondary to the following: drugs, including diuretics, amphotericin B, penicillins, aminoglycosides, and corticosteroids; metabolic acidoses [type I (distal) or type II (proximal) renal tubular acidosis or diabetic ketoacidosis]; post acute tubular necrosis diuresis; osmotic diuresis; salt-wasting nephropathies (interstitial nephritis or Bartter's or Gitelman's syndrome); increased mineralocorticoid activity; and magnesium deficiency.

Other causes include excessive sweating and decreased dietary intake of potassium. Clinical manifestations range from muscle weakness to paralysis, rhabdomyolysis, and cardiac arrhythmias. An ECG can reveal T-wave flattening, ST-segment depression, prolonged QTc interval. In the case of severe hypokalemia, V waves (see color plate) and a trioventricular conduction disturbances can be seen on the ECG.

CLINICAL PRESENTATION

Most cases of hypokalemia are without symptoms. If the serum potassium level is very low, less than 3 mEq per L, the patient may experience muscular weakness or cramping. If the hypokalemia is associated with hypertension, diagnoses such as Conn's syndrome and Liddle's syndrome should be entertained. If relative or outright hypotension exists, then diuretic abuse, Gitelman's syndrome, and Bartter's syndrome are leading diagnoses, in order of descending likelihood.

DIAGNOSIS

In a patient with hypokalemia, a 24-hour urinary potassium loss of less than 25 mEq per day suggests an extrarenal cause. A 24-hour urinary loss of greater than 25 mEq per day implies at least a renal component to the potassium loss. Likewise, a spot urine potassium of below 15 mEq per L implies extrarenal loss, and a value greater than that suggests renal loss. If induced vomiting or diuretic abuse is suspected, a urinary chloride concentration can be helpful. If the urinary chloride is less than 25 mEq per L, volume depletion due to vomiting or diuretic abuse after the drug effect has worn off is likely. If the urinary chloride concentration exceeds 40 mEq per L, an assay for diuretics should be done.

MANAGEMENT

Oral repletion is recommended. For a serum potassium concentration less than 3 mEq per L, 20 to 40 mEq PO every 4 hours for three doses should be given, followed by a repeat serum potassium measurement 4 hours after the last dose. For serum potassium concentrations greater than 3 mEq per L, a slower repletion schedule can be used. As a general rule, for every decrease in serum potassium concentration by 1 mEq per L, there is a 100 to 150 mEq deficit in total body potassium. Intravenous repletion of potassium is less desirable because of discomfort at the site of infusion and the danger of cardiac arrhythmia if infused too quickly. In general, intravenous potassium should be given at a rate of 10 to 20 mEq per hour and should never exceed 40 mEq per hour. Ten milliequivalents of potassium chloride increases the serum potassium level by 0.1 mEq per L. With severe hypokalemia, cardiac monitoring while repleting is necessary. Use normal saline for chloride-responsive hypokalemia in the setting of hypovolemia. For any treatment to be successful, any magnesium deficit must be corrected as well. Magnesium is best given intravenously as magnesium sulfate. Once the patient is out of danger from the electrolyte abnormality, the emphasis switches to treating the underlying cause.

Chapter 113

HYPONATREMIA

Rhuna Shen

OVERVIEW

Hyponatremia is defined as a serum sodium concentration of less than 135 mEq per L. It is the most common electrolyte abnormality observed in hospitalized patients and is seen in approximately 2% of patients. The morbidity associated with it varies widely, depending on the rate of onset, degree of hyponatremia, severity of symptoms, and comorbid conditions. Serious complications can arise from hyponatremia itself and from errors in its management.

PATHOPHYSIOLOGY

Disorders of serum sodium are due to changes in total body water, not the total body sodium. The sodium content of the body is a balance of dietary intake and renal excretion. Normal plasma osmolality is 280 to 300 mOsm per kg. Hyponatremia is a disorder of excess water in relation to sodium. Antidiuretic hormone (ADH) secreted by the posterior pituitary plays an important role in water homeostasis. Secretion of ADH is stimulated by a decreased circulating volume, and ADH then acts on the kidneys to reabsorb water. Hyponatremia is almost always due to increased ADH secretion, either appropriately, as in the case of hypovolemia, or inappropriately, as in the case of the syndrome of inappropriate secretion of ADH (SIADH). The exception is seen in psychogenic polydipsia, in which ADH secretion is depressed by

TABLE 113-1   Causes of Hypotonic Hyponatremia

Impaired Renal Water Excretion			Excessive Water Intake
Decreased ECFV	**Normal ECFV**	**Increased ECFV**	
Renal Na loss:	Thiazide diuretics	CHF	Psychogenic polydipsia
Diuretics	Hypothyroidism	Cirrhosis	Na-free irrigant solu-
Osmotic diuresis	Adrenal insufficiency	Nephrotic syn-	tions (used in
(glucose, urea,	Decreased solute	drome	TURP, laparos-
mannitol)	intake:	Renal failure	copy, or hysteros-
RTA	Beer potomania	(acute or	copy)
Obstruction	Tea-and-toast diet	chronic)	Multiple tap-water
Adrenal insuffi-		Pregnancy	enemas
ciency	SIADH (Table 113-2)		Accidental intake
Extrarenal Na loss:			(swimming lesson)
Diarrhea			
Vomiting			
Blood loss			
Excessive sweating			
Third spacing			

CHF, congestive heart failure; ECFV, extracellular fluid volume; RTA, renal tubular acidosis; SIADH, syndrome of inappropriate secretion of antidiuretic hormone; TURP, transurethral prostatectomy.

excessive free water intake. Unlike hypernatremia, which is always associated with hypertonicity, hyponatremia can be associated with normal, low, or high plasma osmolality.

Hypotonic hyponatremia represents the true excess of water relative to the sodium stores. It is by far the most common form of hyponatremia. The extracellular fluid volume (ECFV) can be increased, normal, or decreased. The final common mechanism for both hypovolemic hyponatremia, as seen in vomiting, diarrhea, bleeding, or renal losses, and hypervolemic hyponatremia, as seen in congestive heart failure, cirrhosis, or nephritic syndrome, is the depletion of effective circulating volume (Table 113-1). The hypovolemic state results in decreased stretch of the carotid sinus baroreceptors. The change in the rate of afferent discharge from these receptors is a potent stimulus for ADH release. In the setting of hyponatremia with an essentially normal ECFV, the most common cause is SIADH (Table 113-2). Hypothyroidism, adrenal insufficiency, thiazide diuretics, and decreased solute intake can cause hypovolemic hypotonic hyponatremia as well. Hypothyroidism is often associated with a decreased cardiac output and a decreased glomerular filtration rate. Although not well understood, it is thought that the former may lead to the secretion of ADH, whereas the latter may directly decrease water excretion by diminishing water delivery to the diluting segment. Cortisol and aldosterone contribute to the hyponatremia seen in adrenal insufficiency. Cortisol deficiency induces ADH secretion by two mechanisms. Cortisol has a negative feedback on corticotropin-releasing hormone, which stimulates ADH release via ACTH. This inhibitory effect is removed with adrenal insufficiency. The lack of cortisol also induces decreased systemic blood pressure and cardiac output, thereby stimulating ADH release. Aldosterone deficiency results in salt wasting and resultant volume depletion, which leads to the hypersecretion of ADH. In the absence of hypothyroidism or adrenal insufficiency, SIADH is the most likely cause of hypotonic hyponatremia. Hyponatremia with normal or

TABLE 113–2   Causes of Syndrome of Inappropriate Secretion of Antidiuretic Hormone

Cancer	CNS Disorders	Pulmonary Conditions	Drugs	Miscellaneous
Lung (small-cell CA)	Acute psychosis	Infections (viral/bacterial pneumonia, TB)	Exogenous hormones:	Postoperative state (thoracic surgery)
Mediastinal CA	Mass lesions		Desmopressin	
Extrathoracic tumors (duodenum CA, pancreas CA, olfactory neuroblastoma)	Stroke	Acute respiratory failure	Oxytocin	Pain
	Hemorrhage		Psychotropic drugs:	Severe nausea
	Trauma		Phenothiazines	HIV
	Inflammatory and demyelinating disease	Pneumothorax	Tricyclics	
		Atelectasis	SSRIs	
		Asthma	Haloperidol	
	Cerebral salt wasting syndrome		Opiates	
			MAOIs	
			Oral antihyperglycemics:	
			Chlorpropamide	
			Carbamazepine	
			Chemotherapy:	
			Cyclophosphamide	
			Vincristine	
			Vinblastine	
			Drugs of abuse:	
			Nicotine	
			"Ecstasy"	

CA, cancer/carcinoma; CNS, central nervous system; HIV, human immunodeficiency virus; MAOI, monoamine oxidase inhibitors; SSRIs, selective serotonin reuptake inhibitors; TB, tuberculosis.

elevated osmolality can be caused by the presence of another effective osmole, such as glucose, mannitol, or glycine, causing free water to move into the extracellular space. For each increase of 100 mg per dL in the serum glucose concentration above 100 mg per dL, the serum sodium is decreased by 1.6 mEq per L. Irrigant solutions used during transurethral prostatectomy, which typically contain mannitol or glycine, either in an isotonic or hypertonic preparation, can cause severe symptomatic hyponatremia. *Pseudohyponatremia* denotes a spurious laboratory value of low sodium when there is concurrent hypertriglyceridemia or hyperparaproteinemia.

The clinical manifestations of hyponatremia are related to central nervous system dysfunction. Cerebral edema occurs when free water moves into the brain as a result of hypotonic hyponatremia. The surrounding cranium limits the swelling of the brain, and intracranial hypertension develops, causing the symptoms of hyponatremia. To compensate, the brain moves solute within hours, inducing water loss and alleviating brain swelling. This effect accounts for the relative asymptomatic nature of most cases of hyponatremia; however, if this process of adaptation develops too quickly, such as in response to rapid treatment, shrinkage of the brain may trigger osmotic demyelination of pontine and extrapontine neurons.

CLINICAL PRESENTATION

The symptoms of hyponatremia are related to cerebral edema, and they occur primarily when the decrease in serum sodium concentration is large and rapid, such as when it occurs over 1 to 3 days. Headache, nausea, vomiting, muscle cramps, lethargy, restlessness, disorientation, and depressed reflexes generally occur when the serum sodium concentration is less than 120 mEq per L. More severe complications may occur when serum sodium is less than 110 mEq per L, and these include seizure, coma, permanent brain damage, respiratory failure, brainstem herniation, and death. Patients with a serum sodium of greater than 125 mEq per L are generally asymptomatic. Up to one-third of the patients with SIADH have a downward resetting of the osmostat and typically stabilize at a new, lower level between 125 and 135 mEq per L. The overly rapid correction of hyponatremia can cause osmotic demyelination with symptoms including paraplegia, quadriplegia, pseudobulbar palsy, seizures, coma, and death. Certain comorbid conditions increase the risk of osmotic demyelination, including liver failure, malnutrition, and potassium depletion.

DIAGNOSIS

The first step in evaluating hyponatremia is the determination of the serum osmolality, which helps to differentiate between hypertonic, isotonic, and hypotonic hyponatremia (Fig. 113–1). The history and physical examination,

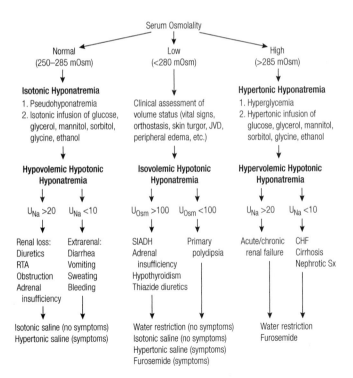

Figure 113–1 Approach to hyponatremia. CHF, congestive heart failure; JVD, jugular venous distention; RTA, renal tubular acidosis; SIADH, syndrome of inappropriate antidiuretic hormone secretion; Sx, symptoms.

paying special attention to volume status (i.e., blood pressure, pulse, orthostatic changes, jugular venous distention, skin turgor, mucous membranes, and peripheral edema), aid in further categorizing the three subgroups of hypotonic hyponatremia. Laboratory tests that should be obtained include the serum and urine osmolality and sodium concentration, blood urea nitrogen, creatinine, and uric acid (usually lower in SIADH). Thyroid or adrenal deficiency should be ruled out before making the diagnosis of SIADH.

MANAGEMENT

The treatment of hyponatremia consists of the gradual correction of hyponatremia to minimize the risk of osmotic demyelination. This correction can be done by water restriction or by the administration of isotonic or hypertonic saline solution. In addition, hormone replacement therapy should be given to patients with hypothyroidism or adrenal insufficiency. Patients exhibiting seizure activity need immediate anticonvulsant therapy and airway protection. Water restriction to the level of less than the urine output is the primary treatment for hypervolemic or euvolemic hyponatremia seen in cases of congestive heart failure, cirrhosis, and SIADH. For patients with true volume depletion, the administration of isotonic saline solution corrects hyponatremia by two mechanisms: volume repletion removes the stimulus to ADH secretion, thereby allowing the excretion of excess water, and normal saline is also slightly hypertonic to the plasma, thereby slowly raising the plasma sodium by 1 to 2 mEq per L for every liter of normal saline infused. Patients with more severe neurologic symptoms require infusion of hypertonic saline, which is usually combined with a loop diuretic to limit ECFV expansion.

Saline infusion is not recommended for patients with SIADH, unless the severity of the symptoms requires more rapid correction. Patients with SIADH have intact sodium excretion but impaired water excretion, thus the administered sodium is excreted in the urine whereas water may be retained, resulting in possible worsening of the hyponatremia. The initial treatment for SIADH should be water restriction. If saline solution must be administered, then the osmolality of the fluid infused should exceed the urine osmolality. Urine osmolality can be fixed at plasma osmolality by simultaneously administering a loop diuretic, such as furosemide (Lasix). Doing so results in depleting the concentrating gradient in the renal medulla; therefore, the gradient down which free water is absorbed is limited to that of the plasma osmolality. Osmotic demyelination is rare, but its prognosis is dismal. It can develop in 1 to several days after overly rapid treatment. Overly rapid correction typically occurs in the following situations: water restriction in primary polydipsia, hypertonic or isotonic saline infusion, cortisol replacement in adrenal insufficiency, and patients with end-stage renal disease being dialyzed against a dialysate with a higher sodium concentration. The recommended rate of correction is 10 to 12 mEq per L per day for asymptomatic patients and 1.2 to 2.0 mEq per L per hour during the first 3 to 4 hours for severely symptomatic patients. The following formulas estimate the effect of 1 L of any infusate on the serum sodium concentration (Table 113–3). Note that potassium is as osmotically active as sodium; therefore, it should be accounted for in the calculation if concurrent potassium repletion is required.

Change in [Na] = Infusate Na^+ – Serum Na^+/Total body weight (TBW) + 1
Or
Change in [Na] = [Infusate Na^+ + Infusate K^+] – Serum Na^+/TBW + 1
TBW = 0.6 × kg weight (for men and children)
TBW = 0.5 × kg weight (for women and elderly men)
TBW = 0.45 × kg weight (for elderly women)

TABLE 113-3 Characteristics of Infusate

Types of Infusate	Na Concentration (mEq/L)
0.45% NaCl ($^{1}/_{2}$ NS)	77
0.9% NaCl (NS)	154
Ringer's lactate	130
3% NaCl	513
5% NaCl	855

NS, normal saline; TBW, total body weight.
The conventional formula for estimating sodium deficit [TBW × (desired [Na] – current [Na])]
  is not recommended.

Chapter 114

HYPERNATREMIA

Rhuna Shen

OVERVIEW

Hypernatremia is defined as a serum sodium concentration higher than 145 mEq per L. It is a common electrolyte disorder that frequently develops in hospitalized patients. The morbidity associated with hypernatremia varies: It can be inconsequential, serious, or life threatening.

PATHOPHYSIOLOGY

Hypernatremia reflects water deficit in relation to total body sodium stores. Serum sodium concentration is closely regulated by water homeostasis and is mediated by thirst, antidiuretic hormone (ADH), and kidneys. Increased serum sodium, and subsequently increased serum osmolality, stimulates posterior pituitary ADH secretion and the hypothalamic thirst mechanism. In a healthy person, this cascade would lead to both water retention and increased water intake. Therefore, hypernatremia usually occurs in a person with impaired thirst mechanism and limited access to water. High-risk patients are those with delirium and dementia, and intubated patients, infants, and frail elderly nursing home and hospitalized patients who rely on their caregivers for access to water. The etiology of hypernatremia can be divided into three broad categories: hypotonic fluid loss, decreased water intake, and iatrogenic hypertonic sodium gain (Table 114–1). Central diabetes insipidus (DI) (pituitary ADH deficiency) can be caused by trauma, autoimmune disease, pituitary surgery, hypoxic encephalopathy, or idiopathic etiologies, whereas acquired nephrogenic DI (renal ADH resistance) is caused by drugs (lithium, demeclocycline, foscarnet, cidofovir, amphotericin B), renal disease, hyper-

TABLE 114-1   Causes of Hypernatremia

Hypotonic Fluid Loss	Decreased Water Intake	Hypertonic Na Gain
Insensible loss: 　Fever/heat 　Burns 　Mechanical ventilation 　Excessive sweating Gastrointestinal loss: 　Vomiting/nasogastric 　　tube suction 　Diarrhea Renal loss: 　Central diabetes insipidus 　Nephrogenic diabetes 　　insipidus 　Osmotic diuresis	Hypothalamic dysfunction: 　Reduced thirst Impaired access to water: 　Comatose patient 　Nursing home or hospi- 　　talized elderly patient 　Infants	Hypertonic NaCl infusion Hypertonic $NaHCO_3$ infusion Hypertonic feeding prepara- 　tions NaCl ingestion Hypertonic saline enemas Intrauterine injection of 　hypertonic saline Hypertonic dialysis Primary hyperaldosteronism Cushing's syndrome

calcemia, and hypokalemia. Approximately 20% to 40% of patients taking lithium develop nephrogenic DI. Net water loss accounts for the majority of cases of hypernatremia (Table 114–1).

The symptoms of hypernatremia result from the acute movement of water out of the brain induced by increased serum osmolality, and therefore a decrease in brain volume. The brain's mechanisms for adapting are twofold: first, water is moved from the cerebrospinal fluid to the brain; second, brain cells increase their uptake of solutes (initially sodium and potassium and later organic osmolytes, such as inositol) to cause the movement of water into the cells.

CLINICAL PRESENTATION

Symptoms and signs of hypernatremia reflect central nervous system dysfunction. Symptoms are more severe when the increase in serum sodium concentration is large or occurs rapidly over a period of hours. Common symptoms are lethargy, weakness, irritability, and confusion, progressing to twitching, seizures, and coma. Assessment is often difficult, because affected patients may have similar symptoms from coexisting neurologic disease. Patients may or may not complain of thirst. Severe symptoms require serum sodium concentration to be higher than 158 mEq per L. Chronic hypernatremia is less likely to induce neurologic symptoms. Patients with sodium concentrations higher than 180 mEq per L have a higher mortality rate. Acute rupture of cerebral veins may occur as a result of acute shrinkage of the brain. This occurrence often leads to focal intracerebral or subarachnoid hemorrhage and irreversible neurologic damage.

DIAGNOSIS

A detailed history and physical examination often provide clues as to the causes of hypernatremia. The history should always include a complete medication list, and the physical examination should focus on the assessment of volume status and neurologic status (Fig. 114–1). Measurement of plasma and urine osmolality is essential. A plasma osmolality of more than 295 mOsm per kg generally induces sufficient ADH secretion to stimulate maximal urine concentration. If the patient is hypovolemic or euvolemic, hypernatremia is likely due to water loss. If urine osmolality is lower than serum osmolality (<300 mOsm/kg), then either central (ADH deficient) or nephrogenic

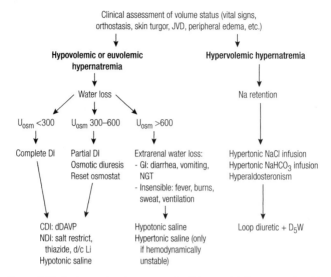

Figure 114-1   Approach to hypernatremia. CDI, central diabetes insipidus; d/c, discontinue; D_5W, dextrose 5% in water; dDAVP, desmopressin acetate; DI, diabetes insipidus; GI, gastrointestinal; JVD, jugular venous distention; Li, lithium; NDI, nephrogenic diabetes insipidus; NGT, nasogastric tube.

(ADH resistant) DI is present. The administration of exogenous ADH (10 μg of desmopressin acetate intranasally or 5 U of vasopressin) raises urine osmolality by 50% or more in central DI, but there is no response in nephrogenic DI. Severe nephrogenic DI in adults is uncommon in the absence of chronic lithium use. A urine osmolality of greater than 600 to 800 mOsm per kg (the point at which the maximum urine-concentrating ability is achieved) indicates intact hypothalamic and renal ADH function. The likely cause of hypernatremia in this setting is gastrointestinal or insensible losses. If the urine osmolality is intermediate, between 300 and 600 mOsm per kg, then possible causes of the hypernatremia include partial DI (central or nephrogenic), osmotic diuresis, or reset osmostat. Hypervolemic hypernatremia is usually due to iatrogenic hypertonic saline infusion. Hyperaldosteronism is less common and rarely symptomatic.

MANAGEMENT

Managing the underlying causes of hypernatremia is as important as correcting hypertonicity itself. Patients presenting with seizures require prompt anticonvulsant therapy and ventilatory support. Correction of chronic hypernatremia should occur slowly to prevent rapid fluid movement into the brain, causing cerebral edema. The preferred rate of correction in asymptomatic patients is less than 12 mEq per L per day. In patients with hypernatremia developing over a period of hours, rapid correction of 1 mEq per L per hour is necessary to improve the prognosis. For hypervolemic hypernatremia, the treatment is the administration of a loop diuretic and 5% dextrose in water. For central DI, desmopressin acetate should be given. For nephrogenic DI, the underlying causes should be treated, such as the discontinuation of lithium; salt restriction and thiazide diuretics are also effective. For hypovolemic and euvolemic hypernatremia, hypotonic fluids are indicated. The preferred route of administration is the oral route or through a feeding tube. Choices of intravenous fluids are 5% dextrose in water, one-half normal saline, and one-quarter normal saline. The sole indication for giving isotonic normal saline to patients with hypernatremia is frank circulatory compromise. The following formulas can be used to estimate the effect of 1 L of any infusate on serum sodium concentration:

$$\text{Change in [Na]} = \text{Infusate Na}^+ - \text{Serum Na}^+/\text{Total body weight (TBW)} + 1$$
$$Or$$
$$\text{Change in [Na]} = [\text{Infusate Na}^+ + \text{Infusate K}^+] - \text{Serum Na}^+/\text{TBW} + 1$$
$$\text{TBW} = 0.6 \times \text{kg weight (for men and children)}$$
$$\text{TBW} = 0.5 \times \text{kg weight (for women and elderly men)}$$
$$\text{TBW} = 0.45 \times \text{kg weight (for elderly women)}$$

The conventional formula for estimating water deficit: TBW $\times$ [1 $-$ (140/ serum [Na])] is not recommended, because it underestimates the amount of hypotonic fluid loss.

Note that potassium is as osmotically active as sodium and therefore should be accounted for in the calculation if concurrent potassium repletion is required (Table 114–2).

TABLE 114–2 Characteristics of Infusate

Types of Infusate	Na Concentration (mEq/L)
D_5W	0
0.2% NaCl ($^1/_4$ NS)	34
0.45% NaCl ($^1/_2$ NS)	77
Ringer's lactate	130
0.9% NaCl (NS)	154

NS, normal saline.

Chapter 115

METABOLIC ACIDOSIS

Jeffrey T. Reynolds

OVERVIEW

A primary metabolic acidosis is a disorder of acid–base homeostasis characterized by a reduced arterial pH, a low serum bicarbonate concentration ($[HCO_3]$), and a compensatory hypocapnia (low partial pressure of carbon dioxide, $PaCO_2$, in the serum). There are two types of metabolic acidosis, anion gap (AG) and nonanion gap. An AG acidosis results from the addition of hydrogen ions (H^+) either from an exogenous source via an ingestion, such as methanol, or from an endogenous source, such as lactic acid produced as a result of underperfusion of a vascular bed. A nonanion gap acidosis results from the loss of base, HCO_3, from the plasma, the most common cause of this being diarrhea.

In a mixed acid–base disturbance, metabolic acidosis is present when the serum bicarbonate is lower than expected in the setting of the primary disturbance and the measured $PaCO_2$. This can take different forms—for example, a patient with obstructive pulmonary disease may have a chronically elevated $PaCO_2$ and a compensatory elevation in serum $[HCO_3]$. Should this patient develop sepsis, his or her serum $[HCO_3]$ would fall and the patient would hyperventilate. The patient's hyperventilation may not be enough to lower the $PaCO_2$ to less than 40 mm Hg, however. Alternatively, a diabetic patient may have an episode of diabetic ketoacidosis (DKA) as the result of a diarrheal illness. The DKA results in an AG acidosis and the bicarbonate loss from the diarrhea, a nonanion gap acidosis. The measured serum $[HCO_3]$ would be lower than expected for either process independently. A metabolic acidosis can be a minor problem due to an easily identifiable process, often responding well to appropriate treatment, or it can be a life-threatening condition that leads to hypotension, ventricular tachycardia and fibrillation, cardiac arrest, and death. The prompt diagnosis and workup of this disorder is mandatory, and rapid and definitive treatment may be necessary to prevent morbidity and mortality to the patient.

PATHOPHYSIOLOGY

A decreased serum bicarbonate concentration can result from either the addition of H^+ ions to, or more commonly, the loss of bicarbonate from, the serum. An acute acid load is partially buffered by the intracellular compartment and bone, so the decrease in bicarbonate is only approximately 40% of the amount of H^+ added to the serum. The net dietary acid load of 50 to 100 mEq H^+ is excreted by the kidneys, mostly in the form of NH_4^+. Transcellular shifts of potassium out of cells in exchange for H^+ moving into cells can be associated with low, normal or high serum K^+ levels, depending on the nature and severity of the primary disorder. With an intact respiratory system, central and peripheral chemoreceptors are stimulated by the acidosis, resulting in increased minute ventilation, decreased arterial PCO_2, and partial correction of the acidemia. Respiratory compensation for metabolic acidosis can be predicted by Winter's formula:

$$\text{Expected } CO_2 = 1.5[HCO_3] + 8 \pm 2$$

It may take 12 to 24 hours for full compensation to be achieved. Metabolic acidosis without an elevated AG is usually due to loss of bicarbonate or gain of H^+ ions without an associated organic anion. When an elevated AG is present, the acidosis is due to the addition of organic acids, such as ketoacids or lactic acid, to the serum.

CLINICAL PRESENTATION

Metabolic acidosis is a common pathway for a number of diverse pathologic processes. Therefore, the clinical presentation may range from asymptomatic to severe hemodynamic compromise and shock. Tachypnea is a cardinal clinical finding for all forms of metabolic acidosis. When respiration is deep and rapid, it is referred to as *Kussmaul's respiration.* Common clinical scenarios resulting in metabolic acidosis include DKA, renal failure, tissue hypoperfusion, diarrhea, and ethanol intoxication. Other causes of metabolic acidosis may be less obvious, such as ingestions of methanol, ethylene glycol, or salicylates. In the case of DKA, notable characteristics of the presentation typically include elevated serum glucose, volume depletion, polyuria, and polydipsia. The differential diagnosis of shock itself is large. Clinically common causes for shock are sepsis and cardiac failure. Sepsis can present with hyperpyrexia or hypopyrexia, leukocytosis, or leukopenia and high cardiac output. Cardiac failure, or cardiogenic shock, generally lacks the signs and symptoms of systemic inflammation and has a low cardiac output.

DIAGNOSIS

The diagnosis of metabolic acidosis requires a low serum bicarbonate with an acidemic pH or a lower than expected bicarbonate in the setting of another acid–base disorder; therefore, arterial blood gas is the first diagnostic step when a low serum $[HCO_3]$ is found. If the arterial blood gas confirms acidemia, the next step is to calculate the serum AG, which differentiates the metabolic acidosis into one of two categories, quickly narrowing the differential diagnosis. If the AG is elevated (generally >10), measure lactic acid, serum and urine ketones, and serum osmolality, as lactic acidosis, DKA, and toxic ingestion of various types of alcohol are common causes. AG metabolic acidosis is identified when the decrease in bicarbonate is roughly equal to the increase in the AG. The anions responsible for an excess AG are often lactic acid or ketoacids from DKA, but organic anions can also be generated in starvation or in ethanol, methanol, ethylene glycol, propylene glycol, or salicylate ingestions, whereas two-thirds of a normal AG is composed of albumin. Therefore, in cases of acidosis that would be expected to produce an AG, the presence of hypoalbuminemia can make the AG appear deceptively low. This should be kept in mind when evaluating chronically ill patients. If the cause of a gap acidosis is not readily apparent, the serum osmolar gap should be determined by subtracting the calculated $[(2 \times Na + BUN)/2.8 + glucose/18]$ from the measured serum osmolality; if greater than 10, this suggests ethanol, ethylene glycol, or methanol. To correct for the presence of ethanol, divide the serum ethanol by 4.6 and subtract it from the osmolar gap; if still higher than 10, another anion is present. Salicylate overdose presents as an AG metabolic acidosis with a normal osmolar gap, combined with a respiratory alkalosis beyond that expected as a compensatory response.

A nongap metabolic acidosis is present when the metabolic acidosis is associated with a normal AG and is caused by net loss of bicarbonate or gain of H^+ with Cl^-. In this setting, first determine whether the acidosis is due to renal [renal tubular acidosis (RTA)] or extrarenal causes by performing an accurate history and physical examination and calculating the urine AG:

$$U_\Delta = U_{NA} + U_K - U_{Cl}$$

If this number is higher than 0, a diagnosis of RTA can be made. Identification of the specific RTA requires an evaluation of the urine pH, fractional excretion of bicarbonate, response to a bicarbonate or NH_4Cl, or evaluation of the plasma aldosterone level. H^+ can be retained as a result of type I or type IV RTA. In each, the kidney cannot adequately acidify the urine. In type 2 RTA, the fractional excretion of bicarbonate is more than 15% when bicarbonate is being given. If the serum K^+ is elevated, type 4 RTA is likely and can be confirmed by a low aldosterone level, or the most common extrarenal etiology of a nongap acidosis is bicarbonate loss through the gastrointestinal (GI) tract from diarrhea, ileostomy, and ileal loop bladder. In massive volume resuscitation, nongap metabolic acidosis can result from dilution of serum bicarbonate with bicarbonate-free fluids, usually normal saline, with Cl^- replacing bicarbonate. A subset of patients with renal failure may also have a nongap metabolic acidosis.

MANAGEMENT

The treatment of metabolic acidosis requires an appropriate workup to identify the underlying process. In the case of an elevated AG, treatment is directed at the underlying process. In DKA, appropriate insulin, fluid resuscitation, and electrolyte therapy should correct the acidosis, although if not initiated early, a partial nongap acidosis can develop owing to loss of ketones in the urine. This results in a net addition of H^+ to serum, neutralizing bicarbonate. The loss of the ketones in the urine results in a loss of substrate, from which bicarbonate could be regenerated; therefore, after correction of the ketoacidosis, it may be necessary to administer a bicarbonate containing fluids to make up the deficit. Lactic acidosis is treated by improving tissue perfusion, usually with volume resuscitation in the form of isotonic fluids or blood and, if necessary, vasopressor medications. Ethanol-related ketoacidosis may require mechanical ventilation if respiratory compensation is not appropriate. Methanol and polyethylene glycol are both treated with ethanol, loaded 0.6 mg per kg over 30 minutes (double rate if being dialyzed) and then titrated to an ethanol level of 100 mg per dL, or fomepizole 15 mg per kg load, then 10 mg per kg every 12 hours to block the alcohol dehydrogenase enzyme. Other therapeutic measures include GI tract decontamination, $NaHCO_3$, hemodialysis, thiamine, and pyridoxine. In nongap acidosis, bicarbonate replacement may be necessary depending on the etiology. In GI tract–related bicarbonate loss, bicarbonate replacement is necessary if the pH is 7.10 or less, or if there is hemodynamic instability or clinically significant hyperkalemia. In RTA, the treatment depends on the type of RTA, but alkali therapy is often appropriate.

Chapter 116

ACUTE RENAL FAILURE

Jeffrey T. Reynolds

OVERVIEW

Acute renal failure (ARF) is common in hospitalized patients and in the outpatient setting. On admission, 5% of non–intensive care unit (ICU) and 30% of ICU patients have ARF, and after admission, 5% of inpatients and 10% to 15% of ICU patients develop ARF. Ten percent of these require dialysis, and of those who survive, 25% require chronic dialysis. In the outpatient setting, chronic renal failure is far more common, but ARF can also occur. *ARF* is defined as an abrupt decrease in glomerular filtration rate (GFR) resulting in an accumulation of urea and creatinine. Urine output (UOP) usually declines but can remain normal owing to decreased reabsorption of the filtered load. An increase in serum creatinine of 1.0 to 1.5 mg per dL per day is consistent with a GFR approaching zero. Oliguric renal failure is azotemia with a UOP of less than 500 mL per day. ARF is usually reversible, but failure to correct the underlying cause can result in end-stage renal failure, and therefore a timely workup and appropriate management are critical.

PATHOPHYSIOLOGY

On average, adult kidneys receive 20% of the cardiac output and filter 180 L of plasma daily. The kidneys are responsible for regulating the concentration of key extracellular ions, maintaining acid–base homeostasis in conjunction with the lungs, controlling blood pressure, and performing important endocrine functions, including the secretion of erythropoietin and conversion of vitamin D to its active form. In ARF, the primary derangements include electrolyte abnormalities, such as hyperkalemia and hyperphosphatemia, the acid–base disorder of metabolic acidosis, and extracellular volume overload. ARF can be due to an isolated disorder, but multifactorial etiologies are common in hospitalized patients. A systematic approach to working up ARF is to consider prerenal, intrinsic renal, and postrenal causes.

Prerenal causes represent more than 50% of cases and are secondary to decreased renal blood flow. Etiologies include hypotension; volume depletion due to inadequate fluid intake or excessive losses, such as from vomiting; diarrhea; hemorrhage; burns; excessive sweating; or Addisonian crisis, third-space shifts from pancreatitis, liver failure, peritonitis, and decreased effective circulating volume in severe congestive heart failure and hepatorenal syndrome. Drugs, such as nonsteroidal antiinflammatory drugs, cyclosporine, angiotensin-converting enzyme inhibitors, and osmotic diuretics, as well as vascular processes, such as embolism, thrombosis, and atherosclerosis of the renal artery, can precipitate ARF in susceptible patients.

Intrinsic renal causes account for 40% to 45% of ARF and include acute tubular necrosis (ATN), interstitial nephritis, and glomerulonephritis. ATN represents 85% of cases of intrinsic causes and is usually due to nephrotoxins, including drugs such as aminoglycosides, intravenous contrast agents, foscarnet, amphotericin B, and chemotherapeutic agents. Other causes of ATN include ischemia from hypovolemia, shock, and sepsis.

Postrenal causes represent 5% of ARF and can result from obstruction of the bilateral ureters secondary to prostatic hypertrophy or tumor, or intratubular obstruction by substrate deposition, such as light chains (multiple myeloma), uric acid (tumor lysis syndrome), and drug crystals (indinavir, sulfadiazine, acyclovir, methotrexate). Uric acid, calcium oxalate, and struvite stones cause pyeloureteral obstruction.

CLINICAL PRESENTATION

The presentation in ARF is variable and depends on the nature of the resulting metabolic derangements. UOP is an important indicator of the degree of renal failure as well as the likely response to therapy and prognosis. A 24-hour UOP of 100 to 400 cc per day represents oliguria, and less than 100 cc per day represents anuria, but renal failure can occur with UOP that is initially within normal limits. Symptoms of uremia include nausea, vomiting, anorexia, pruritus, altered mental status, neuromuscular disorders, asterixis, volume overload, and sometimes hypertension. Diffuse abdominal pain and ileus are common as well. Platelet dysfunction can cause increased risk of bleeding. The electrolyte abnormalities most common in ARF are hyperkalemia and hyperphosphatemia. Hyperkalemia can manifest in weakness, ventricular arrhythmias, and characteristic electrographic changes, including peaked T waves, a widened QRS interval, and a flattened P wave, whereas hyperphosphatemia can cause metastatic calcium phosphate deposition with secondary hypocalcemia, which in turn can cause tetany and perioral paresthesias. Physical examination findings specific for certain etiologic processes include skin changes pointing to infection, thrombotic thrombocytopenic purpura, disseminate intravascular coagulation, atheroemboli, vasculitis, cryoglobulinemia, and septic emboli from endocarditis; severe hypertension pointing to glomerulonephritis, nephrosclerosis, vasculitis, or atheroembolization; dry mucous membranes, orthostatic hypotension, sinus tachycardia, decreased UOP, skin tenting, and peripheral edema pointing to intravascular volume depletion; and arthritic joints and muscular tenderness suggesting rhabdomyolysis.

DIAGNOSIS

Once ARF has been identified by an increasing blood urea nitrogen (BUN) and creatinine (Cr), it is necessary to determine the underlying process quickly and methodically, because a significant proportion of cases will respond favorably to appropriate treatment, whereas delayed or inappropriate treatment may result in irreversible end-stage renal disease. A high BUN/Cr ratio, a low urine sodium, and a low fractional excretion of sodium (FENa) or urea are all markers of prerenal azotemia. An obstruction distal to the bladder can be ruled out by bladder catheterization after voiding, and the confirmation of an obstructive cause is indicated by a normalizing BUN and Cr with the use of continued catheterization. The urinalysis (U/A) provides important information in terms of an etiology. In prerenal states, U/A may be normal, or hyaline casts may be present. In intrinsic renal conditions, the U/A is likely to be abnormal: In ATN, the U/A typically has granular or epithelial cell casts; in interstitial nephritis, the U/A shows white blood cells, hematuria, granular and epithelial cell casts, mild proteinuria, and eosinophils on Wright's stain; and in glomerulonephritis, there is hematuria, marked proteinuria, red blood cell casts, and granular casts. Measuring urine electrolytes helps to differentiate between a prerenal cause and ATN. The FENa is calculated using the following equation: $[(\text{UNa}/\text{SNa})/(\text{SCr}/\text{UCr})] \times 100\%$, where UNa is urinary sodium, SNa is serum sodium, SCr is serum creatinine, and

UCr is urinary creatinine. The FENa is typically less than 1% in prerenal conditions and higher than 1% in ATN. The FENa can be significantly affected by different factors, such as the use of diuretics, which makes an FENa of greater than 1% meaningless, but which makes an FENa of less than 1% even more specific for prerenal state, and conditions such as Addison's disease, which would cause salt wasting and an FENa of greater than 1% despite prerenal physiology. The fractional excretion of urea can be used in patients on diuretics, with less than 35% suggesting a prerenal cause and more than 35% suggesting an intrinsic renal cause.

Renal ultrasonography is usually the first imaging modality to use in ARF and can identify hydronephrosis with a sensitivity of 98%, kidney size and echotexture, cysts, and renal arterial and venous blood flow. Shrunken, echogenic kidneys seen on an ultrasound are consistent with hypertensive nephrosclerosis and other intrinsic renal diseases, but this finding is neither sensitive nor specific. A kidney and urinary bladder x-ray, which is a plain anteroposterior film of abdomen, can easily identify radio-opaque stones. In patients whose anatomies make ultrasound problematic, magnetic resonance angiography provides excellent data regarding renal blood flow and can yield useful information about the renal parenchyma and collecting system as well. Angiography remains the gold standard in evaluating the vascular system, both extrarenally and intrarenally.

MANAGEMENT

Careful volume management requires close monitoring of clinical signs of volume status, and volume replacement must be judicious and based on these observations. Insensible losses must be considered when determining volume management. A Swan-Ganz catheter may be necessary to monitor intravascular volume accurately. A trial of diuretics or low-dose dopamine can be used to convert oliguric to nonoliguric ARF, and although these interventions may make management easier, they do not alter the outcome of the ARF. Hyperkalemia can be prevented or delayed by decreasing potassium intake to below 50 mEq per day. In hyperkalemia, sodium polystyrene sulfonate (Kayexalate) given orally or by a retention enema is often effective, but the shorter-acting therapy of insulin, dextrose, calcium, and bicarbonate may be necessary with hyperkalemic symptoms or electrocardiographic changes. Hypocalcemia and hypomagnesemia should be corrected with replacement therapy. Hyperphosphatemia can lead to hypocalcemia, so phosphate binders can be given, and oral intake of phosphate can be restricted. Drug dosing should be adjusted based on creatinine clearance, but a changing creatinine makes estimates of GFR difficult, and potentially toxic medications may have to be held until a more reliable assessment of GFR can be made. Sodium bicarbonate can be given to help correct a serum pH of 7.1 or less in a nongap metabolic acidosis in ARF, but the sodium load often limits the utility of this option. Uremia, when severe or accompanied with pericarditis, is an indication for hemodialysis. Adequate nutritional support has been shown to improve mortality in ICU patients, and parenteral nutrition is often required to achieve the desired nutritional status. An early renal consultation is appropriate if the case is complicated or if hemodialysis may be required. Pericarditis and other uremic symptoms are an absolute indication for dialysis, whereas volume overload, hyperkalemia, metabolic acidosis, and other severe electrolyte disorders require dialysis when conservative management fails.

Chapter 117

CHRONIC RENAL FAILURE

Ursula C. Brewster

OVERVIEW

Chronic renal failure may develop from an acute insult or from the progression of underlying renal disease. The impact of this illness on a patient's quality of life and mortality is immeasurable. Although the kidneys are still functional, but at a decreased capacity, patients are susceptible to an array of metabolic abnormalities, as well as progression to complete renal failure that would necessitate renal replacement therapy, either dialysis or renal transplantation.

PATHOPHYSIOLOGY

The pathophysiology of chronic renal failure predominantly depends on the underlying etiology. The differential diagnosis includes all the possible causes of renal failure. When a kidney has been injured, it often responds by increasing the filtration rate in the normal nephrons. This adaptive response, although initially keeping the creatinine (Cr) normal or near normal by recruit renal reserve, over time is injurious to the remaining nephrons, leading to progressive renal insufficiency.

CLINICAL PRESENTATION

As renal function declines, patients often become uremic. The symptoms that can develop do not correlate with level of blood urea nitrogen (BUN); that is to say, some patients with only mild elevations in BUN are markedly symptomatic, whereas others with very high levels remain totally asymptomatic. Uremic symptoms include lethargy, anorexia, nausea, vomiting, and neuropathies, among many others. Patients often have abnormalities in electrolytes, volume overload, anemia, and metabolic acidosis as their condition worsens. Initially, these abnormalities are managed by pharmacologic interventions, but ultimately renal replacement therapy will be required.

DIAGNOSIS

The diagnosis of chronic renal failure is largely made on history and physical examination and laboratory test results. Increasing BUN and Cr are the hallmarks. In patients with a history of chronic renal disease, it is important to have prior Cr levels and to examine the trend. One can plot out $1/Cr$ versus time to show a continual decline in glomerular filtration rate (GFR). This graph usually is linear, unless a superimposed acute insult, such as hypoperfusion or a nephrotoxin, is introduced. The utility of this graph lies in the fact that it can help to predict when a patient will need to initiate dialysis, typically when GFR is less than 10 to 15 mL per minute. Additionally, it can be used to assess whether there has been an acute loss of renal function superimposed on the chronic renal insufficiency. Laboratory abnormalities also include hyperkalemia, hyperphosphatemia, anemia, and metabolic acidosis.

MANAGEMENT

There are two aspects to the management of chronic renal disease. The first is the prevention of complete renal failure, and the second is the choice and maintenance of renal replacement therapy once GFR has fallen to a level of less than 10 to 15 mL per minute. Chronic renal failure requires the clinician to be aware of many possible contributing factors, as well as the commonly prescribed nephrotoxins, such as nonsteroidal antiinflammatory drugs and antibiotics. Carefully managing hypertension is critical to patients with chronic renal insufficiency. Although the quality of the data is variable between different types of kidney disease, the general theme is that angiotensin II–converting enzyme inhibitors and angiotensin II receptor blockers have been shown to slow the progression of chronic renal failure. This effect is particularly true in patients with diabetic nephropathy. Calcium channel blockers or beta-blockers can be added if needed to control ongoing hypertension. A blood pressure of 135/85 mm Hg should be targeted. Dietary protein restriction as a means of slowing the rate of loss of kidney function is controversial. It is not universally recommended at this time. As renal failure progresses, there is a reduction in filtered phosphate, leading to hyperphosphatemia. Management of phosphate homeostasis can initially be controlled by dietary restrictions, but it often requires the use of oral phosphate binders, such as calcium carbonate, to prevent renal osteodystrophy from secondary hyperparathyroidism. A normocytic, normochromic anemia often develops in these patients as erythropoietin production is decreased because of a decreased amount of functioning kidney. Administration of exogenous erythropoietin to bring the hemoglobin concentration to 11 g per dL is the goal. There is a balance between the use of erythropoietin injections to raise hematocrit and the adverse effect of its hypertensive effect. Oral or intravenous iron also may be required in those with additional iron deficiency anemia.

Once patients have progressed to the point of needing renal replacement therapy, the choice of dialysis is a difficult one for many patients and clinicians. More and more patients are addressing these questions in advance directives, but patients, families, and clinicians often struggle with the utility of dialysis in those who are terminally ill or elderly. Ideally, many patients with end-stage renal disease could undergo renal transplantation, but not all patients are appropriate because of noncompliance with their health care or underlying medical conditions. This issue is complicated further by the shortage of donor kidneys, making dialysis the only option for many. The next decision is between peritoneal dialysis, which many patients can do in the comfort of their own homes, or hemodialysis, requiring frequent trips to large dialysis centers. The comorbid conditions, as well as compliance and confidence of patients, weigh in to this decision. For those in whom peritoneal dialysis would be appropriate, a dialysis catheter is placed directly into the abdominal cavity and requires only 1 to 2 weeks to heal before it can be used safely. Patients who may do well with peritoneal dialysis include those with remaining residual renal function, no prior abdominal surgeries, compliance with medical care, and a constant living environment. Additionally, peritoneal dialysis may be the method of choice in a patient who cannot tolerate the large volume shifts that occur on hemodialysis. For those requiring hemodialysis, arteriovenous fistulas or synthetic grafts should be placed well before patients require treatment to allow them to heal to the point they can be used safely. If emergency hemodialysis is required, internal jugular or femoral vein catheters are used. Once on dialysis, all the complications discussed in those with chronic renal insufficiency are just as important to control, but there are the additional concerns of monitoring the vascular access for patency, preventing infection, and providing adequate nutrition.

Chapter 118

HEMATURIA AND NEPHROLITHIASIS

Ursula C. Brewster

OVERVIEW

Hematuria is defined as the presence of more than four red blood cells per high-power field of urine sediment; however, pathologic hematuria can range from this small amount up to gross hematuria. In microscopic hematuria, the red blood cells are only visible under the microscope, whereas in macroscopic hematuria the urine is red, pink, or cola colored. There are benign causes of hematuria; however, these should be diagnoses of exclusion, as the other causes are harbingers of more significant disease.

Nephrolithiasis is a cause of hematuria four times more common in men than in women, and it can carry significant morbidity with it. Most stones smaller than 8 mm in diameter pass on their own, whereas those that do not may require more invasive procedures to prevent urinary obstruction and renal failure. Most stones are comprised of calcium oxalate (75%), with uric acid (10–15%), struvite (15–20%), and cystine (1%) constituting the remainder.

PATHOPHYSIOLOGY

Hematuria may develop from a renal or extrarenal site. Renal causes are divided into glomerular and extraglomerular sites. Hematuria secondary to glomerulonephritis (GN) can be from a primary renal disease, as in the case of immunoglobulin A nephropathy, postinfectious GN, membranoproliferative GN, and rapidly progressive GN, or from a secondary GN, as seen in systemic lupus erythematosus, Henoch-Schönlein purpura, Goodpasture's syndrome, hepatitis B and C, and systemic vasculitis. Familial syndromes, such as thin glomerular basement membrane disease or Alport's syndrome, also may be associated with hematuria.

Nonglomerular renal causes of hematuria include papillary necrosis from sickle cell disease, and analgesic or alcohol use. Neoplasms, such as renal cell carcinoma, Wilms' tumor, or multiple myeloma, also may lead to hematuria. Vascular events, such as renal infarction, renal vein thrombosis, and arteriovenous malformations, may lead to significant bleeding. If the history demonstrates a familial pattern, then polycystic kidney disease and medullary sponge kidney are diagnostic possibilities. Drug-induced acute interstitial nephritis, most commonly associated with the use of semisynthetic penicillins, can cause hematuria.

The most common extrarenal etiology, renal calculi, can cause bleeding at any point along the urinary tract. An increased concentration of calcium and oxalate or decreased urine volume can lead to stone formation, whereas decreased levels of citrate and magnesium, which are known to be potent inhibitors of stone formation, can lead to the development of calculi. In addition, an alkaline pH and urine with increased amounts of uric acid promote stone development. Neoplasms such as transitional cell carcinoma may cause bleeding from the urinary bladder, ureter, or renal pelvis, whereas squamous cell carcinoma is more commonly found in the urethra. Bacterial infections causing cystitis, prostatitis, or urethritis commonly lead to microscopic or macroscopic hematuria. Trauma and foreign body or exercise-induced hematuria also must be considered. Chemotherapeutic agents, such as cyclophosphamide, may be associated with hemorrhagic cystitis with gross hematuria.

CLINICAL PRESENTATION

Hematuria may present with severe flank pain radiating to the groin, as in the case of calculi, or as an incidental finding on a routine urinalysis. A history of dysuria and increased frequency may be suggestive of a urinary tract infection, whereas hesitancy and a weak stream are more suggestive of lower tract obstruction from benign prostatic hypertrophy or tumor. Hematuria secondary to glomerular causes typically presents with hypertension. Arthritis and rashes usually accompany hematuria secondary to autoimmune and inflammatory disorders. A history of a recent upper respiratory infection may suggest postinfectious GN. It is important to inquire about medication, travel, and family history. The physical examination should focus attention on blood pressure measurement and the presence of peripheral edema, as these may be suggestive of glomerular disease and protein-losing states. A thorough skin examination should be done, as rashes associated with autoimmune diseases, such as systemic lupus erythematosus and systemic vasculitis, may be subtle. A boggy, tender prostate would point to prostatitis leading to hematuria, although benign prostatic hypertrophy alone rarely causes hematuria. In addition, the presence of a vaginal or penile discharge in the setting of hematuria may point to the existence of a urethritis secondary to a sexually transmitted disease.

DIAGNOSIS

Diagnosis is made by gross observation, urine dipstick analysis, or microscopic examination of the urinary sediment. Glomerular causes typically produce hematuria, proteinuria, and dysmorphic red blood cells on microscopic examination. The finding of true red blood cell casts is diagnostic of a glomerular origin for the hematuria. If a glomerular etiology is suspected, then the further workup includes obtaining serum complement levels. If complement levels are low, cryoglobulins, antinuclear antibody, antistreptolysin O titers, and hepatitis serologies should be sent. If complement levels are normal, serum and urine protein electrophoresis, hemoglobin S screening in patients of African-American heritage, antineutrophil cytoplasmic antibody, and coagulation studies should be checked. Renal biopsy is usually reserved for patients with significant proteinuria, for those who are developing renal failure, or for diagnostic certainty in the form of a tissue diagnosis. A urinary tract infection, especially the first episode, requires no further workup, except for checking a repeat urine culture to ensure sterilization of the urine. If a patient's presentation is consistent with urinary calculi, the urine should be screened and analyzed to determine the makeup of the stone. Evaluation of the urinalysis, serum calcium, serum intact parathyroid hormone level, uric acid, blood urea nitrogen, and creatinine also may aid in obtaining a diagnosis. Radiographic evaluation with an abdominal flat plate x-ray may show radio-opaque calculi, such as calcium oxalate or struvite stones. Renal ultrasound is a useful, noninvasive test for hematuria in the absence of glomerular injury and may reveal renal neoplasms, cysts, hydronephrosis, and occasionally stones. The renal ultrasound is useful in those patients with chronic renal insufficiency who cannot undergo an intravenous pyelogram (IVP) because of the risk of acute renal failure associated with intravenous contrast dye. IVP is often the first test in young patients with hematuria, as it can show medullary sponge kidney that would not be found on ultrasound. Cystoscopy is used when the renal ultrasound and IVP are negative. Generally, cystoscopy is recommended for those patients with hematuria who are older than 50 years of age or who are at an increased risk for neoplasms owing to a history of benzene exposure, smoking, or treatment with cyclophosphamide. Cystoscopy is recommended in all patients who have unexplained, persistent, or intermittent gross hematuria.

MANAGEMENT

The management of hematuria depends on identifying the source of blood loss and treating its underlying cause. Acute therapy is typically supportive. If a coagulopathy is present, it should be reversed. If clots are present in the urine, blood loss may be significant, and the hematocrit and hemodynamic parameters should be monitored. Increasing urine volume through increased oral intake or intravenous fluids may help prevent clot formation and flush out existing clots. Urinary calculi are predominantly managed with intravenous fluids to increase urinary volume and pain medication as needed. Antibiotic therapy is only indicated if there is clinical evidence of infection, such as a fever, leukocytosis, or positive urinalysis suggesting a coexistent infection. Admission to the hospital is not routine and should be reserved for those patients with a complicated clinical course or evidence of obstruction or infection. If a stone is 8 mm or larger in diameter, it is unlikely to pass on its own, and urologic consultation is warranted. In addition, emergency urologic consultation should be considered for fever, obstruction, or probable failure of spontaneous passage of the stone. Extracorporeal shock wave lithotripsy is used to treat stones in the renal pelvis or upper ureter that are unlikely to pass on their own. Although this method can be used in stones located in the lower tract, the success rate is less, only 70% to 80%, and in these cases ureteroscopy with basket retrieval of the stone is generally preferred. If infection in the setting of an obstruction is suspected, placement of a percutaneous nephrostomy tube or retrograde ureteral stent is indicated.

Chapter 119

GLOMERULONEPHRITIS

Vadjista Broumand

OVERVIEW

Glomerulonephritis (GN) is the term applied to a group of diseases characterized by inflammatory changes in glomerular capillaries and accompanying signs and symptoms of an acute nephritic syndrome. These signs include hematuria, proteinuria, and diminished renal function, and in some cases they are associated with fluid retention, hypertension, and edema. The *acute nephritic syndrome* is a medical emergency, and the use of this term implies rapid destruction of glomeruli. It is distinct from the term *chronic glomerulonephritis*, which is applied to patients in whom no specific diagnosis for their renal disease is made. This latter diagnosis is the third most common cause of end-stage renal disease in the United States and Europe.

PATHOPHYSIOLOGY

Both humeral and cell-mediated immune mechanisms play a part in the pathogenesis of glomerular inflammation. Two basic mechanisms of antibody-mediated glomerular injury have been identified: (i) Antibodies bind to a structural component of the glomerulus, and (ii) circulating antigen-antibody complexes escape clearance by the reticuloendothelial system and are deposited in the glomerulus. The role played by cellular immunity is less clear. First, monocytes and macrophages remove immune deposits from the glomerulus and, in the process, can cause injury by the release cytokines. Second and less clear is the role played by T-cells' responding directly to antigens presented in the glomerulus.

Glomerular damage in GN occurs in two phases. During the acute phase, as immune processes take place in the glomeruli, a variety of mediators of tissue injury, such as complement, coagulation factors, growth factors, and cytokines, is activated. A secondary component of the acute phase is the result of cell proliferation with overproduction of extracellular matrix in the glomerulus. Renal damage after the acute phase of GN is mediated by nonimmune mechanisms that develop as a result of loss of filtering surface with accompanying increases in glomerular pressures in the remaining nephrons.

CLINICAL PRESENTATION

Most forms of acute GN present with hematuria, proteinuria, and renal failure. Proteinuria in acute GN is generally less than 3.5 g per day. As renal function deteriorates, there is a progressive loss in the ability to excrete sodium. The resulting positive sodium balance causes edema and hypertension. The edema is seen in the periorbital region, ankles, and scrotum. The hypertension can be quite severe and causes progression of the renal injury, hence worsening of the hypertension and damage to other end organs. In previously normotensive individuals, even modest increases in blood pressure can lead to end-organ damage.

The differential diagnosis of the acute nephritic syndrome is broad. Some specific aspects of the more common forms are discussed.

Acute postinfectious GN is often associated with a streptococcal infection due to *Streptococcus pyogenes*. The renal manifestations commonly present 1 to 3 weeks after pharyngitis or impetigo. Other infectious causes include systemic *Staphylococcus aureus* infection, infective endocarditis, and shunt infections.

Immunoglobulin (Ig) A nephropathy or Berger's disease is the most common form of GN worldwide. Fifty percent of patients present with gross hematuria, with one-half of the patients presenting 24 to 48 hours after the onset of an upper respiratory infection. Gastrointestinal symptoms are seen in 10% of patients, and a flulike illness is apparent in 15% of cases. The prognosis of IgA nephropathy is variable but generally good. Predictors of progression include a raised serum creatinine at the time of diagnosis, urine protein excretion of more than 2 g per day, male gender, hypertension, and sclerotic glomeruli or extensive tubulointerstitial disease on biopsy.

The term *rapidly progressive GN* (RPGN) refers to the rate of loss of renal function. Patients can progress to end-stage renal disease within days to weeks.

Examination of the renal biopsy reveals glomerular crescent formation. For this reason, it is also termed *crescentic GN*. This, however, is a histopathologic designation, and on immunofluorescent examination there appear to be three distinct types. Type 1 RPGN has linear fluorescent staining of the glomerular basement membrane (GBM), in effect a renal-limited Goodpasture's syndrome. Type 2 RPGN is associated immune deposits in the glomeruli and is thought to be a renal-limited immune complex vasculitis. Type 3 RPGN is a pauciimmune GN, lacking immune deposits on immunofluorescent staining, with necrotizing vasculitis. Often, the patients are antineutrophil cytoplasmic antibody positive. This type of acute GN is thought to be renal-limited Wegener's granulomatosis.

Anti-GBM nephritis presents with or without pulmonary hemorrhage. If patients with acute GN have pulmonary hemorrhage and high titers of anti-GBM antibodies, they meet the criteria for Goodpasture's syndrome.

The most common type of renal vasculitis is a microscopic polyangiitis or polyarteritis nodosa. Systemic signs of vasculitis, such as fever, malaise, and weight loss, usually accompany polyarteritis nodosa. If associated with upper or lower respiratory tract symptoms, the clinical diagnosis is Wegener's granulomatosis.

Some renal diseases can demonstrate both nephritic and nephrotic features. An example of this is mesangiocapillary GN (MCGN), formerly referred to as *membranoproliferative GN*. Although MCGN presents more frequently as nephrotic syndrome, many patients show nephritic features as well. There are at least two major morphologic forms of MCGN. Type I MCGN shares many features with lupus nephritis, including mesangial and subendothelial immune-complex deposits, hypocomplementemia, and glomerular cell proliferation. The disorder is usually idiopathic, but many adults have associated infection with hepatitis C virus, presenting after 10 to 15 years of chronic hepatitis C, with high concentrations of cryoglobulins. Type II MCGN, or intramembranous dense–deposit disease, is less common than type I, associated with hypocomplementemia and C3 nephritic factor.

DIAGNOSIS

The diagnosis of acute GN starts with the history and physical examination, and a microscopic examination of the urine. The urinalysis is characterized by dysmorphic red blood cells and red blood cell casts in the urinary sediment. Once the diagnosis of acute GN is made, the serologic workup helps to differentiate between the different causes of acute GN. Important initial tests include serum complements, antistreptolysin O titers, antinuclear antibody, serum immunoglobulins, anti-GBM antibody, antineutrophil cytoplasmic antibody, C3 nephritic factor, cryoglobulins, venereal disease research laboratory, and a hepatitis panel.

A logical starting point is the testing of serum complements. Low serum complements support the diagnosis of immune-mediated GN, and normal serum complements support the diagnosis of nonimmune-mediated GN, the so-called pauciimmune GN. The premise is that the bound or trapped antibody in immune GN activates the complement cascade, whereas there is no activation in the pauciimmune GN. Forms of GN that have low complements result from systemic diseases, such as systemic lupus erythematosus, subacute bacterial endocarditis, cryoglobulinemia, and shunt nephritis, or primary renal diseases, such as acute poststreptococcal GN and mesangiocapillary GN. Forms of GN that have normal complements can also be divided into systemic diseases, such as polyarteritis nodosa, Wegner's granulomatosis, Henoch-Schönlein purpura, and Goodpasture's syndrome, and primary renal diseases, such as IgA nephritis and anti-GBM disease. Once the distinction between immune and pauciimmune GN has been made, subsequent serologic tests can be ordered, as dictated by the clinical scenario. It is generally frowned on to order tests in a "shotgun" fashion, because false-positive test results from tests ordered for inappropriate reasons can confuse or delay the diagnosis.

MANAGEMENT

The general principles of management of acute GN are early recognition of the syndrome, early diagnosis of the specific disease, early involvement of the renal team, and management of immediate life-threatening sequelae of the disease. General long-term therapies include blood pressure control with angiotensin-converting enzyme II inhibitors (ACE-IIs) or angiotensin II receptor blockers (ARBs), control of cholesterol if elevated, blood sugar control if diabetic, and strict counseling about tobacco abuse cessation. Some examples of treatment approaches to specific forms of acute GN follow.

Treatment of postinfectious GN is generally supportive, with the use of antihypertensives, salt restriction, and diuretics as needed. The prognosis in children is very favorable, with 90% experiencing complete recovery, 2.5% recovering but with some renal insufficiency, and 2.5% progressing to end-stage renal disease. Fewer than 5% of adults progress to develop a rapidly progressive GN.

Treatment for IgA nephropathy is largely symptomatic. Several studies evaluating the use of steroids, immunosuppressive agents, platelet inhibitors, and large doses of fish oil had varying and largely inconclusive results. Control of blood pressure with ACE-II/ARB to decrease intraglomerular pressure is recommended.

RPGN is a medical emergency, and success of therapy depends on early intervention. Management recommendations are beyond the scope of this text.

Treatment for Goodpasture's syndrome includes pulse steroids followed by high-dose oral steroids, 1 mg per kg per day, for several months; plasma exchange daily until anti-GBM antibodies are no longer detectable; and cyclophosphamide, 2 mg per kg per day. Dialysis can be avoided in more than 70% of patients if they are treated early in the course of the disease, again stressing the importance of early diagnosis and involvement of the renal team.

Patients with vasculitis can benefit from pulse steroids. Substantial improvement in renal function can occur in approximately 75% of patients treated with steroids alone, and this increases to 80% to 85% when cyclophosphamide is added.

The treatment of idiopathic MCGN with steroids and cytotoxic drugs has not shown consistent benefit, and the decision to treat or not should be left to the nephrology team. The use of ACE-II/ARB is beneficial for their renal protection effects.

Type I and type II patterns of lupus nephritis require no specific treatment. Patients with extensive type III and all type IV lesions should receive immunosuppressive therapy. Type V should be treated if superimposed proliferative lesions exist. In all types of lupus nephritis, especially those with associated hypertension, ACE-II/ARB are indicated for their renal protective effects. In type VI lupus nephritis, lowering intraglomerular pressure with an ACE-II/ARB may ameliorate progressive renal dysfunction.

Chapter 120

PROTEINURIA AND NEPHROTIC SYNDROME

Ursula C. Brewster

OVERVIEW

Nephrotic range proteinuria is defined as urinary protein loss of more than 3.5 g per 24 hours. The nephrotic syndrome is nephrotic range proteinuria accompanied by hypoalbuminemia, hypercholesterolemia, and peripheral edema. Other associated findings include hypercoagulability that is presumed due to the loss of antithrombin III in the urine, lipiduria that results for unclear reasons, and ascites that results from low serum oncotic pressure. The study and understanding of the diseases that cause the nephrotic syndrome are complicated by the nomenclature. The names are based on the histopathology seen on light microscopy, for example, *membranous nephropathy*. If a disease entity has been linked to the renal histopathology, such as systemic lupus erythematosus, it is called *secondary membranous glomerulonephritis* (GN). If physicians cannot find a systemic disease process affecting the patient that is known to be associated with the renal lesion, the renal disease is called *idiopathic*. It is therefore more appropriate to study disease processes and understand how they may affect the kidney as opposed to memorizing the alphabet soup of kidney disease.

The nephrotic syndrome can develop from primary, therefore idiopathic, renal diseases, such as minimal change disease, membranous GN, focal segmental glomerulosclerosis (FSGS), and mesangiocapillary GN (MCGN), previously referred to as *membranoproliferative GN*, or secondary to systemic diseases, such as diabetes mellitus and amyloidosis.

PATHOPHYSIOLOGY

Nephrotic syndrome has many causes, but the end result is an increase in glomerular permeability that leads to a loss of protein in the urine. In the normal kidney, there is a barrier to size and charge that prevents proteins from being filtered across the glomerulus into Bowman's space. In the damaged glomerulus, one or both of these mechanisms may be affected. In addition to protein, albumin, antithrombin III, and immunoglobulins may also spill into the urine. Previously, peripheral edema was thought to be due to reduced oncotic pressure, leading to hypovolemia and increased sodium retention. Recent evidence suggests that these patients may also be total body volume overloaded and have a low natriuretic response to atrial natriuretic peptide. Alterations in coagulation factors from hyperfiltration of proteins, such as antithrombin III, lead to hypercoagulability. A low plasma albumin leads to increased hepatic synthesis of lipoproteins, leading to hyperlipidemia.

CLINICAL PRESENTATION

Most patients with nephrotic syndrome have no symptoms at the time of presentation. Proteinuria is often detected on routine urinalysis, leading to further workup. The complications of the disease, such as peripheral edema, thromboembolic complications, hyperlipidemia, and ascites, may be the presenting signs and symptoms.

DIAGNOSIS

Once protein has been detected on a urinalysis, further workup consists of a 24-hour urine collection for protein and a search for probable causes. Alternatively, a spot urine sample can be sent for protein and creatinine. The ratio of urine protein to urine creatinine results in a number that corresponds to the number of grams of protein lost in the urine per 24 hours. The most important step in the diagnosis of nephrotic syndrome is a carefully directed history and physical examination. Patients with primary nephrotic syndrome often have a history and physical examination that reveal no obvious pathology. Causes of secondary nephrotic syndrome include diabetic nephropathy, connective tissue diseases, malignancy, human immunodeficiency virus disease, hepatitis, and drugs, both prescription and illicit. It should be noted that only one of these diseases can present with isolated nephrotic range proteinuria. With the exception of a pediatric patient presenting with minimal change disease, a renal biopsy is necessary for diagnostic purposes.

Minimal change disease is a classic cause of primary nephrotic syndrome. It is usually acute in onset and often presents with normal renal function. It is the major cause of nephrotic syndrome in children but is only responsible for 20% of adult cases. Light microscopy is normal in minimal change disease and is the reason for its name. Immunofluorescence staining is equally unrevealing. Electron microscopy shows the pathologic change that is the fusion of foot processes, termed *effacement.*

Idiopathic membranous GN is the primary cause of nephrotic syndrome in adults, with 50% of cases carrying this diagnosis. In addition to the findings of the nephrotic syndrome, patients often present with hypertension and mild renal insufficiency. Renal vein thrombosis is relatively common, but reported incidence varies between studies. Secondary causes of membranous GN include hepatitis B, systemic lupus erythematosus and other connective tissue diseases, malignancy, and medications. Light microscopy shows thickened capillary loops.

Idiopathic FSGS constitutes 10% of adult cases, with a mean age of onset at 21 years. Secondary causes include human immunodeficiency virus disease, heroin use, morbid obesity, and vesicoureteral reflux. Patients often present with hypertension, renal insufficiency, proteinuria, and hematuria. Although the light microscopy findings vary somewhat between different causes of FSGS, the general theme is one of glomeruli that are partially sclerotic and scattered randomly throughout the renal parenchyma.

Idiopathic MCGN is divided into types I, II, and III depending on the type and location of the immune deposits. All three activate the complement cascade, although the components that predominate on immunofluorescence staining differ between the three. The common clinical presentation is subnephrotic range proteinuria and asymptomatic hematuria. Progression to renal failure follows a variable course in each type. Secondary causes of MCGN include infections, connective tissue diseases, and hepatitis B and C. The major cause of the renal pathology in these diseases is deposition of cryoglobulins (immunoglobulins that precipitate in the cold). The complement cascade is also activated in secondary MCGN. As opposed to idiopathic MCGN, the clinical presentation is weighted toward nephrotic range proteinuria. Hematuria is often present as well, but not as consistently as in idiopathic MCGN. The light microscopy in both idiopathic and secondary MCGN shows a thickened glomerular basement membrane and lobulation of glomeruli. Immunofluorescence staining and electron microscopy distinguish individual types.

MANAGEMENT

As proteinuria is a predictor of progression to end-stage renal disease, management consists of finding and treating the underlying primary disease, and reducing protein excretion. In primary renal disease, steroids may be effective. A good example of this is pediatric minimal change disease. Often, a trial of steroids is used before subjecting a pediatric patient to a renal biopsy, and a positive response is considered diagnostic. Pediatric patients with minimal change disease generally respond well to steroids, with up to 80% having resolution of their proteinuria. Of the responders, up to 60% may have a recurrence and require repeat therapy.

Adults with nephrotic syndrome should be evaluated for secondary causes with history, physical examination, and serologic studies. Ultimately, most adults with nephrotic syndrome will undergo a renal biopsy for diagnostic certainty, prognosis, and guiding therapy. The response of idiopathic forms of renal disease to immunosuppressive and cytotoxic therapy is highly variable and depends on disease. The reason for these differences is unclear.

In general, management should focus on the diagnosis of a primary systemic disease. If no primary systemic disease is found, or while waiting for therapy to be effective, efforts should be made to reduce proteinuria to the lowest possible level. Agents such as angiotensin-converting enzyme inhibitors, angiotensin II receptor blockers, and nonsteroidal antiinflammatory drugs should be used to reduce the level of proteinuria. Blood pressure control is also a cornerstone of management. Although control of blood pressure below 140/90 mm Hg has not been shown to slow the rate of progression of renal disease in the population of renal patients as a whole, in patients with glomerular diseases and proteinuria, lower is probably better. The lowest blood pressure tolerated by the patient should be the goal. A low-protein diet of 0.7 g per kg per day also has been shown to decrease protein excretion, but whether it slows progression of renal disease is debated. Control of hypercholesterolemia may also benefit renal survival. The role of antiplatelet agents remains uncertain.

Chapter 121

DIABETES INSIPIDUS

Eric N. Taylor

OVERVIEW

Diabetes insipidus (DI) is a condition in which the kidney is unable to concentrate the urine because of defects in the action or production of antidiuretic hormone (ADH, or vasopressin). These defects produce a state of hypotonic polyuria and excessive water intake. DI may occur in complete or partial forms. DI frequently starts early in life, with a median age of onset of 24 years, and is more common in men than in women.

PATHOPHYSIOLOGY

DI is caused by the failure of the hypothalamic-pituitary axis to release adequate amounts of ADH (central DI), or by the failure of the kidney to produce concentrated urine despite adequate levels of ADH (nephrogenic DI). Any pathologic process involving the hypothalamic-pituitary axis can cause central DI. Causes include pituitary surgery, head trauma, neoplasia (e.g., dysgerminomas, craniopharyngiomas, suprasellar pituitary tumors, metastatic carcinomas of the breast, lymphoma, or leukemia), vascular lesions (e.g., aneurysms, cerebrovascular accidents, Sheehan's syndrome), infections (e.g., meningoencephalitis, tuberculosis, syphilis), and infiltrative granulomatous diseases (e.g., sarcoid and histiocytosis). In 60% of patients with neoplastic or infiltrative lesions of the hypothalamus or pituitary causing DI, dysfunction of the anterior pituitary is also present. In 30% of patients, central DI is idiopathic. There are also genetic forms of central DI. Nephrogenic DI may also be acquired or genetic, with the acquired form being far more common and usually associated with certain drugs. Lithium is the most common culprit, although demeclocycline, methoxyflurane, and amphotericin B can also cause nephrogenic DI. Acquired nephrogenic DI can also result from electrolyte disturbances (hypercalcemia and severe hypokalemia) and obstructive uropathy. DI can occur during pregnancy secondary to increased levels of placental vasopressinase.

CLINICAL PRESENTATION

In DI, the inability of the kidney to concentrate the urine leads to polyuria, thirst, and secondary polydipsia. If water consumption can adequately replace urinary water loss, hypernatremia and hypertonicity will not develop. Notably, hypernatremia is not a requisite feature of DI. In extreme cases, the volume of urine can be on the order of 16 to 24 L of urine per day, requiring a patient to urinate every half-hour to hour. More commonly, urine volume is increased to a lesser extent, on the order of 3 to 6 L per day. The urine is typically pale in color. Hypotonic polyuria causes the serum osmolality to rise, which in turn causes thirst. Cold fluids are often preferred. Because the hypothalamic thirst center ensures that polydipsia is tightly coupled with polyuria, dehydration in DI is usually undetectable, except for a slight elevation of the serum sodium. When the replacement of excreted water is insufficient; DI leads to severe dehydration, resulting in weakness, psychosis, tachycardia, prostration, hypotension, fever, and even death. In these cases, the serum osmolality rises and the serum sodium levels can exceed 175 mmol per L.

DIAGNOSIS

The polyuria of DI must be distinguished from other causes of polyuria, such as primary polydipsia, solute diuresis, and resolving acute renal failure. A urine osmolality of less than 150 mmol per kg usually rules out solute diuresis (from mannitol or glycosuria) as a cause of polyuria. Formal dehydration testing is usually unnecessary in patients with severe polyuria and can result in hypotension and severe hypernatremia. Dehydration testing can be useful to diagnose partial forms of DI and can also be used to differentiate DI from other causes of polyuria. During dehydration testing, the patient is restricted from drinking fluids. Urine osmolality is measured hourly and plasma osmolality every 4 to 6 hours. Fluid deprivation is maintained until plasma osmolality reaches 295 mmol per kg or urine osmolality varies less than 5% over 3 hours. In patients with complete DI, the urine osmolality remains less than that of plasma. In partial DI, the urine osmolality is greater than that of plasma, but the urine is not optimally concentrated. The urinary response to the administration of ADH differentiates central and nephrogenic DI.

MANAGEMENT

Desmopressin, an ADH analog, is the drug of choice for the treatment of patients with central DI. It does not have pressor effects and acts for 10 to 24 hours when given intranasally (10–20 µg), subcutaneously (1–4 µg), or intravenously (1–4 µg). There is an oral form available (50–800 µg/day), with the greater dose due to relatively poor enteral bioavailability. Patients with partial central DI are sometimes treated with chlorpropamide or carbamazepine, which act to stimulate ADH release. Nephrogenic DI can be treated by salt restriction. The kidney must excrete a set amount of osmoles each day, and if the dietary load of osmoles is reduced, less urine has to be excreted for a given urine osmolality. Nonsteroidal antiinflammatory medications and diuretic therapy, primary hydrochlorothiazide, have also been used. Intravascular volume depletion and a diminished glomerular filtration rate result in enhanced reabsorption of fluid in the proximal part of the nephron. The management of patients with DI who do not consume sufficient amounts of water because of altered mental status or acute illness is particularly difficult. These patients can rapidly develop severe hypernatremia and can progress to circulatory collapse. In these cases, intake and output of fluids, measurement of body weight, vital signs, and serum creatinine must be monitored. Exogenous fluid intake must approximate urine volume and fluid loss from other sources. One of the most important recommendations to make to a patient with DI, and to their family, is that when oral intake is impaired, immediate medical care must be sought.

INDEX

Page numbers followed by *f* indicate figures; numbers followed by *t* indicate tables.

INFECTIOUS DISEASES
Human Immunodeficiency Virus

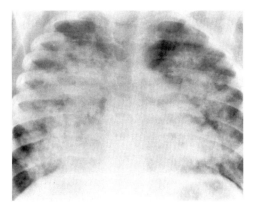

Pneumocystis carinii pneumonia. (From Eisenberg RL, ed. *Clinical imaging: an atlas of differential diagnosis*, 4th ed. Philadelphia: Lippincott Williams & Wilkins, 2003, with permission.)

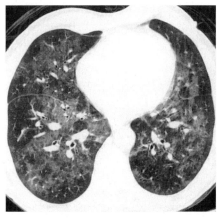

Pneumocystis carinii pneumonia/high-resolution computed tomography scan. (From Muller NL, Fraser RS, Leek S, et al., eds. *Diseases of the lung: radiologic and pathologic correlations*. Philadelphia: Lippincott Williams & Wilkins, 2003, with permission.)

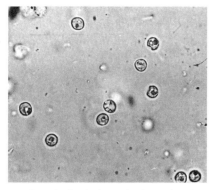

Pneumocystis carinii/bronchoalveolar lavage/methenamine silver. (From Koneman EW, Allen SD, Janda WM, et al. *Color atlas and textbook of diagnostic microbiology.* Philadelphia: Lippincott–Raven Publishers, 1997, with permission.)

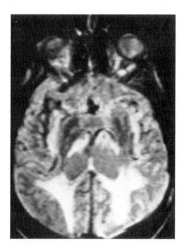

Progressive multifocal leukoencephalopathy. (From Eisenberg RL, ed. *Clinical imaging: an atlas of differential diagnosis,* 4th ed. Philadelphia: Lippincott Williams & Wilkins, 2003, with permission.)

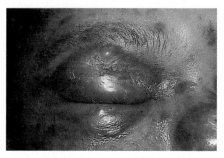

Disseminated Kaposi's sarcoma. (From Mannis MJ, Macsai MS, Huntley AC. *Eye and skin disease.* Philadelphia: Lippincott–Raven Publishers, 1996, with permission.)

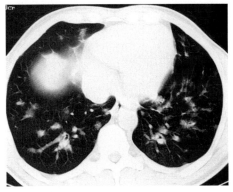

Disseminated Kaposi's sarcoma/computed tomography scan. (From Pope TL, Jr. *Aunt Minnie's atlas of imaging-specific diagnosis*, 2nd ed. Philadelphia: Lippincott Williams & Wilkins, 2003, with permission.)

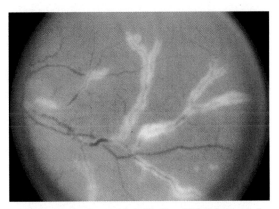

Cytomegalovirus retinitis. (From Mannis MJ, Macsai MS, Huntley AC. *Eye and skin disease*. Philadelphia: Lippincott–Raven Publishers, 1996, with permission.)

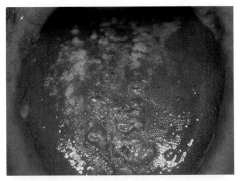

Oral thrush/candida. (From Smith DS. *Field guide to bedside diagnosis*. Philadelphia: Lippincott Williams & Wilkins, 1999, with permission.)

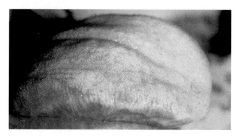

Oral hairy leukoplakia. (From Smith DS. *Field guide to bedside diagnosis*. Philadelphia: Lippincott Williams & Wilkins, 1999, with permission.)

Endocarditis

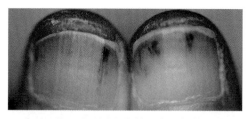

Splinter hemorrhages. (From Smith DS. *Field guide to bedside diagnosis*. Philadelphia: Lippincott Williams & Wilkins, 1999, with permission.)

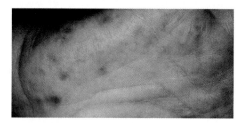

Osler's nodes. (From Smith DS. *Field guide to bedside diagnosis*. Philadelphia: Lippincott Williams & Wilkins, 1999, with permission.)

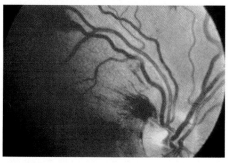

Roth spots. (From Smith DS. *Field guide to bedside diagnosis*. Philadelphia: Lippincott Williams & Wilkins, 1999, with permission.)

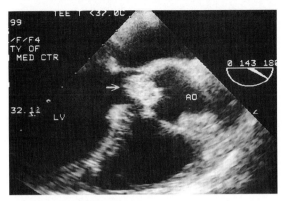

Aortic valve vegetations (*arrow*)/transesophageal echocardiogram. AO, aorta; LV, left ventricle. (From Humes DH, ed. *Kelley's textbook of internal medicine*, 4th ed. Philadelphia: Lippincott Williams & Wilkins, 2000, with permission.)

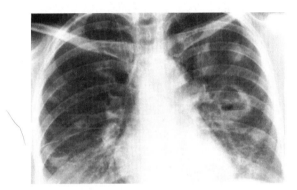

Septic pulmonary emboli/tricuspid endocarditis. (From Eisenberg RL, ed. *Clinical imaging: an atlas of differential diagnosis*, 4th ed. Philadelphia: Lippincott Williams & Wilkins, 2003, with permission.)

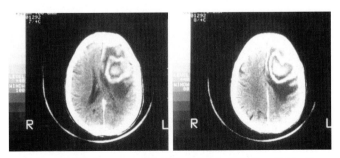

Brain abscess/staphylococcus endocarditis. L, left; R, right. (From Vahjen G. Yale University Health Services, Radiology Department.)

Pneumonia

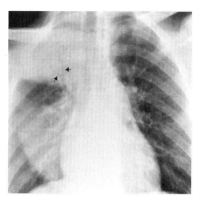

Pneumococcal pneumonia with air bronchograms (*arrows*). (From Eisenberg RL, ed. *Clinical imaging: an atlas of differential diagnosis*, 4th ed. Philadelphia: Lippincott Williams & Wilkins, 2003, with permission.)

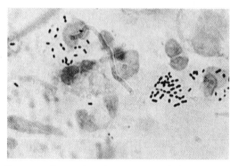

Pneumococci in sputum/lancet-shaped gram-positive diplococci. (From Koneman EW, Allen SD, Janda WM, et al. *Color atlas and textbook of diagnostic microbiology*. Philadelphia: Lippincott–Raven Publishers, 1997, with permission.)

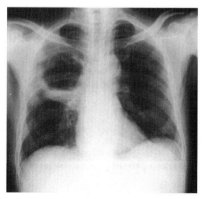

Klebsiella lung abscess. (From Vahjen G. Yale University Health Services, Radiology Department.)

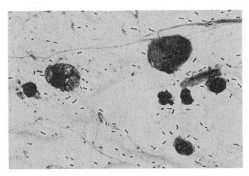

Klebsiella pneumoniae in sputum/gram-negative bacilli with halo. (From Koneman EW, Allen SD, Janda WM, et al. *Color atlas and textbook of diagnostic microbiology*. Philadelphia: Lippincott–Raven Publishers, 1997, with permission.)

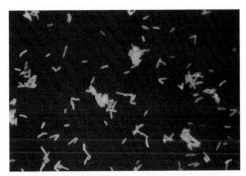

Legionella smear. (From Stoller JK, Ahmad M, Longworth DC, eds. *Cleveland Clinic intensive review of internal medicine*, 2nd ed. Philadelphia: Lippincott Williams & Wilkins, 2000, with permission.)

Sexually Transmitted Disease

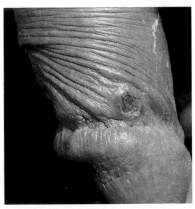

Syphilis chancre. (From Mannis MJ, Macsai MS, Huntley AC. *Eye and skin disease*. Philadelphia: Lippincott–Raven Publishers, 1996, with permission.)

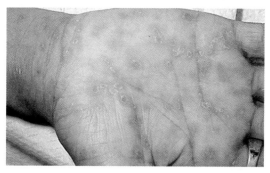

Secondary syphilis/palmar papulosquamous syphilids. (From Mannis MJ, Macsai MS, Huntley AC. *Eye and skin disease*. Philadelphia: Lippincott–Raven Publishers, 1996, with permission.)

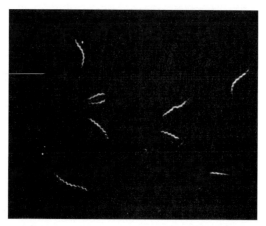

Treponema pallidum on dark-field microscopic examination. (From Humes DH, ed. *Kelley's textbook of internal medicine*, 4th ed. Philadelphia: Lippincott Williams & Wilkins, 2000, with permission.)

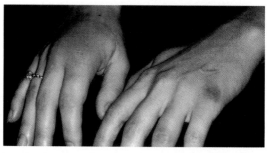

Disseminated gonococcemia. (From Smith DS. *Field guide to bedside diagnosis*. Philadelphia: Lippincott Williams & Wilkins, 1999, with permission.)

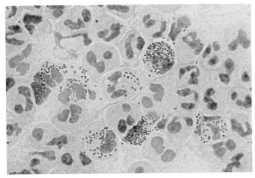

Gonococci/gram-negative intracellular diplococci/urethral smear. (From Koneman EW, Allen SD, Janda WM, et al. *Color atlas and textbook of diagnostic microbiology.* Philadelphia: Lippincott–Raven Publishers, 1997, with permission.)

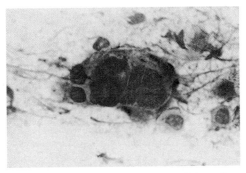

Herpes simplex/Tzanck smear/multinucleated giant cell. (From Koneman EW, Allen SD, Janda WM, et al. *Color atlas and textbook of diagnostic microbiology.* Philadelphia: Lippincott–Raven Publishers, 1997, with permission.)

Sepsis

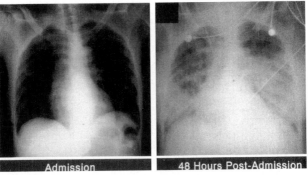

Acute respiratory distress syndrome. (From Humes DH, ed. *Kelley's textbook of internal medicine*, 4th ed. Philadelphia: Lippincott Williams & Wilkins, 2000, with permission.)

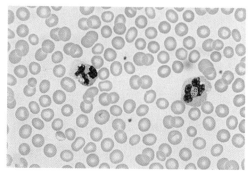

Intracellular bacteria in sepsis. (From Lee GR, Foerster J, Lukens J, et al., eds. *Wintrobe's clinical hematology*, 10th ed. Philadelphia: Williams & Wilkins, 1999, with permission.)

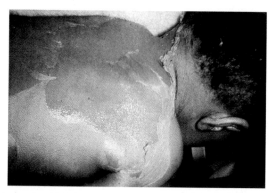

Staphylococcal scalded skin syndrome. (From Koneman EW, Allen SD, Janda WM, et al. *Color atlas and textbook of diagnostic microbiology*. Philadelphia: Lippincott–Raven Publishers, 1997, with permission.)

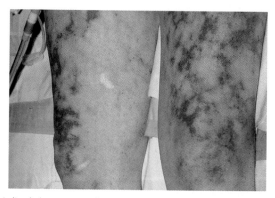

Purpuric livedo/pneumococcal sepsis. (From Smith DS. *Field guide to bedside diagnosis*. Philadelphia: Lippincott Williams & Wilkins, 1999, with permission.)

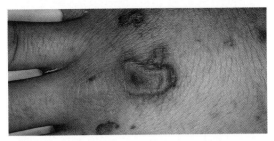

Gun-metal purpura/meningococcemia. (From Smith DS. *Field guide to bedside diagnosis.* Philadelphia: Lippincott Williams & Wilkins, 1999, with permission.)

Tuberculosis

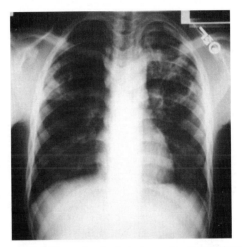

Upper lobe cavitary infiltrates/mediastinal adenopathy. (From Vahjen G. Yale University Health Services, Radiology Department.)

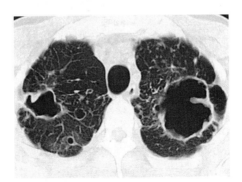

Upper lobe cavities/computed tomography scan. (From Humes DH, ed. *Kelley's textbook of internal medicine,* 4th ed. Philadelphia: Lippincott Williams & Wilkins, 2000, with permission.)

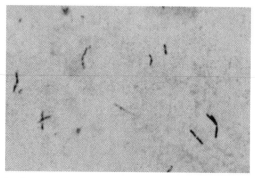

Acid-fast bacilli/*Mycobacterium tuberculosis*. (From Koneman EW, Allen SD, Janda WM, et al. *Color atlas and textbook of diagnostic microbiology*. Philadelphia: Lippincott–Raven Publishers, 1997, with permission.)

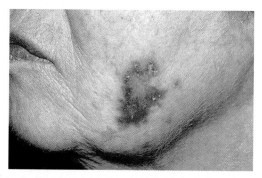

Lupus vulgaris. (From Mannis MJ, Macsai MS, Huntley AC. *Eye and skin disease*. Philadelphia: Lippincott–Raven Publishers, 1996, with permission.)

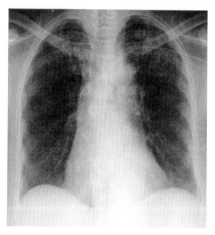

Miliary tuberculosis. (From Pope TL, Jr. *Aunt Minnie's atlas of imaging-specific diagnosis*, 2nd ed. Philadelphia: Lippincott Williams & Wilkins, 2003, with permission.)

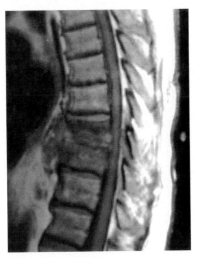

Tuberculosis of the spine/T1-weighted magnetic resonance image. (From Pope TL, Jr. *Aunt Minnie's atlas of imaging-specific diagnosis*, 2nd ed. Philadelphia: Lippincott Williams & Wilkins, 2003, with permission.)

CARDIOLOGY

Acute Myocardial Infarction

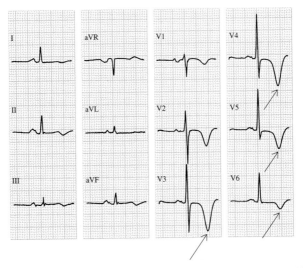

Hyperacute T waves in acute anterior myocardial infarction. (From Wagner GS, ed. *Mariott's practical electrocardiography*, 10th ed. Philadelphia: Lippincott Williams & Wilkins, 2001, with permission.)

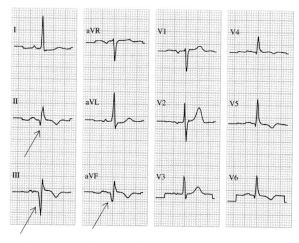

Q waves (*arrows*) in inferior myocardial infarction. (From Wagner GS, ed. *Mariott's practical electrocardiography*, 10th ed. Philadelphia: Lippincott Williams & Wilkins, 2001, with permission.)

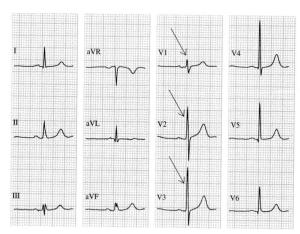

R waves (*arrows*) in acute posterior myocardial infarction. (From Wagner GS, ed. *Mariott's practical electrocardiography*, 10th ed. Philadelphia: Lippincott Williams & Wilkins, 2001, with permission.)

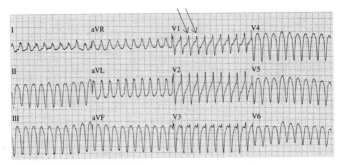

Ventricular tachycardia. Arrows indicate broad (≥0.04 sec) initial R waves in lead V_1. (From Wagner GS, ed. *Mariott's practical electrocardiography*, 10th ed. Philadelphia: Lippincott Williams & Wilkins, 2001, with permission.)

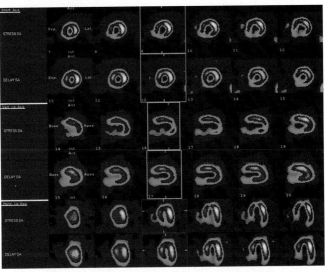

Unstable angina on T1 single-photon emission computed tomography scan. Note apical, inferoseptal ischemia. (From Pohost GM, O'Rourke RA, Berman DS, Shah PM, eds. *Imaging in cardiovascular disease*. Philadelphia: Lippincott Williams & Wilkins, 2000, with permission.)

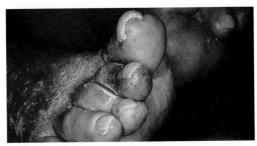

Arterial embolism/blue toes. (From Smith DS. *Field guide to bedside diagnosis*. Philadelphia: Lippincott Williams & Wilkins, 1999, with permission.)

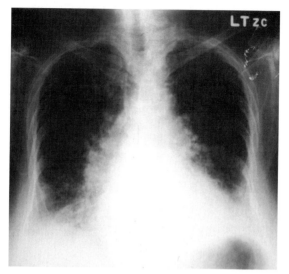

Pulmonary edema. (From Vahjen G. Yale University Health Services, Radiology Department.)

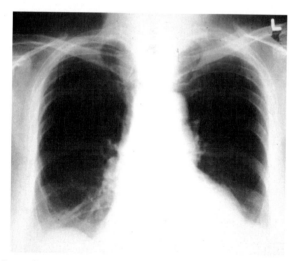

Cardiomegaly postdiuresis/follow-up of above patient. (From Vahjen G. Yale University Health Services, Radiology Department.)

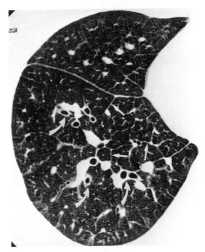

Pulmonary edema. High-resolution computed tomography scan shows smooth thickening of interlobular septa (*straight arrows*) and bronchovascular bundles (*curved arrows*). (From Muller NL, Fraser RS, Leek S, et al., eds. *Diseases of the lung: radiologic and pathologic correlations*. Philadelphia: Lippincott Williams & Wilkins, 2003, with permission.)

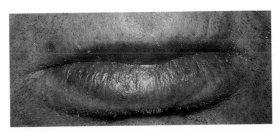

Central cyanosis. (From Smith DS. *Field guide to bedside diagnosis*. Philadelphia: Lippincott Williams & Wilkins, 1999, with permission.)

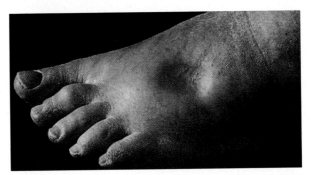

Pitting edema. (From Smith DS. *Field guide to bedside diagnosis*. Philadelphia: Lippincott Williams & Wilkins, 1999, with permission.)

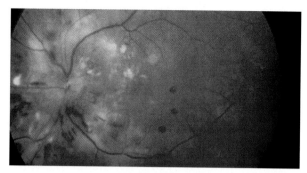

Hypertensive retinopathy/accelerated. (From Smith DS. *Field guide to bedside diagnosis*. Philadelphia: Lippincott Williams & Wilkins, 1999, with permission.)

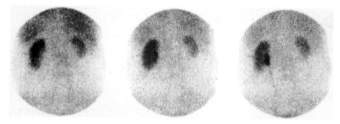

Renal artery stenosis/captopril renal scan. (From Vahjen G. Yale University Health Services, Radiology Department.)

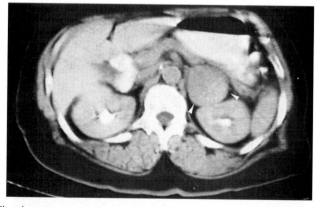

Pheochromocytoma on a computed tomography scan. Large pear-shaped mass (*arrowheads*) anterior to the left kidney. (From Eisenberg RL, ed. *Clinical imaging: an atlas of differential diagnosis*, 4th ed. Philadelphia: Lippincott Williams & Wilkins, 2003, with permission.)

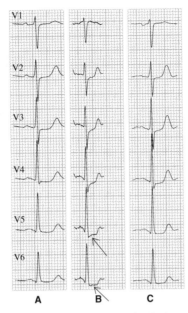

A–C: Electrocardiographic stress test/anterior ischemia. Arrows indicate horizontal ST-segment depression. (From Wagner GS, ed. *Mariott's practical electrocardiography*, 10th ed. Philadelphia: Lippincott Williams & Wilkins, 2001, with permission.)

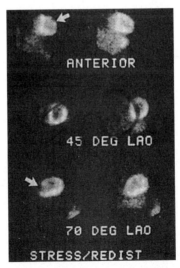

Thallium stress test/anterior ischemia. Defects are seen (*arrows*) in the anterolateral and apical walls in the anterior view and in the anterior wall in the 70-degree left anterior oblique (LAO) view. (From Humes DH, ed. *Kelley's textbook of internal medicine*, 4th ed. Philadelphia: Lippincott Williams & Wilkins, 2000, with permission.)

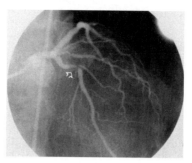

Left anterior descending artery stenosis/coronary arteriogram. Arrows indicate stenosis. (From Humes DH, ed. *Kelley's textbook of internal medicine*, 4th ed. Philadelphia: Lippincott Williams & Wilkins, 2000, with permission.)

Pericardial Effusion/Tamponade

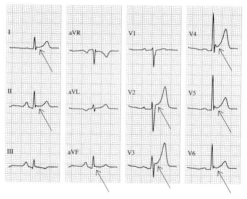

Acute pericarditis/diffuse ST-segment elevation. Arrows indicate widespread ST-segment elevation. (From Wagner GS, ed. *Mariott's practical electrocardiography*, 10th ed. Philadelphia: Lippincott Williams & Wilkins, 2001, with permission.)

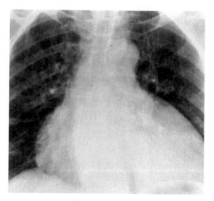

Water-bottle heart/coxsackievirus/chest x-ray. (From Eisenberg RL, ed. *Clinical imaging: an atlas of differential diagnosis*, 4th ed. Philadelphia: Lippincott Williams & Wilkins, 2003, with permission.)

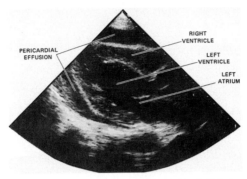

Pericardial effusion/echocardiogram. (From Humes DH, ed. *Kelley's textbook of internal medicine*, 4th ed. Philadelphia: Lippincott Williams & Wilkins, 2000, with permission.)

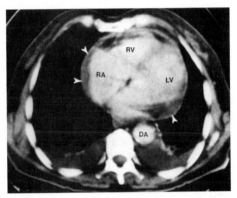

Pericardial effusion/computed tomography scan. DA, descending aorta; LV, left ventricle; RA, right atrium; RV, right ventricle. (From Eisenberg RL, ed. *Clinical imaging: an atlas of differential diagnosis*, 4th ed. Philadelphia: Lippincott Williams & Wilkins, 2003, with permission.)

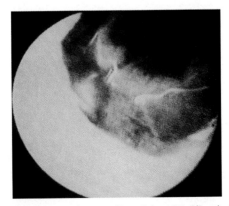

Fibrinous pericarditis/pericardioscopy. (From Pohost GM, O'Rourke RA, Berman DS, Shah PM, eds. *Imaging in cardiovascular disease*. Philadelphia: Lippincott Williams & Wilkins, 2000, with permission.)

Aortic Aneurysm/Dissection

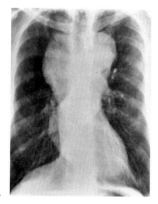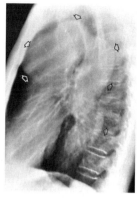

A,B: Thoracic aortic aneurysm/chest x-ray. **B:** Note marked dilatation of both the ascending and descending portions of the thoracic aorta (*arrows*), producing anterior and posterior mediastinal masses, respectively. (From Eisenberg RL, ed. *Clinical imaging: an atlas of differential diagnosis*, 4th ed. Philadelphia: Lippincott Williams & Wilkins, 2003, with permission.)

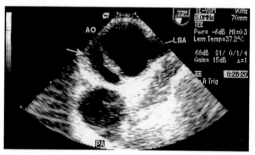

Thoracic aorta dissection/transesophageal echocardiograph. Ao, aorta; LSA, left subclavian artery; PA, pulmonary artery. (From Pohost GM, O'Rourke RA, Berman DS, Shah PM, eds. *Imaging in cardiovascular disease*. Philadelphia: Lippincott Williams & Wilkins, 2000, with permission.)

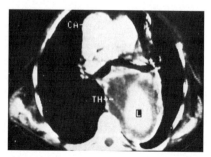

Thoracic aortic aneurysm with mural thrombus (TH)/computed tomography scan. L, descending aorta; OA, ascending aorta. (From Eisenberg RL, ed. *Clinical imaging: an atlas of differential diagnosis*, 4th ed. Philadelphia: Lippincott Williams & Wilkins, 2003, with permission.)

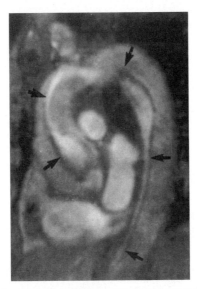

Thoracic aorta dissection (*arrows*)/magnetic resonance image. (From Humes DH, ed. *Kelley's textbook of internal medicine*, 4th ed. Philadelphia: Lippincott Williams & Wilkins, 2000, with permission.)

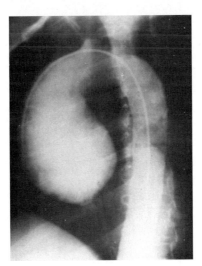

Thoracic aortic aneurysm/angiogram/Marfan's syndrome. (From Eisenberg RL, ed. *Clinical imaging: an atlas of differential diagnosis*, 4th ed. Philadelphia: Lippincott Williams & Wilkins, 2003, with permission.)

Arrhythmia

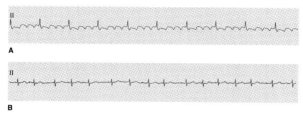

Atrial flutter **(A)** and fibrillation **(B)**. (From Wagner GS, ed. *Mariott's practical electrocardiography*, 10th ed. Philadelphia: Lippincott Williams & Wilkins, 2001, with permission.)

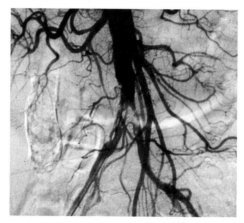

Distal aorta saddle embolism. (From Humes DH, ed. *Kelley's textbook of internal medicine*, 4th ed. Philadelphia: Lippincott Williams & Wilkins, 2000, with permission.)

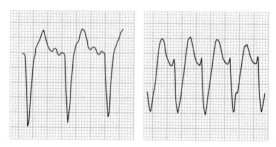

Left bundle branch block **(A)** versus ventricular tachycardia **(B)**. (From Wagner GS, ed. *Mariott's practical electrocardiography*, 10th ed. Philadelphia: Lippincott Williams & Wilkins, 2001, with permission.)

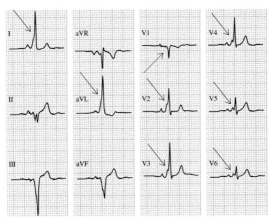

Delta waves (*arrows*) in Wolf-Parkinson-White syndrome. (From Wagner GS, ed. *Mariott's practical electrocardiography*, 10th ed. Philadelphia: Lippincott Williams & Wilkins, 2001, with permission.)

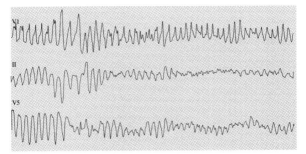

Torsades de pointes in hypokalemia. (From Wagner GS, ed. *Mariott's practical electrocardiography*, 10th ed. Philadelphia: Lippincott Williams & Wilkins, 2001, with permission.)

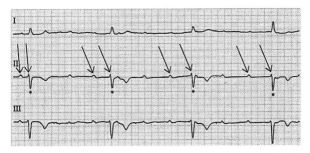

Third-degree atrioventricular block. Arrows indicate the varying PR interval relations and asterisks indicate the ventricular escape beats. (From Wagner GS, ed. *Mariott's practical electrocardiography*, 10th ed. Philadelphia: Lippincott Williams & Wilkins, 2001, with permission.)

Valvular Heart Disease

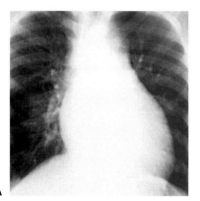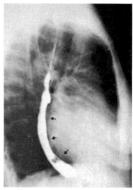

A,B: Aortic stenosis/apex displacement. **B:** Lateral view shows bulging of the lower half of the posterior cardiac silhouette, causing a broad indentation on the barium-filled esophagus (*arrows*). (From Eisenberg RL, ed. *Clinical imaging: an atlas of differential diagnosis*, 4th ed. Philadelphia: Lippincott Williams & Wilkins, 2003, with permission.)

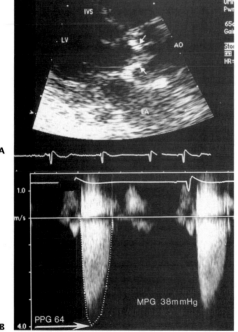

Aortic stenosis/ echocardiogram. **A:** Arrow indicates thickened aortic leaflets with restricted mobility. **B:** Image shows continuous wave Doppler with peak pressure gradient of 64 mm Hg and mean gradient of 38 mm Hg. (From Humes DH, ed. *Kelley's textbook of internal medicine*, 4th ed. Philadelphia: Lippincott Williams & Wilkins, 2000, with permission.)

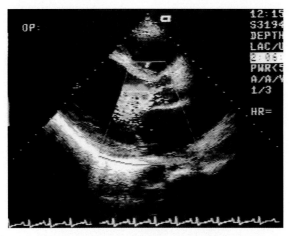

Aortic regurgitation/color Doppler. (From Pohost GM, O'Rourke RA, Berman DS, Shah PM, eds. *Imaging in cardiovascular disease*. Philadelphia: Lippincott Williams & Wilkins, 2000, with permission.)

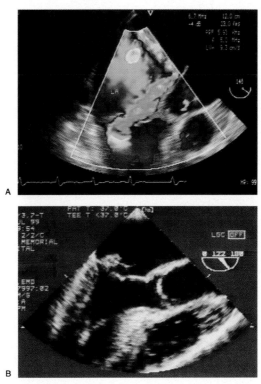

A,B: Mitral regurgitation with flail leaflet/echocardiogram. (From Pohost GM, O'Rourke RA, Berman DS, Shah PM, eds. *Imaging in cardiovascular disease*. Philadelphia: Lippincott Williams & Wilkins, 2000, with permission.)

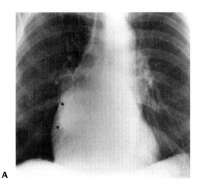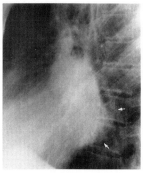

A,B: Mitral stenosis/left atrial enlargement (*arrows*). (From Eisenberg RL, ed. *Clinical imaging: an atlas of differential diagnosis*, 4th ed. Philadelphia: Lippincott Williams & Wilkins, 2003, with permission.)

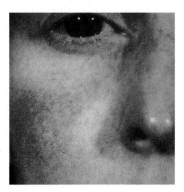

Mitral stenosis/malar flush. (From Smith DS. *Field guide to bedside diagnosis*. Philadelphia: Lippincott Williams & Wilkins, 1999, with permission.)

PULMONARY AND CRITICAL CARE

Pulmonary Embolism

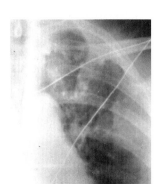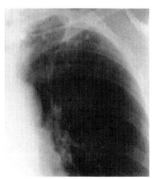

A: Westermark's sign. Baseline chest x-ray. **B:** Oligemia. (From Eisenberg RL, ed. *Clinical imaging: an atlas of differential diagnosis*, 4th ed. Philadelphia: Lippincott Williams & Wilkins, 2003, with permission.)

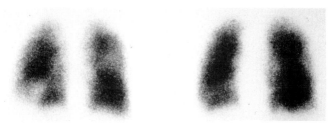

High-probability perfusion scan. (From Vahjen G. Yale University Health Services, Radiology Department.)

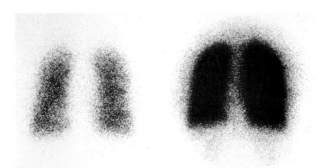

Ventilation scan mismatch on patient above. (From Vahjen G. Yale University Health Services, Radiology Department.)

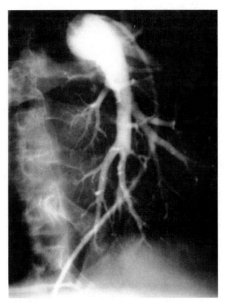

Pulmonary embolism/pulmonary arteriogram. (From Vahjen G. Yale University Health Services, Radiology Department.)

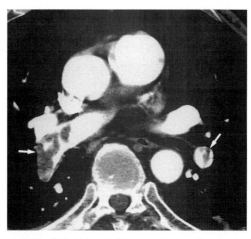

Pulmonary embolism/spiral computed tomography scan. Arrows show filling defects within the right interlobar and left lower lobe pulmonary arteries. (From Muller NL, Fraser RS, Leek S, et al., eds. *Diseases of the lung: radiologic and pathologic correlations.* Philadelphia: Lippincott Williams & Wilkins, 2003, with permission.)

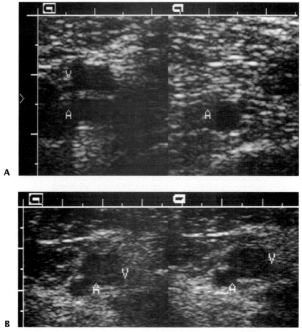

A,B: Noncompressible leg vein in deep venous thrombosis/ultrasound. A, artery; V, vein. (From Humes DH, ed. *Kelley's textbook of internal medicine*, 4th ed. Philadelphia: Lippincott Williams & Wilkins, 2000, with permission.)

Sarcoidosis

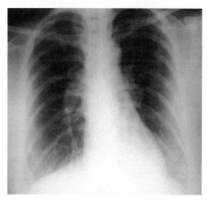

Bilateral hilar adenopathy/chest x-ray. (From Vahjen G. Yale University Health Services, Radiology Department.)

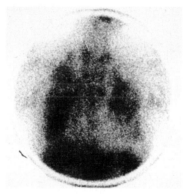

Pulmonary sarcoidosis/gallium scan. (From Vahjen G. Yale University Health Services, Radiology Department.)

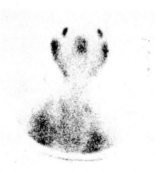

Sarcoidosis parotid involvement/"panda sign." (From Vahjen G. Yale University Health Services, Radiology Department.)

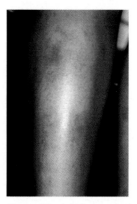

Erythema nodosum. (From Humes DH, ed. *Kelley's textbook of internal medicine*, 4th ed. Philadelphia: Lippincott Williams & Wilkins, 2000, with permission.)

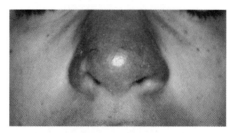

Lupus pernio. (From Smith DS. *Field guide to bedside diagnosis*. Philadelphia: Lippincott Williams & Wilkins, 1999, with permission.)

Chronic Obstructive Pulmonary Disease and Interstitial Lung Disease

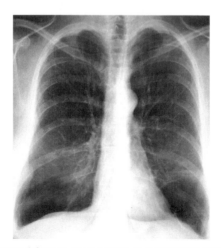

Alpha$_1$-antitrypsin deficiency. (From Pope TL, Jr. *Aunt Minnie's atlas of imaging-specific diagnosis*, 2nd ed. Philadelphia: Lippincott Williams & Wilkins, 2003, with permission.)

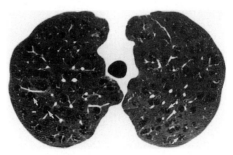

Emphysema/high-resolution computed tomography scan. Arrows indicate pulmonary vessels. (From Muller NL, Fraser RS, Leek S, et al., eds. *Diseases of the lung: radiologic and pathologic correlations*. Philadelphia: Lippincott Williams & Wilkins, 2003, with permission.)

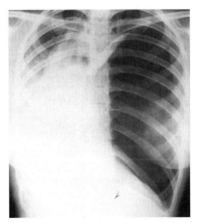

Tension pneumothorax. (From Eisenberg RL, ed. *Clinical imaging: an atlas of differential diagnosis*, 4th ed. Philadelphia: Lippincott Williams & Wilkins, 2003, with permission.)

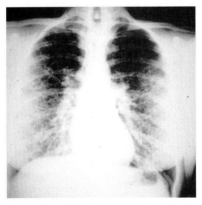

Interstitial lung disease. (From Vahjen G. Yale University Health Services, Radiology Department.)

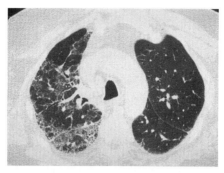

Pulmonary fibrosis/high-resolution computed tomography scan. (From Humes DH, ed. *Kelley's textbook of internal medicine*, 4th ed. Philadelphia: Lippincott Williams & Wilkins, 2000, with permission.)

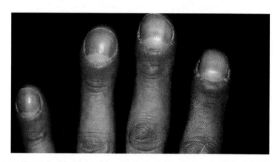

Clubbing. (From Smith DS. *Field guide to bedside diagnosis*. Philadelphia: Lippincott Williams & Wilkins, 1999, with permission.)

GASTROENTEROLOGY

Acute Abdominal Pain

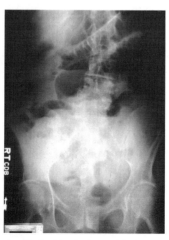

Small bowel obstruction/air-fluid levels. (From Vahjen G. Yale University Health Services, Radiology Department.)

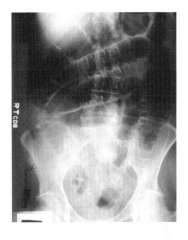

Ileus. (From Vahjen G. Yale University Health Services, Radiology Department.)

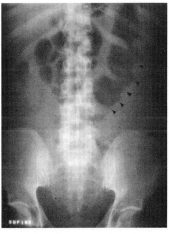

Mesenteric ischemia (*arrowheads*). (From Yamada T, Alpers DH, Owyang C, et al., eds. *Atlas of gastroenterology: self-assessment guide.* Philadelphia: Lippincott–Raven Publishers, 1997, with permission.)

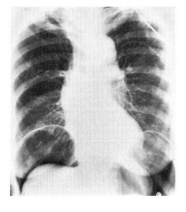

Free air under the diaphragms. (From Eisenberg RL, ed. *Clinical imaging: an atlas of differential diagnosis,* 4th ed. Philadelphia: Lippincott Williams & Wilkins, 2003, with permission.)

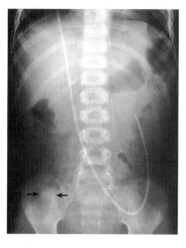

Appendicitis/laminated calcification in the right lower quadrant (*arrows*). (From Pope TL, Jr. *Aunt Minnie's atlas of imaging-specific diagnosis*, 2nd ed. Philadelphia: Lippincott Williams & Wilkins, 2003, with permission.)

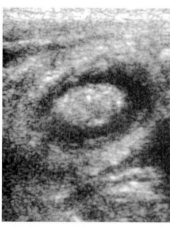

Appendicitis/ultrasound. (From Pope TL, Jr. *Aunt Minnie's atlas of imaging-specific diagnosis*, 2nd ed. Philadelphia: Lippincott Williams & Wilkins, 2003, with permission.)

Cirrhosis

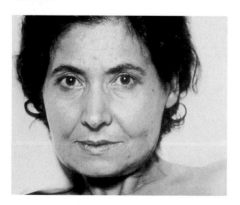

Jaundice. (From Smith DS. *Field guide to bedside diagnosis*. Philadelphia: Lippincott Williams & Wilkins, 1999, with permission.)

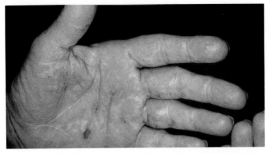

Palmar xanthoma/biliary cirrhosis. (From Smith DS. *Field guide to bedside diagnosis*. Philadelphia: Lippincott Williams & Wilkins, 1999, with permission.)

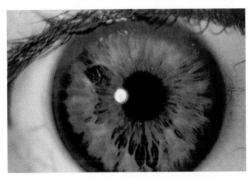

Kayser-Fleischer ring/Wilson's disease. (From Humes DH, ed. *Kelley's textbook of internal medicine*, 4th ed. Philadelphia: Lippincott Williams & Wilkins, 2000, with permission.)

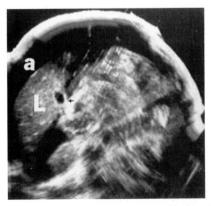

Ascites/ultrasound. a, ascitic fluid; L, liver. (From Eisenberg RL, ed. *Clinical imaging: an atlas of differential diagnosis*, 4th ed. Philadelphia: Lippincott Williams & Wilkins, 2003, with permission.)

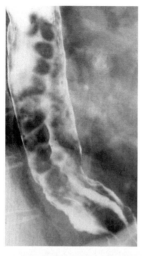

Esophageal varices on barium swallow. (From Eisenberg RL, ed. *Clinical imaging: an atlas of differential diagnosis*, 4th ed. Philadelphia: Lippincott Williams & Wilkins, 2003, with permission.)

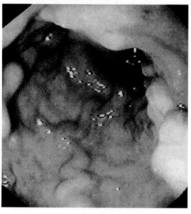

Rectal varices/portal hypertension. (From Stoller JK, Ahmad M, Longworth DC, eds. *Cleveland Clinic intensive review of internal medicine*, 2nd ed. Philadelphia: Lippincott Williams & Wilkins, 2000, with permission.)

Inflammatory Bowel Disease

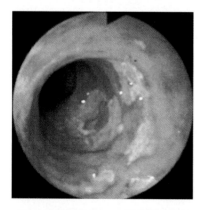

Crohn's terminal ileum/ colonoscopy. (From Yamada T, Alpers DH, Owyang C, et al., eds. *Atlas of gastroenterology: self-assessment guide*. Philadelphia: Lippincott–Raven Publishers, 1997, with permission.)

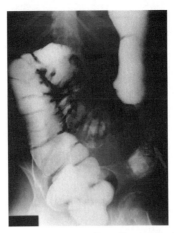

Crohn's segmental colitis/barium enema. (From Humes DH, ed. *Kelley's textbook of internal medicine*, 4th ed. Philadelphia: Lippincott Williams & Wilkins, 2000, with permission.)

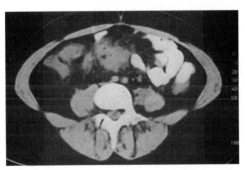

Right lower quadrant inflammatory mass/Crohn's disease/computed tomography scan. (From Humes DH, ed. *Kelley's textbook of internal medicine*, 4th ed. Philadelphia: Lippincott Williams & Wilkins, 2000, with permission.)

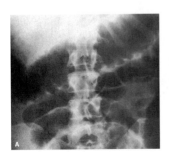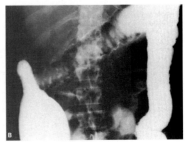

A,B: Toxic megacolon/ulcerative colitis. (From Yamada T, Alpers DH, Owyang C, et al., eds. *Atlas of gastroenterology: self-assessment guide*. Philadelphia: Lippincott–Raven Publishers, 1997, with permission.)

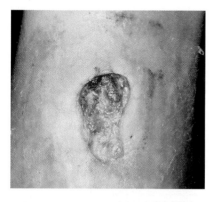

Pyoderma gangrenosum. (From Smith DS. *Field guide to bedside diagnosis.* Philadelphia: Lippincott Williams & Wilkins, 1999, with permission.)

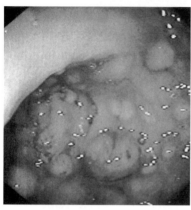

Clostridium difficile colitis/ sigmoidoscopy. (From Humes DH, ed. *Kelley's textbook of internal medicine,* 4th ed. Philadelphia: Lippincott Williams & Wilkins, 2000, with permission.)

Cholecystitis

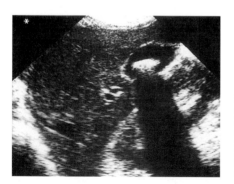

Gallstone with postacoustic shadowing/ultrasound. (From Humes DH, ed. *Kelley's textbook of internal medicine,* 4th ed. Philadelphia: Lippincott Williams & Wilkins, 2000, with permission.)

Acute cholecystitis/ hepatobiliary scan/ gallbladder not visible. (From Humes DH, ed. *Kelley's textbook of internal medicine*, 4th ed. Philadelphia: Lippincott Williams & Wilkins, 2000, with permission.)

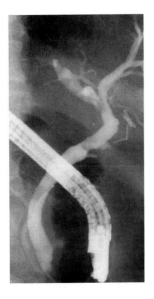

Common bile duct stone/endoscopic retrograde cholangiopancreatography. (From Humes DH, ed. *Kelley's textbook of internal medicine*, 4th ed. Philadelphia: Lippincott Williams & Wilkins, 2000, with permission.)

Peptic Ulcer Disease

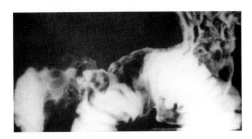

Duodenal ulcer on upper gastrointestinal tract. (From Vahjen G. Yale University Health Services, Radiology Department.)

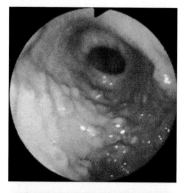

Lymphocytic gastritis/*Helicobacter pylori*/upper endoscopy. (From Yamada T, Alpers DH, Owyang C, et al., eds. *Atlas of gastroenterology: self-assessment guide.* Philadelphia: Lippincott–Raven Publishers, 1997, with permission.)

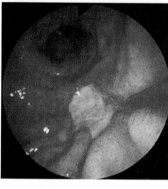

Nonsteroidal antiinflammatory drug–induced gastric ulcer. (From Yamada T, Alpers DH, Kaplowitz N, et al. *Textbook of gastroenterology*, 4th ed. Philadelphia: Lippincott Williams & Wilkins, 2003, with permission.)

Esophagitis

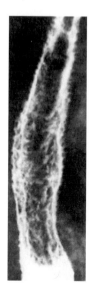

Candida esophagitis on barium swallow. (From Eisenberg RL, ed. *Clinical imaging: an atlas of differential diagnosis*, 4th ed. Philadelphia: Lippincott Williams & Wilkins, 2003, with permission.)

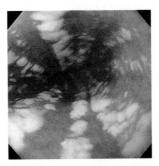

Candida esophagitis/endoscopy. (From Yamada T, Alpers DH, Kaplowitz N, et al. *Textbook of gastroenterology*, 4th ed. Philadelphia: Lippincott Williams & Wilkins, 2003, with permission.)

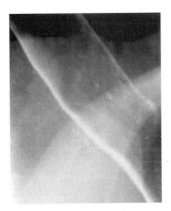

Reflux esophagitis with distal erosions on barium swallow. (From Eisenberg RL, ed. *Clinical imaging: an atlas of differential diagnosis*, 4th ed. Philadelphia: Lippincott Williams & Wilkins, 2003, with permission.)

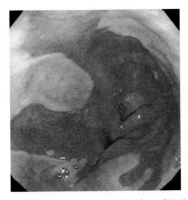

Barrett's esophagus/endoscopy. (From Yamada T, Alpers DH, Kaplowitz N, et al. *Textbook of gastroenterology*, 4th ed. Philadelphia: Lippincott Williams & Wilkins, 2003, with permission.)

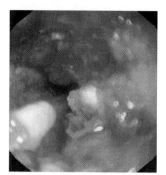

Circumferential esophageal cancer/endoscopy. (From Yamada T, Alpers DH, Kaplowitz N, et al. *Textbook of gastroenterology*, 4th ed. Philadelphia: Lippincott Williams & Wilkins, 2003, with permission.)

HEMATOLOGY AND ONCOLOGY

Mediastinal Mass

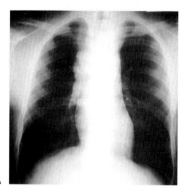

A

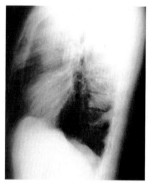

B

A,B: Anterior mediastinal mass/Hodgkin's disease/chest x-ray. (From Vahjen G. Yale University Health Services, Radiology Department.)

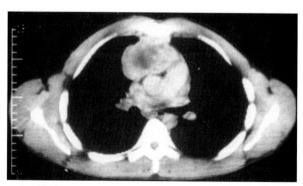

Anterior mediastinal mass/computed tomography scan. (From Vahjen G. Yale University Health Services, Radiology Department.)

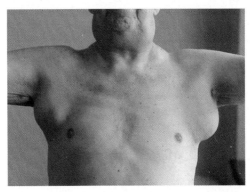

Axillary lymphadenopathy/lymphoma. (From Handin RI, Lux SE, Stossel TP. *Blood: principles and practice of hematology*, 2nd ed. Philadelphia: Lippincott Williams & Wilkins, 2003, with permission.)

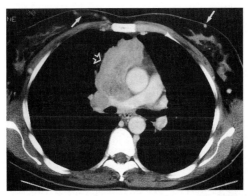

Superior vena cava syndrome/small cell cancer (*open arrow*)/computed tomography scan. Solid arrows show dilatation of collateral veins of the chest wall. (From Humes DH, ed. *Kelley's textbook of internal medicine*, 4th ed. Philadelphia: Lippincott Williams & Wilkins, 2000, with permission.)

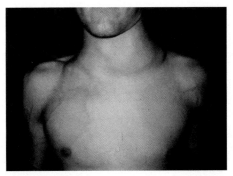

Superior vena cava syndrome venous engorgement. (From Handin RI, Lux SE, Stossel TP. *Blood: principles and practice of hematology*, 2nd ed. Philadelphia: Lippincott Williams & Wilkins, 2003, with permission.)

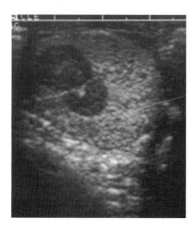

Testicular mass/ultrasound. (From Humes DH, ed. *Kelley's textbook of internal medicine*, 4th ed. Philadelphia: Lippincott Williams & Wilkins, 2000, with permission.)

Lung Cancer

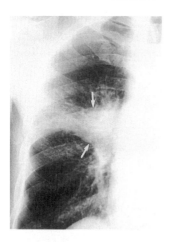

Squamous cell cancer/obstructive pneumonitis. (From Muller NL, Fraser RS, Leek S, et al., eds. *Diseases of the lung: radiologic and pathologic correlations.* Philadelphia: Lippincott Williams & Wilkins, 2003, with permission.)

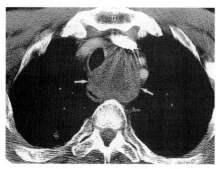

Small cell cancer/ mediastinal adenopathy/ high-resolution computed tomography scan. Arrows show lymph node enlargement in left paratracheal area. (From Muller NL, Fraser RS, Leek S, et al., eds. *Diseases of the lung: radiologic and pathologic correlations.* Philadelphia: Lippincott Williams & Wilkins, 2003, with permission.)

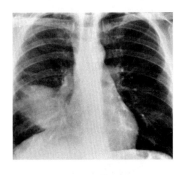

Bronchoalveolar cancer. (From Eisenberg RL, ed. *Clinical imaging: an atlas of differential diagnosis*, 4th ed. Philadelphia: Lippincott Williams & Wilkins, 2003, with permission.)

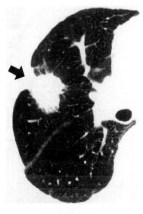

Adenocarcinoma/high-resolution computed tomography scan. Arrow indicates pleural puckering. (From Muller NL, Fraser RS, Leek S, et al., eds. *Diseases of the lung: radiologic and pathologic correlations*. Philadelphia: Lippincott Williams & Wilkins, 2003, with permission.)

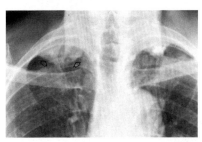

Pancoast's tumor. Note increased opacification in the right apex (*arrows*). (From Eisenberg RL, ed. *Clinical imaging: an atlas of differential diagnosis*, 4th ed. Philadelphia: Lippincott Williams & Wilkins, 2003, with permission.)

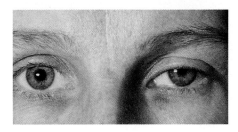

Horner's syndrome. (From Smith DS. *Field guide to bedside diagnosis*. Philadelphia: Lippincott Williams & Wilkins, 1999, with permission.)

Breast Cancer

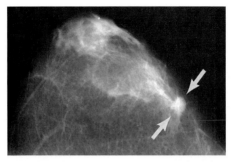

Spiculated mass (*arrows*)/mammogram. (From Humes DH, ed. *Kelley's textbook of internal medicine*, 4th ed. Philadelphia: Lippincott Williams & Wilkins, 2000, with permission.)

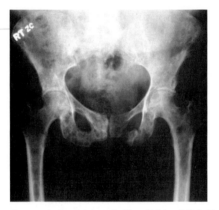

Metastatic breast cancer before treatment. (From Vahjen G. Yale University Health Services, Radiology Department.)

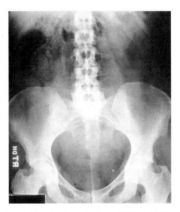

Metastatic breast cancer after treatment. (From Vahjen G. Yale University Health Services, Radiology Department.)

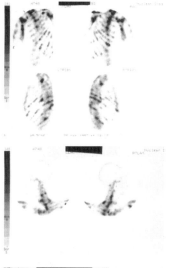

Metastatic prostate cancer before Lupron. (From Vahjen G. Yale University Health Services, Radiology Department.)

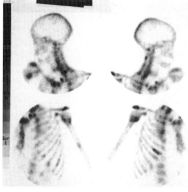

Metastatic prostate cancer after Lupron. (From Vahjen G. Yale University Health Services, Radiology Department.)

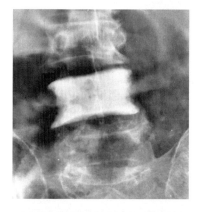

Ivory vertebrae. (From Eisenberg RL, ed. *Clinical imaging: an atlas of differential diagnosis*, 4th ed. Philadelphia: Lippincott Williams & Wilkins, 2003, with permission.)

Colon Cancer

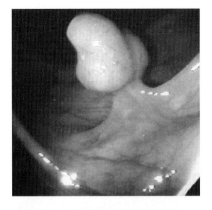

Adenomatous polyp/ colonoscopy. (From Humes DH, ed. *Kelley's textbook of internal medicine*, 4th ed. Philadelphia: Lippincott Williams & Wilkins, 2000, with permission.)

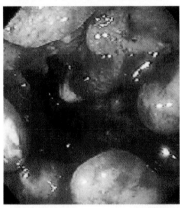

Circumferential ulcerated mass/ adenocarcinoma/colonoscopy. (From Stoller JK, Ahmad M, Longworth DC, eds. *Cleveland Clinic intensive review of internal medicine*, 2nd ed. Philadelphia: Lippincott Williams & Wilkins, 2000, with permission.)

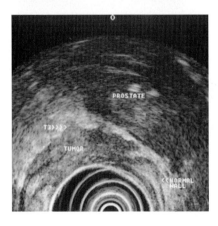

Colon cancer/endoscopic ultrasound. (From Humes DH, ed. *Kelley's textbook of internal medicine*, 4th ed. Philadelphia: Lippincott Williams & Wilkins, 2000, with permission.)

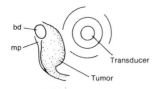

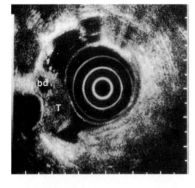

Ampullary cancer/endoscopic ultrasound. bd, bile duct; mp, muscularis propria; T, tumor. (From Yamada T, Alpers DH, Owyang C, et al., eds. *Atlas of gastroenterology: self-assessment guide.* Philadelphia: Lippincott–Raven Publishers, 1997, with permission.)

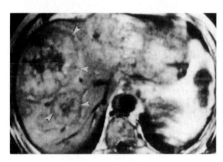

Liver metastases/colon cancer/enhanced magnetic resonance image. On a delayed-phase contrast scan, the masses demonstrate central enhancement and peripheral washout (*arrowheads*). (From Eisenberg RL, ed. *Clinical imaging: an atlas of differential diagnosis,* 4th ed. Philadelphia: Lippincott Williams & Wilkins, 2003, with permission.)

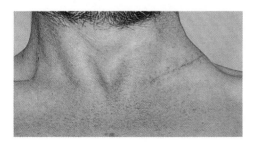

Virchow's node. (From Smith DS. *Field guide to bedside diagnosis.* Philadelphia: Lippincott Williams & Wilkins, 1999, with permission.)

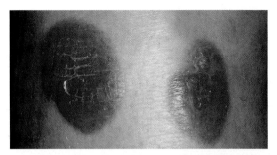

Leukemia cutis/plum nodule. (From Smith DS. *Field guide to bedside diagnosis.* Philadelphia: Lippincott Williams & Wilkins, 1999, with permission.)

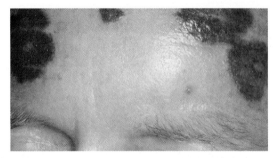

Sweet's syndrome/acute myelogenous leukemia. (From Smith DS. *Field guide to bedside diagnosis.* Philadelphia: Lippincott Williams & Wilkins, 1999, with permission.)

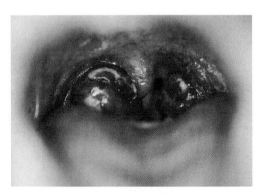

Bilateral tonsillar enlargement/M5a acute myelogenous leukemia. (From Handin RI, Lux SE, Stossel TP. *Blood: principles and practice of hematology*, 2nd ed. Philadelphia: Lippincott Williams & Wilkins, 2003, with permission.)

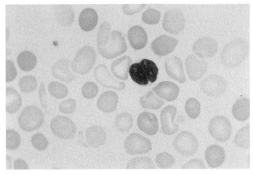

Small cleaved-cell lymphoma/peripheral smear. (From Handin RI, Lux SE, Stossel TP. *Blood: principles and practice of hematology*, 2nd ed. Philadelphia: Lippincott Williams & Wilkins, 2003, with permission.)

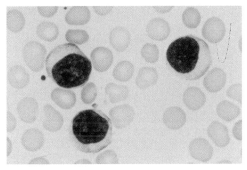

Chronic lymphocytic leukemia peripheral smear. (From Handin RI, Lux SE, Stossel TP. *Blood: principles and practice of hematology*, 2nd ed. Philadelphia: Lippincott Williams & Wilkins, 2003, with permission.)

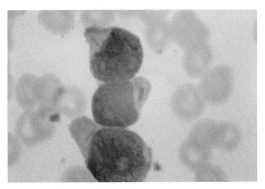

M1 myeloblastic leukemia with Auer rods/marrow. (From Handin RI, Lux SE, Stossel TP. *Blood: principles and practice of hematology*, 2nd ed. Philadelphia: Lippincott Williams & Wilkins, 2003, with permission.)

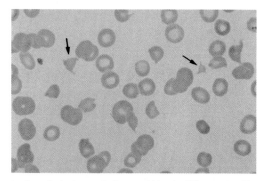

Schistocytes/hemolysis. Arrows indicate red blood cell fragments. (From Stoller JK, Ahmad M, Longworth DC, eds. *Cleveland Clinic intensive review of internal medicine*, 2nd ed. Philadelphia: Lippincott Williams & Wilkins, 2000, with permission.)

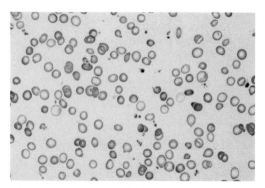

Hypochromic microcytic smear in iron deficiency. (From Stoller JK, Ahmad M, Longworth DC, eds. *Cleveland Clinic intensive review of internal medicine*, 2nd ed. Philadelphia: Lippincott Williams & Wilkins, 2000, with permission.)

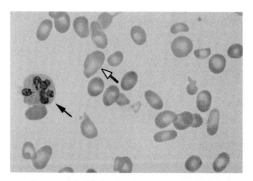

Hypersegmented neutrophils (*dark arrow*), macrocytosis/megaloblastic smear. Open white arrow indicates oval macrocyte. (From Stoller JK, Ahmad M, Longworth DC, eds. *Cleveland Clinic intensive review of internal medicine*, 2nd ed. Philadelphia: Lippincott Williams & Wilkins, 2000, with permission.)

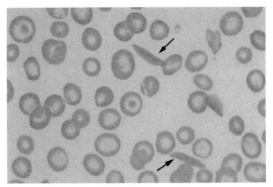

Sickle cells (*arrows*). (From Stoller JK, Ahmad M, Longworth DC, eds. *Cleveland Clinic intensive review of internal medicine*, 2nd ed. Philadelphia: Lippincott Williams & Wilkins, 2000, with permission.)

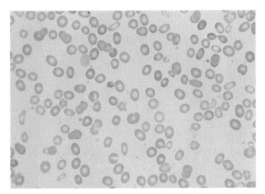

Oval macrocytes, acanthocytes/refractory anemia with ringed sideroblasts. (From Lee GR, Foerster J, Lukens J, et al., eds. *Wintrobe's clinical hematology*, 10th ed. Philadelphia: Williams & Wilkins, 1999, with permission.)

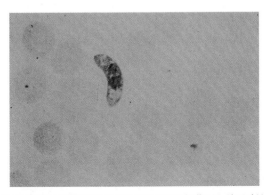

Plasmodium falciparum/banana gametocyte. (From Stoller JK, Ahmad M, Longworth DC, eds. *Cleveland Clinic intensive review of internal medicine*, 2nd ed. Philadelphia: Lippincott Williams & Wilkins, 2000, with permission.)

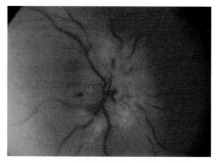

Papilledema. (From Smith DS. *Field guide to bedside diagnosis*. Philadelphia: Lippincott Williams & Wilkins, 1999, with permission.)

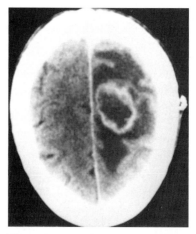

Glioblastoma multiforme. (From Eisenberg RL, ed. *Clinical imaging: an atlas of differential diagnosis*, 4th ed. Philadelphia: Lippincott Williams & Wilkins, 2003, with permission.)

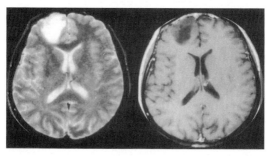

Frontal astrocytoma. (From Humes DH, ed. *Kelley's textbook of internal medicine*, 4th ed. Philadelphia: Lippincott Williams & Wilkins, 2000, with permission.)

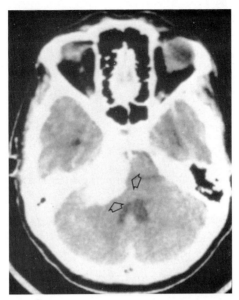

Meningioma. Arrows show dense enhancing lesion that is more broadly based along the petrous bone than a typical acoustic neuroma. (From Eisenberg RL, ed. *Clinical imaging: an atlas of differential diagnosis*, 4th ed. Philadelphia: Lippincott Williams & Wilkins, 2003, with permission.)

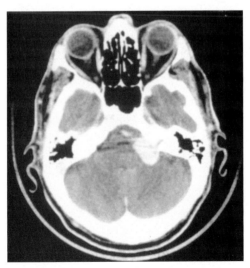

Acoustic neuroma. (From Vahjen G. Yale University Health Services, Radiology Department.)

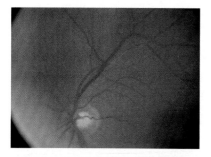

Amaurosis fugax/retinal artery embolism. (From Smith DS. *Field guide to bedside diagnosis.* Philadelphia: Lippincott Williams & Wilkins, 1999, with permission.)

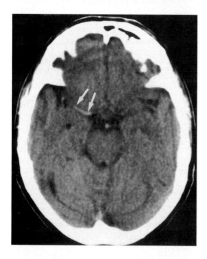

Hyperdense middle cerebral artery (MCA) thrombus (*arrows*)/acute MCA stroke/computed tomography scan. (From Batjer HH, Caplan LR, Friberg L, et al, eds. *Cerebrovascular disease.* Philadelphia: Lippincott–Raven Publishers, 1997, with permission.)

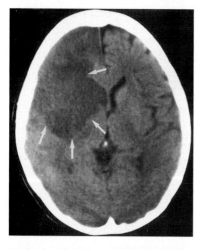

Middle cerebral artery stroke 1 week later/computed tomography scan. Arrows indicate more mass effect in region of infarction. (From Batjer HH, Caplan LR, Friberg L, et al, eds. *Cerebrovascular disease.* Philadelphia: Lippincott–Raven Publishers, 1997, with permission.)

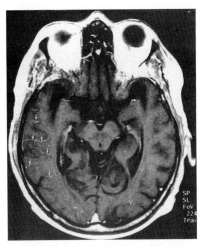

Middle cerebral artery (MCA) stroke/T1-weighted magnetic resonance image. Arrows indicate extensive intravascular enhancement within MCA branches in temporal sulci. (From Batjer HH, Caplan LR, Friberg L, et al, eds. *Cerebrovascular disease.* Philadelphia: Lippincott–Raven Publishers, 1997, with permission.)

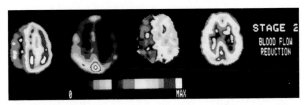

Transient ischemic attack/reduced left cerebral flow/positron-emission tomography scan. (From Batjer HH, Caplan LR, Friberg L, et al, eds. *Cerebrovascular disease.* Philadelphia: Lippincott–Raven Publishers, 1997, with permission.)

Intracerebral Hemorrhage

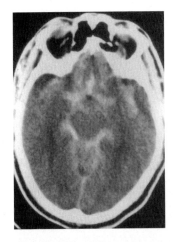

Posterior communicating artery aneurysm/computed tomography scan. (From Eisenberg RL, ed. *Clinical imaging: an atlas of differential diagnosis,* 4th ed. Philadelphia: Lippincott Williams & Wilkins, 2003, with permission.)

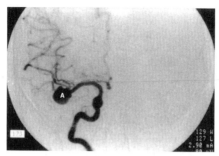

Middle cerebral artery bifurcation aneurysm (A)/angiogram. (From Eisenberg RL, ed. *Clinical imaging: an atlas of differential diagnosis*, 4th ed. Philadelphia: Lippincott Williams & Wilkins, 2003, with permission.)

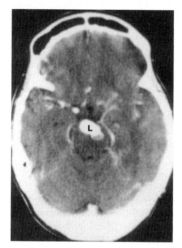

Basilar artery aneurysm (L)/contrast-enhanced computed tomography scan. (From Eisenberg RL, ed. *Clinical imaging: an atlas of differential diagnosis*, 4th ed. Philadelphia: Lippincott Williams & Wilkins, 2003, with permission.)

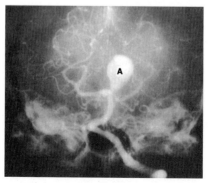

Basilar artery aneurysm (A)/angiogram. (From Eisenberg RL, ed. *Clinical imaging: an atlas of differential diagnosis*, 4th ed. Philadelphia: Lippincott Williams & Wilkins, 2003, with permission.)

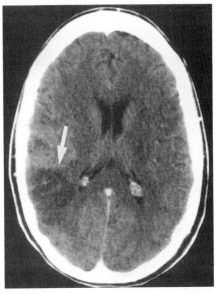

Subarachnoid hemorrhage (*arrow*)/computed tomography scan. (From Batjer HH, Caplan LR, Friberg L, et al, eds. *Cerebrovascular disease*. Philadelphia: Lippincott–Raven Publishers, 1997, with permission.)

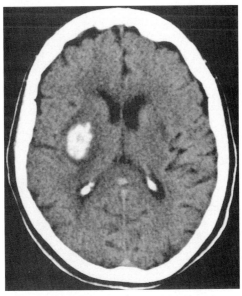

Thalamic hypertensive hemorrhage/contrast-enhanced computed tomography scan. (From Batjer HH, Caplan LR, Friberg L, et al, eds. *Cerebrovascular disease*. Philadelphia: Lippincott–Raven Publishers, 1997, with permission.)

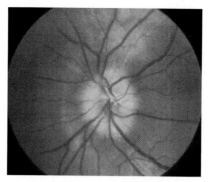

Acute optic neuritis. (From Smith DS. *Field guide to bedside diagnosis*. Philadelphia: Lippincott Williams & Wilkins, 1999, with permission.)

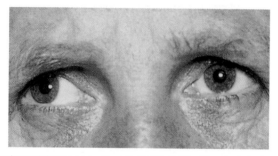

Internuclear ophthalmoplegia. (From Smith DS. *Field guide to bedside diagnosis*. Philadelphia: Lippincott Williams & Wilkins, 1999, with permission.)

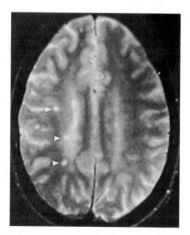

White matter signal enhancement (*arrowheads*) on magnetic resonance imaging. (From Eisenberg RL, ed. *Clinical imaging: an atlas of differential diagnosis*, 4th ed. Philadelphia: Lippincott Williams & Wilkins, 2003, with permission.)

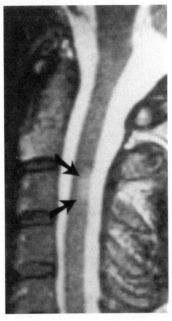

Spinal cord plaque (*arrows*) on magnetic resonance imaging. (From Eisenberg RL, ed. *Clinical imaging: an atlas of differential diagnosis*, 4th ed. Philadelphia: Lippincott Williams & Wilkins, 2003, with permission.)

RHEUMATOLOGY AND ALLERGY

Vasculitis/Lupus

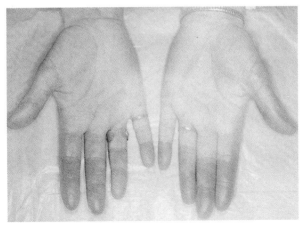

Raynaud's phenomenon. (From Stoller JK, Ahmad M, Longworth DC, eds. *Cleveland Clinic intensive review of internal medicine*, 2nd ed. Philadelphia: Lippincott Williams & Wilkins, 2000, with permission.)

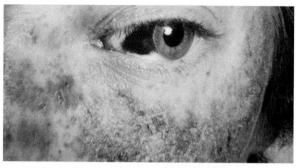

Malar rash/thrombocytopenia. (From Smith DS. *Field guide to bedside diagnosis*. Philadelphia: Lippincott Williams & Wilkins, 1999, with permission.)

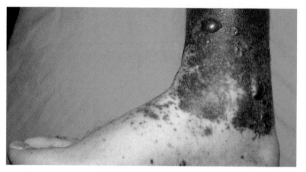

Palpable purpura/leukocytoclastic vasculitis. (From Smith DS. *Field guide to bedside diagnosis*. Philadelphia: Lippincott Williams & Wilkins, 1999, with permission.)

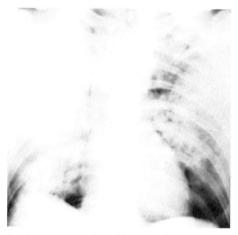

Goodpasture's pulmonary hemorrhage. (From Eisenberg RL, ed. *Clinical imaging: an atlas of differential diagnosis*, 4th ed. Philadelphia: Lippincott Williams & Wilkins, 2003, with permission.)

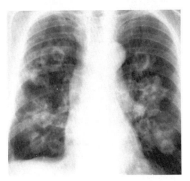

Wegener's thick-walled cavities on chest x-ray. (From Eisenberg RL, ed. *Clinical imaging: an atlas of differential diagnosis*, 4th ed. Philadelphia: Lippincott Williams & Wilkins, 2003, with permission.)

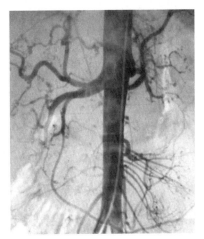

Polyarteritis nodosa on angiogram. (From Eisenberg RL, ed. *Clinical imaging: an atlas of differential diagnosis*, 4th ed. Philadelphia: Lippincott Williams & Wilkins, 2003, with permission.)

Rheumatoid Arthritis

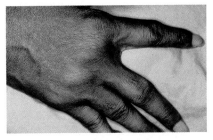

Rheumatoid arthritis hand deformities. (From Smith DS. *Field guide to bedside diagnosis*. Philadelphia: Lippincott Williams & Wilkins, 1999, with permission.)

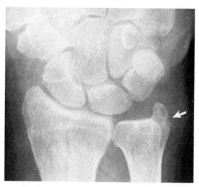

Ulnar erosion (*arrow*) in the wrist. (From Eisenberg RL, ed. *Clinical imaging: an atlas of differential diagnosis*, 4th ed. Philadelphia: Lippincott Williams & Wilkins, 2003, with permission.)

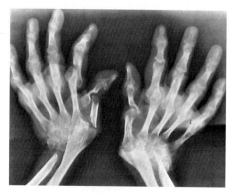

Destructive rheumatoid arthritis deformities in a hand film. (From Eisenberg RL, ed. *Clinical imaging: an atlas of differential diagnosis*, 4th ed. Philadelphia: Lippincott Williams & Wilkins, 2003, with permission.)

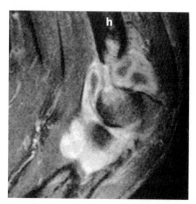

Synovial enhancement of knee in a magnetic resonance image. h, humerus. (From Eisenberg RL, ed. *Clinical imaging: an atlas of differential diagnosis*, 4th ed. Philadelphia: Lippincott Williams & Wilkins, 2003, with permission.)

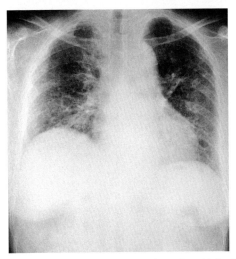

Rheumatoid lung/reticular pattern and honeycombing. (From Muller NL, Fraser RS, Leek S, et al., eds. *Diseases of the lung: radiologic and pathologic correlations*. Philadelphia: Lippincott Williams & Wilkins, 2003, with permission.)

Osteoarthritis

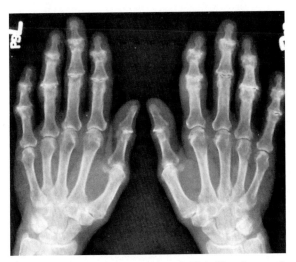

Osteoarthritis hand film. (From Eisenberg RL, ed. *Clinical imaging: an atlas of differential diagnosis*, 4th ed. Philadelphia: Lippincott Williams & Wilkins, 2003, with permission.)

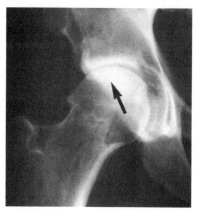

Sclerosis/hip x-ray. Arrow indicates superolateral migration of the femoral head. (From Humes DH, ed. *Kelley's textbook of internal medicine*, 4th ed. Philadelphia: Lippincott Williams & Wilkins, 2000, with permission.)

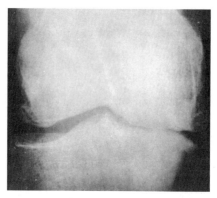

Osteoarthritis knee/x-ray. (From Humes DH, ed. *Kelley's textbook of internal medicine*, 4th ed. Philadelphia: Lippincott Williams & Wilkins, 2000, with permission.)

Gout

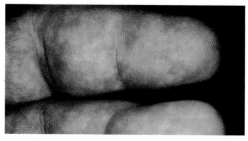

Tophi. (From Smith DS. *Field guide to bedside diagnosis*. Philadelphia: Lippincott Williams & Wilkins, 1999, with permission.)

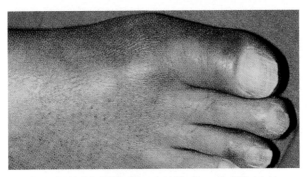

Podagra. (From Smith DS. *Field guide to bedside diagnosis*. Philadelphia: Lippincott Williams & Wilkins, 1999, with permission.)

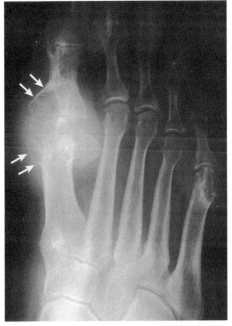

Gout erosion in metatarsophalangeal joint (*arrows*). (From Pope TL, Jr. *Aunt Minnie's atlas of imaging-specific diagnosis*, 2nd ed. Philadelphia: Lippincott Williams & Wilkins, 2003, with permission.)

Psoriatic Arthritis

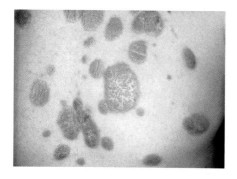

Psoriasis plaque. (From Humes DH, ed. *Kelley's textbook of internal medicine*, 4th ed. Philadelphia: Lippincott Williams & Wilkins, 2000, with permission.)

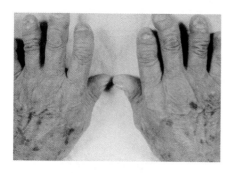

Psoriasis arthritis mutilans. (From Sontheimer RD, Provost TT. *Cutaneous manifestations of rheumatic diseases*, 2nd ed. Philadelphia: Williams & Wilkins, 2004, with permission.)

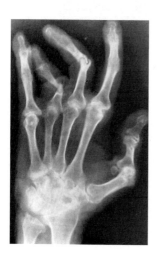

Psoriasis hand film. (From Eisenberg RL, ed. *Clinical imaging: an atlas of differential diagnosis*, 4th ed. Philadelphia: Lippincott Williams & Wilkins, 2003, with permission.)

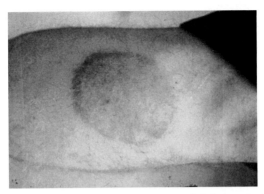

Erythema migrans/Lyme disease. (From Humes DH, ed. *Kelley's textbook of internal medicine*, 4th ed. Philadelphia: Lippincott Williams & Wilkins, 2000, with permission.)

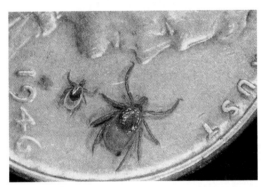

Ixodes ticks on a penny. (From Koneman EW, Allen SD, Janda WM, et al. *Color atlas and textbook of diagnostic microbiology*. Philadelphia: Lippincott–Raven Publishers, 1997, with permission.)

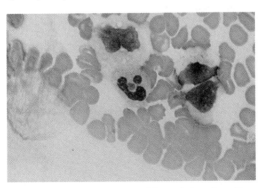

Human granulocytic ehrlichiosis/neutrophil blue inclusion. (From Koneman EW, Allen SD, Janda WM, et al. *Color atlas and textbook of diagnostic microbiology*. Philadelphia: Lippincott–Raven Publishers, 1997, with permission.)

ENDOCRINOLOGY

Adrenal Disease

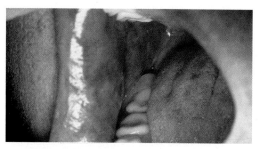

Addison's buccal hyperpigmentation. (From Smith DS. *Field guide to bedside diagnosis*. Philadelphia: Lippincott Williams & Wilkins, 1999, with permission.)

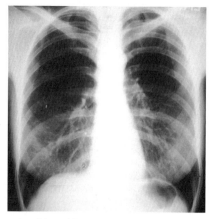

Addison's disease/small heart/chest x-ray. (From Vahjen G. Yale University Health Services, Radiology Department.)

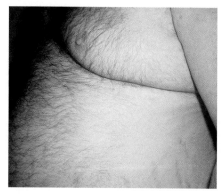

Cushing's syndrome/purple striae/truncal obesity. (From Smith DS. *Field guide to bedside diagnosis*. Philadelphia: Lippincott Williams & Wilkins, 1999, with permission.)

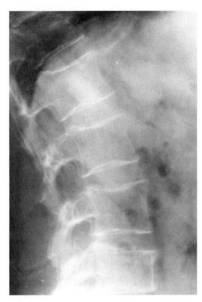

Osteoporosis/Cushing's syndrome. (From Eisenberg RL, ed. *Clinical imaging: an atlas of differential diagnosis*, 4th ed. Philadelphia: Lippincott Williams & Wilkins, 2003, with permission.)

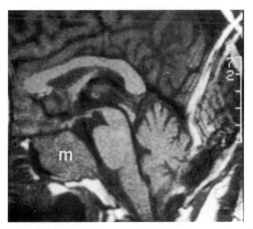

Pituitary macroadenoma (m)/magnetic resonance image. (From Eisenberg RL, ed. *Clinical imaging: an atlas of differential diagnosis*, 4th ed. Philadelphia: Lippincott Williams & Wilkins, 2003, with permission.)

Thyroid Disease

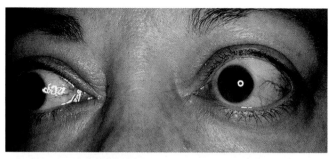

Grave's disease/exophthalmos. (From Smith DS. *Field guide to bedside diagnosis*. Philadelphia: Lippincott Williams & Wilkins, 1999, with permission.)

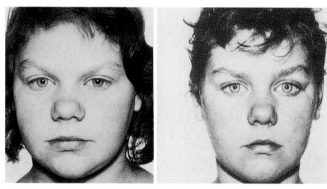

A   **B**

Hypothyroid face before **(A)** and after **(B)** treatment. (From Smith DS. *Field guide to bedside diagnosis*. Philadelphia: Lippincott Williams & Wilkins, 1999, with permission.)

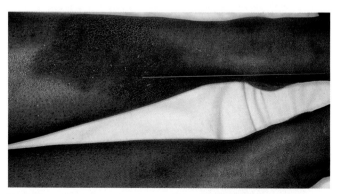

Pretibial myxedema. (From Smith DS. *Field guide to bedside diagnosis*. Philadelphia: Lippincott Williams & Wilkins, 1999, with permission.)

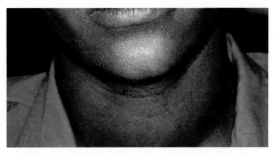

Goiter. (From Smith DS. *Field guide to bedside diagnosis*. Philadelphia: Lippincott Williams & Wilkins, 1999, with permission.)

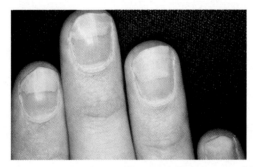

Thyroid onycholysis. (From Smith DS. *Field guide to bedside diagnosis*. Philadelphia: Lippincott Williams & Wilkins, 1999, with permission.)

Diabetes

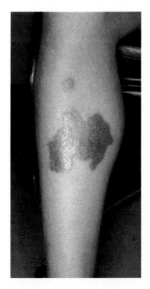

Necrobiosis lipoidica diabeticorum. (From Humes DH, ed. *Kelley's textbook of internal medicine*, 4th ed. Philadelphia: Lippincott Williams & Wilkins, 2000, with permission.)

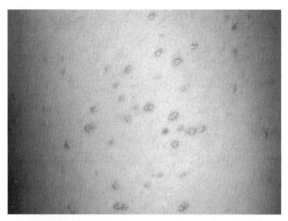

Eruptive xanthomas. (From Humes DH, ed. *Kelley's textbook of internal medicine*, 4th ed. Philadelphia: Lippincott Williams & Wilkins, 2000, with permission.)

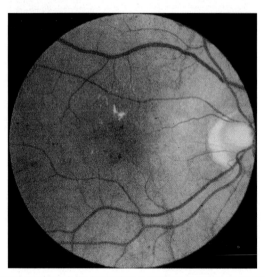

Diabetic retinopathy with dot hemorrhages and hard exudates. (From Stoller JK, Ahmad M, Longworth DC, eds. *Cleveland Clinic intensive review of internal medicine*, 2nd ed. Philadelphia: Lippincott Williams & Wilkins, 2000, with permission.)

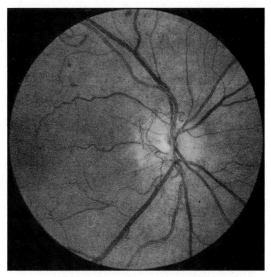

Diabetic retinopathy/disc neovascularization. (From Stoller JK, Ahmad M, Longworth DC, eds. *Cleveland Clinic intensive review of internal medicine*, 2nd ed. Philadelphia: Lippincott Williams & Wilkins, 2000, with permission.)

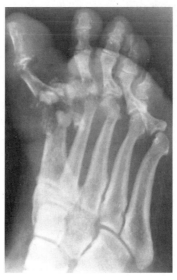

Osteomyelitis in the great toe in diabetes. (From Eisenberg RL, ed. *Clinical imaging: an atlas of differential diagnosis*, 4th ed. Philadelphia: Lippincott Williams & Wilkins, 2003, with permission.)

RENAL AND ELECTROLYTE

Electrolyte Disorders

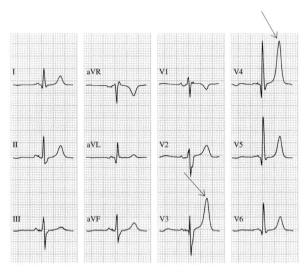

Hyperkalemia (serum potassium, 7.1 mmol/L) with prominent peaked T waves (*arrows*)/electrocardiogram. (From Wagner GS, ed. *Mariott's practical electrocardiography*, 10th ed. Philadelphia: Lippincott Williams & Wilkins, 2001, with permission.)

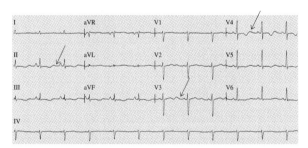

Hypokalemia (serum potassium, 1.7 mmol/L) with markedly prolonged QT interval (*arrows*)/electrocardiogram. (From Wagner GS, ed. *Mariott's practical electrocardiography*, 10th ed. Philadelphia: Lippincott Williams & Wilkins, 2001, with permission.)

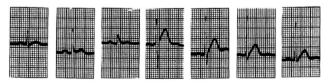

Hypercalcemia (serum calcium, 17 mg/dL) with short ST segment/ electrocardiogram. (From Humes DH, ed. *Kelley's textbook of internal medicine*, 4th ed. Philadelphia: Lippincott Williams & Wilkins, 2000, with permission.)

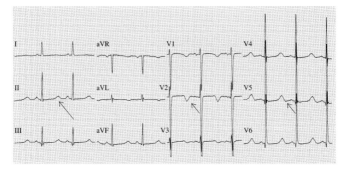

Hypocalcemia (serum calcium, 4.7 mg/dL) with prolonged QT interval (*arrows*)/ electrocardiogram. (From Wagner GS, ed. *Mariott's practical electrocardiography*, 10th ed. Philadelphia: Lippincott Williams & Wilkins, 2001, with permission.)

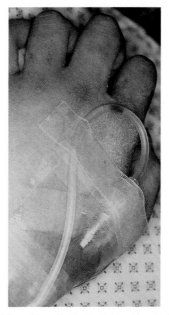

Uremic frost/renal failure. (From Smith DS. *Field guide to bedside diagnosis*. Philadelphia: Lippincott Williams & Wilkins, 1999, with permission.)